Contraception today

THE INTERNATIONAL CONGRESS, SYMPOSIUM AND SEMINAR SERIES

I•C•S•S

VOLUME 14

ISSN: 0969-2622

Contraception today

Edited by
C. Coll Capdevila, L. Iglesias Cortit
and G. Creatsas

The Proceedings of the 4th Congress of
the European Society of Contraception

The Parthenon Publishing Group
International Publishers in Medicine, Science & Technology
NEW YORK LONDON

Published in the USA by
The Parthenon Publishing Group Inc.
One Blue Hill Plaza
PO Box 1564, Pearl River
New York 10965, USA

Published in the UK and Europe by
The Parthenon Publishing Group Limited
Casterton Hall, Carnforth
Lancs. LA6 2LA, UK

First published 1997

Library of Congress Cataloging-in-Publication Data
European Society of Contraception. World Congress (4th : 1996 : Barcelona, Spain)
Contraception today : the proceedings of the 4th Congress of the European Society of Contraception / edited by C. Coll Capdevila, L. Iglesias Cortit, G. Creatsas.
p. cm. -- (The International congress, symposium, and seminar series. ISSN 0969-2622 ; v. 14)
Includes bibliographical references and index.
ISBN 1-85070-767-7
1. Contraception--Congresses. 2. Birth control--Congresses. I. Coll Capdevila, C. II. Iglesias Cortit, Luis. III. Creatsas, G. IV. Title. V. Series.
[DNLM: 1. Contraception--congresses. 2. Contraceptive Devices --congresses. 3. Contraceptive Agents--congresses. W1 IN736I v. 14 1998 / WP 630 E89c 1998]
RG136.A2E95 1996
613.9'4--dc21 97-48549
CIP

British Library Cataloguing in Publication Data
Contraception today : the proceedings of the 4th Congress of the European Society of Contraception. - (The international congress, symposium and seminar series ; v. 14)
1. Contraception - Congresses 2. Birth control - Congresses
I. Coll Capdevila, C. II. Iglesias Cortit, L. III. Creatsas, G.
613.9'4

ISBN 1-85070-767-7

Typeset by H&H Graphics, Blackburn, UK

Printed and bound by Bookcraft (Bath) Ltd., Midsomer Norton, UK

Contents

Intrauterine contraception

Barrier methods

Abortion in Europe

Central and Eastern Europe

List of principal contributors

A. Alcaraz
Department of Urology
Hospital Clinic
C/Villarroel N°170
08036 Barcelona
Spain

E. Aubeny
Centre d'Orthologenie
Hôpital Broussais
96 rue Didot
75014 Paris
France

I. Batár
Department of Obstetrics and Gynecology
University Medical School
Debrecen
Hungary

R.J.C.M. Beerthuizen
Department of Obstetrics and Gynecology
Streekzeikenhuis Koningin Beatrix
PO Box 9005
7100 GG Winterswijk
The Netherlands

G. Benagiano
Istituto Superiore di Sanita
Viale Regina Elena 299
00161 Rome
Italy

W. Bounds
Margaret Pyke Family Planning Centre
73 Charlotte Street
London W1P 1LB
UK

C. Coll Capdevila
Conseil de Cent, 170, 3A
08015 Barcelona
Spain

G. Creatsas
Department of Obstetrics and Gynecology
University of Athens
Aceteion Maternity Hospital
9 Kanari Street
10671 Athens
Greece

P.G. Crosignani
1 Department of Obstetrics and Gynecology
University of Milan
Milan
Italy

S. Dexeus
Free University of Barcelona
Institut Dexeus
Paseo Boranova 67
08017 Barcelona
Spain

M. Filshie
Department of Obstetrics and Gynecology
B Floor, East Block
Queen's Medical Centre
Nottingham NG7 2UH
UK

G. Freundl
NP-Research Projects at the Heinrich-Heine-University of Dusseldorf
Urdenbacher Allee, 83
D-40593 Dusseldorf
Germany

A.R. Genazzani
Department of Obstetrics and Gynecology
University of Pisa
Via Roma, 67
56100 Pisa
Italy

E.A. Hassan
Pindarou 1A
14565 Ekali
Greece

J. Henry-Suchet
Cabinet Gynecologique Marignan
10 Rue de Marignan
75008 Paris
France

L. Iglesias Cortit
Family Planning Center
Barcelona
Spain

A.A. Kubba
The Churchill Clinic
80 Lambeth Road
London SE1 7PW
UK

G. Lazdane
Dzirciema Str. 16
LV-1007 Riga
Latvia

F. Martinez
Department of Obstetrics and Gynecology
Institut Dexeus
Paseo Bonanova 67
08017 Barcelona
Spain

V. Odlind
Department of Obstetrics and Gynecology
University of Uppsala
751 85 Uppsala
Sweden

E.J. Oloto
Academic Division of Obstetrics and Gynaecology
St. James's University Hospital
Beckett Street
Leeds LS9 7TF
UK

J. Orfila
Place V. Pauchet - BP3006
80030 Amiens
France

C.M.M. Pyper
Holmwood
Foxcombe Road
Oxford OX1 5DL
UK

B. Rojnik
Family Health International
Research Triangle Park
PO Box 13950
NC 27709
USA

H. Salzer
Gynäkologisch-geburtshilfliche Abteilung des Wilhelminenspitales der Stadt Wien
Vienna
Austria

H.P.G. Schneider
Department of Obstetrics and Gynecology
University of Münster
D-48129 Münster
Germany

F. Soler
ACODIPLAN
C/Valencia 494, entr. 4°B
08013 Barcelona
Spain

H.E. Van Kets
International Study Group for Intrauterine Drug Delivery
University Hospital Ghent
Department of Obstetrics and Gynecology
De Pintelaan 185
B-9000 Ghent
Belgium

R.H.W. van Lunsen
Department of Sexology and Psychosomatic Gynecology
Academic Medical Center
University of Amsterdam
Meibergdreef 9
1105 AZ Amsterdam
The Netherlands

M. Vekemans
Université Libre de Bruxelles et Centre Hospitalier
rue Haute 322
B-1000 Bruxelles
Belgium

J.M. Viladoms i Fuster
Centro Medico Teknon
c/Marquesa de Vilallonga 12, d-21
08017 Barcelona
Spain

A. Volpe
Clinica Ginecologica e Ostetrica
Via del Pozzo 71
41100 Modena
Italy

A.M.C. Webb
North Mersey Community (NHS) Trust
Abacus
16 Lord Street
Liverpool L2 1TA
UK

D. Wildemeersch
Piers de Raveschootlaan 125
B-8300 Knokke-Heist
Belgium

1 Benefits of family planning

G. Benagiano and I. Shah

INTRODUCTION

A question which is often asked, at least in the industrialized world, is whether contraception has changed women's lives and, if so, in what ways. An answer to this question is not straightforward, as, depending on the point of view, one could say: 'in everything or in nothing'[1] it all depends on the parameters one utilizes and the end points one chooses. The discussion on the impact of contraception on the lives of women can be organized around four main points:

(1) The acquired freedom to easily choose the number of children women wish to have, and the spacing between births;

(2) The improvements in women's health brought about by the availability of modern contraceptives;

(3) The impact of contraception on the struggle to promote the condition of women;

(4) The differences, and they are major, between the north and the south of the world in this respect.

FREEDOM OF CHOICE

Figure 1 shows the reaction of women to contraception. The number of women who practice contraception and use effective methods depends on their desire for small families.

In Figure 1, countries are ranked according to the stated average number of children desired (almost seven for Cameroon and just above two for France)[1]; clearly, there is a general trend towards greater use of contraception where fewer children are wanted. Modern contraceptives have, therefore, offered the opportunity to women to realize their reproductive goals.

In this respect, if we look at the evolution of fertility in two, fairly similar European countries, France and Italy (Figure 2), we can conclude that the problem of 'population growth' had already been resolved by French and Italian women, or, for that matter, by most European couples, in the 1950s[2]. One could further conclude that there was no need for organized family planning or modern contraception to promote the freedom of women to choose, or, to use more forceful words, to promote their right to empower in these matters. Indeed,

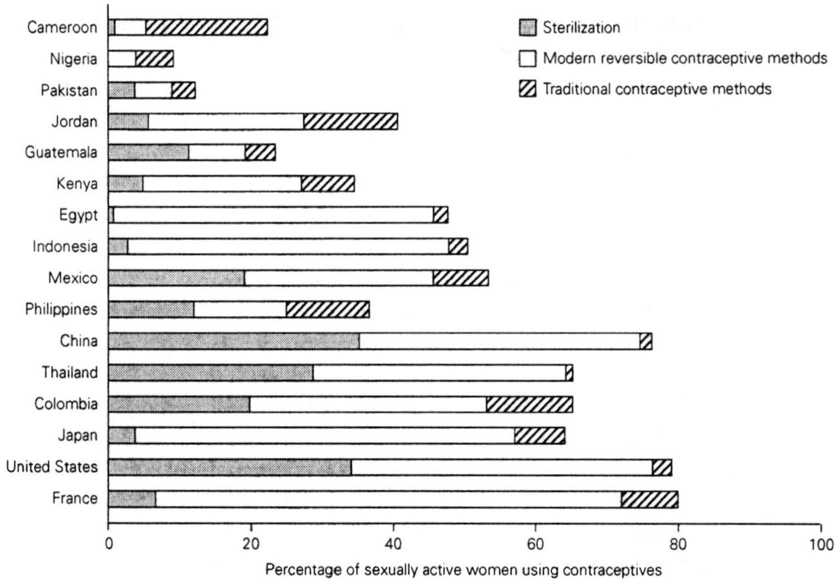

Figure 1 Comparison of birth control methods in various countries. In countries where desired family size is small, more women practice birth control and use effective methods

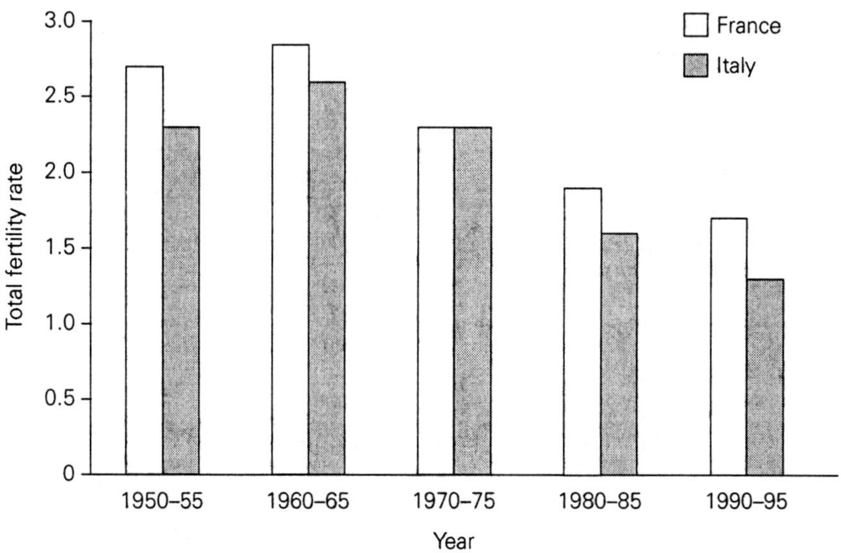

Figure 2 Total fertility rates for France and Italy, 1950–1995. Data from the UN World Population Prospects for 1994 (1995)

total fertility rates decreased in these two countries from slightly above two children per couple for the period 1950–55, to below replacement levels today[2]. In Italy, especially, which has the lowest birth rate of all countries compared, one could argue for the need to encourage child bearing, not birth limitation. This is, however, a very superficial way to look at the situation, which is actually far more complex. For example, a large number of clandestine abortions in several European countries in the 1960s had major implications on women's health[3].

The lack of modern and effective methods of contraception has, therefore, carried a price in terms of health. It is precisely this passage from abortion to contraception that represents the first positive effect of family planning on women's well-being. There is no question that contraception is the cornerstone of our fight to reduce abortion, although the relationship between contraception and abortion is fairly complex. Data from several industrialized countries show that, where contraception is well-established and utilized by the vast majority of people, and where it is associated with a proper sex education, the need to resort to an abortion has substantially decreased[4]. Denmark and The Netherlands are the best examples of this. Even in Italy, following legalization, abortions decreased from about 235 000 in 1984 to some 150 000 in 1993 (Figure 3)[5]. In addition, the ratio of abortion to live birth decreased from 38 to 27%. Finally, abortion rates among women of reproductive age decreased from 17 to 10.5 per 1000 (Figure 3).

The situation is different in England where both the number of legal abortions and the ratio of abortions to live births continued to increase until 1991[6] (Figure 4). It is difficult to determine the reasons for this trend. However, looking at the incredibly low numbers and rates in the 1970s, one may conclude a high degree of underreporting during that period. In France, the number of abortions per 100 live births has remained fairly constant at about 22.5 from 1985 onward, but started to decline during 1992 and 1993[6] (Figure 5). In order for contraception to successfully decrease the need for abortion, there has to be active promotion. Thus, in general, one can conclude that family planning has created the conditions for a major reduction in the need to resort to abortion.

HEALTH BENEFITS OF FAMILY PLANNING

It is interesting to note that, given motivation and education, the reduction in the incidence of abortion can occur with almost any contraceptive mix. Figure 6 shows the percentage utilization of the various contraceptive methods in Italy and France[7] and, although Italians seem to prefer more traditional methods, they none the less seem to manage their fertility very well.

The choice of a contraceptive method can also influence the health status of women. The press talks frequently of the negative consequences, which are usually exaggerated, of hormonal contraceptives but, unfortunately, the positive consequences are normally ignored. Among the well-established, non-

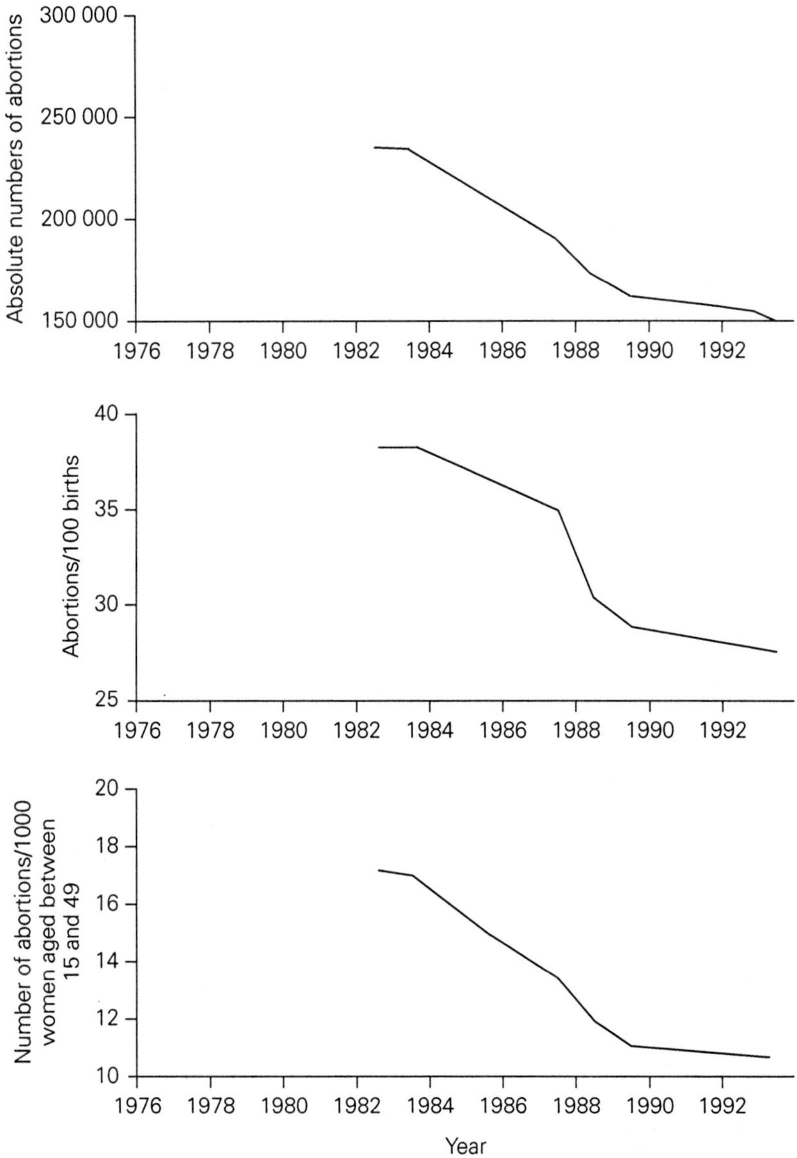

Figure 3 Abortion rates in Italy

contraceptive benefits of oral contraceptives, one can list reductions in: the need for voluntary pregnancy termination and sterilization; the risk of endometrial cancer (approximately 50%)[8] and of ovarian cancer (up to 65%)[9]; and the frequency of benign breast disease[10], ectopic pregnancy[11], salpingitis[11] and rheumatoid arthritis[12]. There is also a probable reduction in the incidence

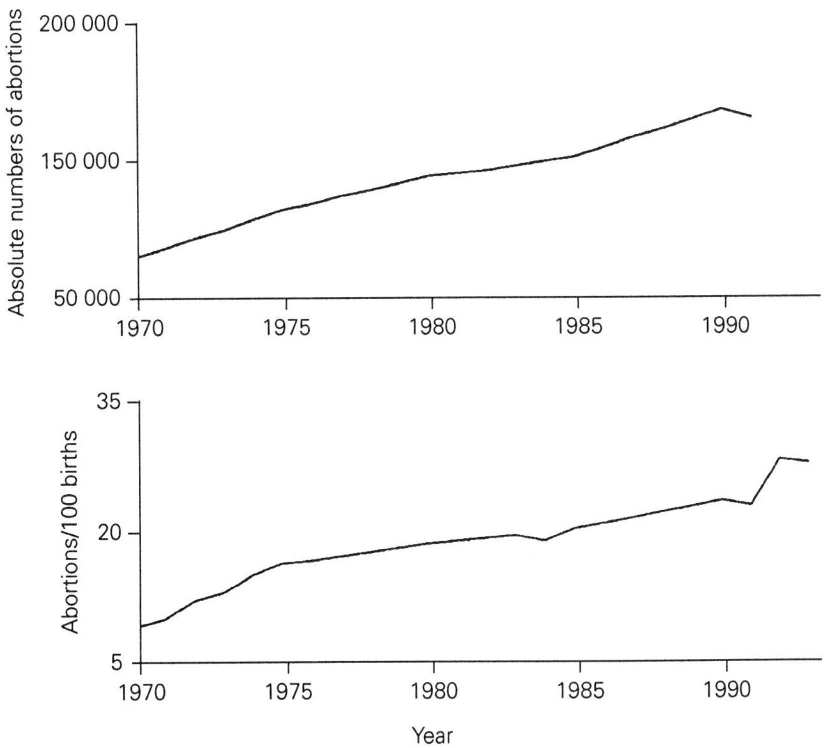

Figure 4 Evolution of abortion in England

of endometriosis[13], uterine leiomyomata[14] and ovarian cysts[15]. Finally, oral contraceptives probably afford protection against atherosclerosis[16].

LEVELS AND TRENDS IN CONTRACEPTIVE USE

On a global scale, modern contraception has achieved impressive gains for humanity and its future. In the late 1960s only about 10% of couples in developing countries, or about 30 million people, used any contraceptive method at all, and the rate is now more than 50%, thus exceeding 500 million users[17]. Indeed, contraceptive practice, measured in terms of its prevalence (or the percentage of those 'currently' using contraception among couples in which the woman is of childbearing age), has been estimated for the period 1960–65 at 30% for the world as a whole and below 10% for the less developed regions. In 1990, this figure had risen to 57% for the world overall. The rise in contraceptive practice has been most spectacular in developing countries, where 53% of couples were utilizing a method of family planning in 1990. Contraceptive practice was already high in the more developed regions in 1960-65 (67%), increasing to 72% in

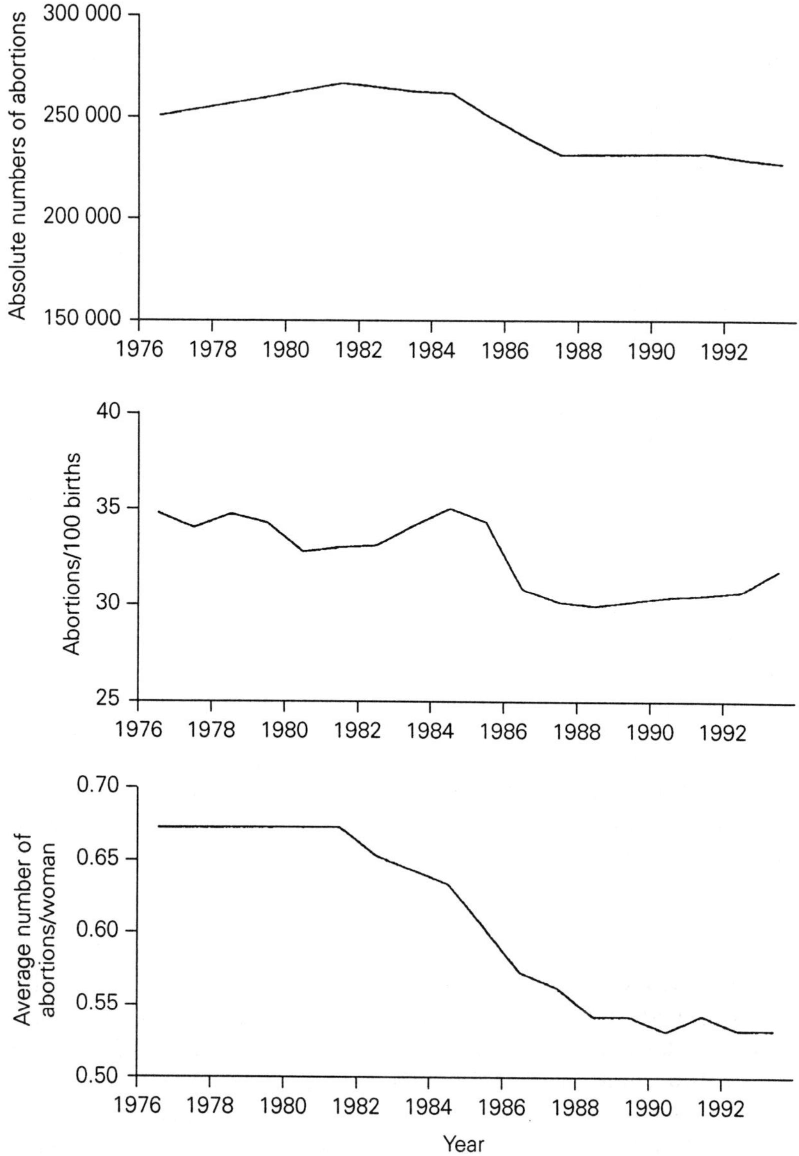

Figure 5 Abortion rates in France

1990. With over 50% of couples using a contraceptive method in 1990, contraception – a 'novelty' three decades ago – has become a reproductive norm in much of the world. Only in sub-Saharan Africa does the prevalence remain below 18% in most countries. However, it is expected to rise to 26% by the year 2000[17].

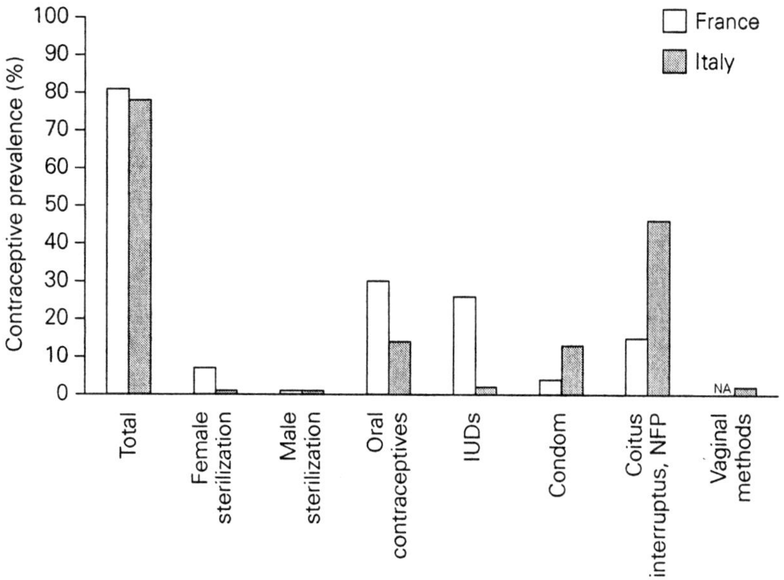

Figure 6 Contraceptive prevalence by method in France and Italy. IUDs, intrauterine devices; NFP, natural family planning; NA, not available

These achievements can rightly be called the 'contraceptive revolution' because, as so beautifully stated by La Rochefoucauld, certain revolutions are so generalized that they completely change the way people feel and think and, thereby, the world's fortunes. The availability of modern contraceptives has done exactly that: it has changed the way people think and act.

CONTRACEPTION AND THE EMPOWERING OF WOMEN

It seems obvious, retrospectively, that a revolution of this magnitude could not have happened without controversy and resistance, which is already evident in the way contraception is defined. On one hand, there are those who, in defining contraception, underline that this is a technology which separates the two great meanings of sexual intercourse, the 'union between man and woman' and 'the creation of new life'. On the other hand, there are others who point out that contraception is the tool utilized by couples to regulate their fertility, a fundamental human right.

Family planning itself has come under criticism because, from an expression designed to promote the right of women and men to have the number of children they wish, it has developed – in the second part of the 20th century – to represent the instrument to achieve population control and stabilization.

In order to understand the inner reason for this controversy, we must recognize that family planning touches upon a fundamental issue, that of gender equality.

Ambivalence towards gender equality goes back to the deepest roots of our culture[18]. In Western countries, the situation improves daily and we must thank women like Arletta Jakobs in the Netherlands, Margaret Sanger in the USA, Marie Stopes in the UK and Marie Andrée Lagroua in France, who risked contempt and even jail in order to promote contraception and women's equality. By contrast, in many developing countries, the struggle to achieve gender equality is far from being successfully achieved. We must ensure, therefore, that women become at least equal partners with men in any decisions about family size. In a world of almost total male domination of politics, economics, religion and the law, it will not be easy to bring about these changes.

The concept of reproductive health has forced a new reality upon world attention, the recognition that the global population problem is a problem for individual couples, being a health and development problem and not only a demographic one.

Women suffer because of reproduction much more than men. Indeed, when it comes to 'disease burden' in the area of reproduction there is no comparison in terms of health consequences between women and men. Between the ages of 15 and 45 years, practically one-third of the global burden of disease for women relates to reproduction, whereas the percentage for men is approximately 10 (Figure 7)[19].

NORTH–SOUTH DIFFERENTIALS

Education of women accounts for much of the North–South differential in reproductive health and gender equality. Through education, women and men can be convinced that pregnancy in young adolescents, births that are too closely spaced or occur at advanced age and high parities, pose substantial risks to children, mothers or both. For example, in the absence of obstetric care, giving birth before the age of 18 years increases the likelihood of mortality due to childbirth by three-fold[19]. Child-bearing during adolescence has emerged as an issue of increasing concern throughout the world. There is growing awareness that early child-bearing poses a health risk for the mother and the child and may truncate a girl's education, threatening her economic prospects, earning capacity and overall well-being. It is estimated that, worldwide, about 15 million women aged 15–19 years give birth each year, and that about 11% of all babies are currently born to adolescents[20].

Women's education influences reproductive health in many different ways. Data from Mexico show that, even if one takes into account the social and economic differences that go with differences in education, 'education saves lives'. Figure 8 shows a four-fold decrease in maternal mortality with increasing levels of education[21]. In this connection, the World Health Organization estimates that 100 000 maternal deaths could be avoided each year if all women who wish not to have more babies could, indeed, avoid pregnancy[19].

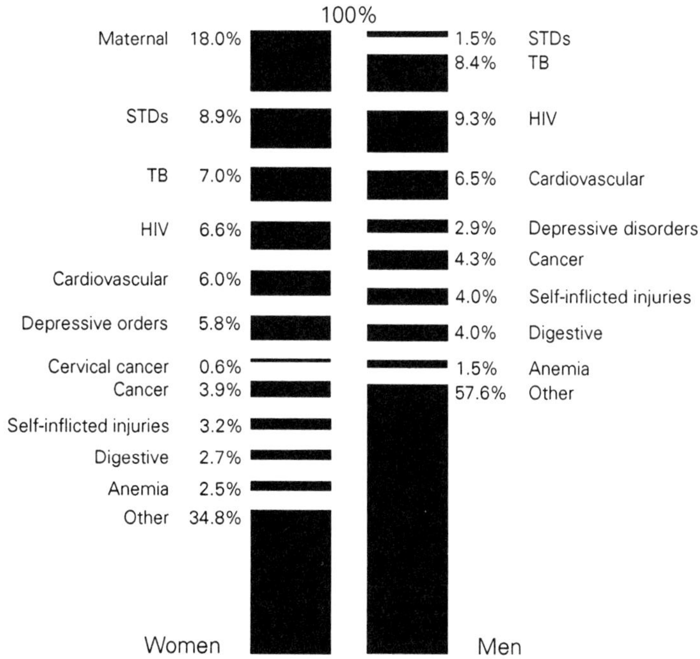

Figure 7 Disease burden in men and women aged 15–44 years. From reference 19. STDs, sexually transmitted diseases; TB, tuberculosis; HIV, Human Immunodeficiency Virus

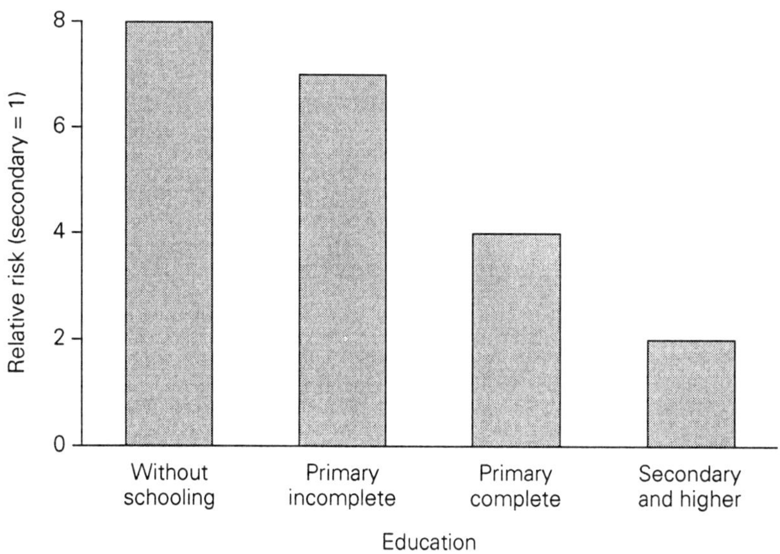

Figure 8 Educational attainment and maternal mortality, Mexico (1990). From reference 21

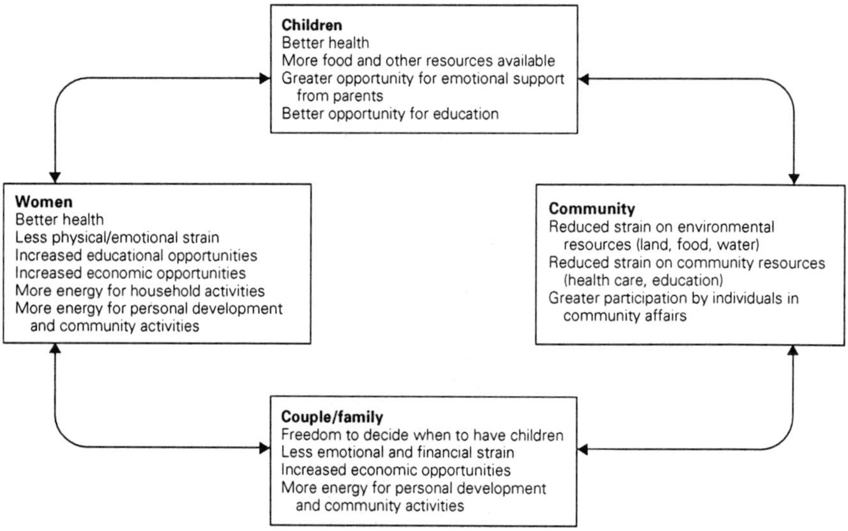

Figure 9 Benefits of family planning

CONCLUSIONS

The major advantages of family planning for communities, families, couples, children and women are summarized in Figure 9. Focusing on the box for women, family planning means, above all, better health with less physical and emotional stress. It means greater energy for personal development and social activities[22].

Can we hope to realize all of this throughout the world as it has been accomplished in Western countries? Yes, but we must create a second revolution, this time in the developing world. The challenge before of us is daunting, but we must have the strength to meet it.

REFERENCES

1. The Alan Guttmacher Institute. *Hopes and Realities*. New York: The Alan Guttmacher Institute 1995; 27–36
2. Monnier A, de Guibert-Lantoinc, G. The Demographic Situation of Europe and the Developed Countries Overseas: an Annual Report. *Population: An English Selection* 1995; 7: 187–202
3. Benagiano G. Benefits from family planning. *Eur J Contracep Reprod Health Care* 1996; 1: 225–30
4. Grunseit A, Kippax S. *Effects of Sex Education on Young People's Sexual Behaviour.* Unpublished review commissioned by the Global Programme on AIDS. Geneva: The World Health Organization 1993
5. Relazione del Ministero della Sanità sull'attuazione della Legge contenente norme

per la tutela sociale della maternità e per l'interruzione volontaria della gravidanza. Rome: Istituto poligrafico dello Stato, 1995

6. Monnier A, de Guilbert-Lantoine, C. The demographic situation of Europe and the developed countries overseas: an annual report. *Population: An English Selection* 1996: 235–50
7. United Nations. *Levels and Trends of Contraceptive Use as assessed in 1994*. New York: United Nations, 1996
8. Schesselman JJ. Oral contraceptives and neoplasia of the uterine corpus. *Contraception* 1991; 43: 557–79
9. Hankinson S, Colditz FA, Spencer DJ, *et al.* A quantitative assessment of oral contraceptive use and risk for ovarian cancer. *Obstet Gynecol* 1992; 80: 708–14
10. British Royal College of General Practitioners: Oral Contraceptive Study. Effect on hypertension and benign breast disease of progesterone component. *Lancet* 1977; 1: 624–7
11. Panser LA, Phipps WR. Type of oral contraceptives in relation to acute initial episodes of pelvic inflammatory disease. *Contraception* 1991; 43: 91–9
12. Hazes JMW, Dijkmans BAC, Vandenbroucke JP, *et al.* Reduction of the risk of rheumatoid arthritis among women who take oral contraceptives. *Arthritis Rheum* 1991; 34: 498–9
13. Kirshon B, Poindexter AN. Contraception: a risk factor for endometriosis. *Obstet Gynecol* 1988; 71: 829–31
14. Ross RK, Pike MC, Vessey MP, *et al.* Risk factors for uterine fibroids: reduced risks associated with oral contraceptives. *Br Med J* 1986; 293: 359–62
15. Lanes SF, Birmann B, Walker AM, *et al.* Oral contraceptive type and functional ovarian cysts. *Am J Obstet Gynecol* 1992; 166: 956–61
16. Clarkson TB, Shively CA, Morgan TM, *et al.* Oral contraceptives and coronary atherosclerosis of cynomolgus monkeys. *Obstet Gynecol* 1990; 75: 17–22
17. Shah IH. The advance of the contraceptive revolution. *World Health Statist* 1994; 47: 9–15
18. Wrangham R, Peterson D. *Demonic Males*. Boston, USA: Houghton Mifflin 1996
19. The World Bank. *World Development Report 1993: Investing in Health*. New York: Oxford University Press 1993
20. Senderowitz J. *Adolescent Health: Reassessing the Passage to Adulthood*. Discussion paper 272. Washington: the World Bank 1995
21. Lozano R, Hernandez B, Langer A. Factores Sociales y Económicos de la Mortalidad Materna en México. In del Carmen Elu M, Langer A, eds. *Maternidad sin Riesgos en México*. Mexico City: IMES/Comité Promoter de la Inciativa por una Maternidad sin Riesgos en Mexico, 1994
22. Division of Family Health of WHO. *Health Benefits of Family Planning*. Geneva: World Health Organization 1995

This paper has been reproduced from *Eur J Contracept Reprod Health Care* 1996; 1: 225–30

2 Clinical overview of hormonal contraception with special emphasis on long-term effects

P.G. Crosignani, F. Parazzini, C. La Vecchia, S. Meroni and E. Ricci

INTRODUCTION

Oral contraceptives (OCs) are the most widely used contraceptive methods in Western Europe, and, with the exception of intrauterine devices (common in China) OCs are the most widely used reversible contraceptive methods. This is primarily attributable to their high efficacy. Among reversible contraceptive methods, OCs have the lowest expected failure rates (Table 1) and are also prescribed for menstrual pain relief. In addition, OCs reduce the frequency of functional ovarian cysts, benign breast disease, metrorrhagia, endometriosis, amenorrhea, hyper-menorrhea, premenstrual syndrome and other menstrual cycle disorders[1]. These indications are well recognized, and very few data have been added in the literature in the last few years on the 'efficacy' of the pill.

Most research conducted in the last decade on the clinical effects of OCs has been focused on their potential long-term effect on cardiovascular diseases or carcinogenesis[2]. In this paper we review the main evidence of this research (a more detailed analysis is also available)[3,4].

CARDIOVASCULAR DISEASE

There is general evidence to show that the risk of heart and cerebrovascular disease is higher among women who have used oral contraceptives[5,6]. Overall, the relative risk is increased about 2-fold in current OC users, both for cardiovascular and cerebrovascular diseases[7]. The elevated risk seems to be restricted to current users, and no material association is observed in ex-users. For example, in the American Nurses' Health Study cohort[8], the relative risks for past users were 0.8 for major coronary diseases, 1.0 for stroke and 0.9 for all cardiovascular conditions. There was no evidence of a trend in the risk with duration of use or time since last use.

The role of OCs is apparently independent from that of other risk factors for cardiovascular disease[9–12], with the possible exception of smoking. In fact, there is, for example, some evidence that the relative risk (although clearly not the

Table 1 Failure rates during the first year of use (USA). Modified from Trussell J, *et al. Fam Plann* 1990; 21: 51

Method of contraception	*Percentage of women with pregnancy – lowest rate expected*
Combination pill	0.1
Intrauterine devices	0.8
Female sterilization	0.2
Male sterilization	0.1
Spermicides	3.0
Periodic abstinence	
calendar	9.0
ovulation method	3.0
symptothermal	2.0
Withdrawal	4.0
Diaphragm and spermicides	6.0
Condom	2.0

absolute excess risk) is similar in subsequent age groups[11]. Conversely, some studies have suggested that the relative risk in OC users/heavy smokers compared with non-smokers/non-oral contraceptive users is markedly elevated, thus indicating a multiplicative interaction on the relative risk. Such grossly elevated risk estimates are clearly of major concern for women exposed simultaneously to both risk factors. In clinical practice, this indicates that the avoidance of OC use in smokers would avoid, and has indeed avoided[13], most of the excess risk of cardiovascular diseases associated with OCs.

From the point of view of public health, these indications for selective prescription have probably been even more important for reducing vascular risk than the changes in composition (in particular, the reduced estrogen content) of newer formulations. Recently, it has been suggested that there is a greater risk of cardiovascular disease with third-generation oral contraceptives than with second-generation ones. Available data are, however, scanty and not completely consistent[14].

BREAST CANCER

Over the last few years a substantial amount of epidemiological data has been published on the OC/breast cancer issue, but the topic is still open. The overall evidence from published studies of the relationship between ever OC use and breast cancer risk is reassuring. Reviews and meta-analysis, based on several thousand cases, have estimated relative risks around unity[3,4,15–21]. There are, however, indications that current OC use is related to some excess breast cancer risk (about 20–30%), but there appears to be no association between breast cancer risk and past OC use.

A 20–30% excess risk clearly has different implications for younger women, whose baseline incidence of the disease is extremely low, compared to women aged 35–40 years or older, whose risk of breast cancer is no longer negligible. These considerations have practical implications for prescribing to women who are reaching the menopause, as well as women's individual informed choices.

Another relevant issue on which further data have become available in the last decade concerns the variation in breast cancer risk with different types of OCs. After making an allowance for duration of use, the World Health Organization (WHO) Collaborative Study on Neoplasms and Steroid Contraceptives[22] found that there was a slight indication that preparations containing high doses of estrogen and progestin were associated with breast cancer risk more than lower-dose ones, although the differences in risk were small. No appreciable difference was observed in breast cancer risk between products containing mestranol or estradiol, and between preparations containing progestins derived from 19-nortestosterone and 17α-hydroxyprogesterone. However, there is some indication from an American case-control study of breast cancer in young women[23] that any association may be stronger for higher-potency pills. Any difference in breast cancer risk between different types of preparation, if present, is likely to be limited and, hence, difficult to quantify.

ENDOMETRIAL CANCER

There is general evidence that ever OC use reduces the risk of endometrial cancer by about 50%[3,4,15]. The reduced risk seems to persist for at least 15–20 years after discontinuing use[24], but the limited number of elderly women who have used OCs does not allow a definitive estimate of the protection afforded after longer periods and/or according to duration of exposure. The protection afforded by OCs against endometrial cancer has been interpreted in terms of a relative increase in progestin levels. However, in an American population-based case–control study[25], the progestin potency of OCs was found to be unrelated to the risk of endometrial cancer. In contrast, the results of the WHO Collaborative Study of Neoplasia and Steroid Contraceptives[26] suggested that the protection was stronger for users of high-dose progestin preparations.

OVARIAN CANCER

Oral contraceptive use decreases the risk of ovarian cancer, with the estimated protection being approximately 40% in ever users, and increasing with duration of use. The favorable effect of OCs on ovarian cancer risk seems to persist for at least 10–15 years after OC use has ceased[27,28], and it is not confined to any particular type of OC formulation[29]. There is some suggestion that lower-dose estrogen formulations may be slightly less protective: in the WHO Collaborative Study on Neoplasms and Steroid Contraceptives[30], the relative risk of ovarian cancer was 0.7 for high-dose preparations and 0.8 for low-dose ones. Moreover, available data do not provide definitive evidence of an association between low-dose estrogen OCs and ovarian cancer for longer periods or in relation to latency or recency of use.

CERVICAL CANCER

Several studies have suggested a positive association between cervical cancer and OCs. Although published data are not totally consistent, available evidence indicates an approximately 50% higher risk of invasive cervical cancer among long-term OC users, which is not explained by potentially confounding effects of major covariates, including indicators of sexual habits[3,15].

Interpretation of these findings in biological terms is largely tentative. There are some suggestions that the relative risk is higher in the short term, and decreases with time since first and last use. OCs increase the risk of invasive cervical cancer, but not of intraepithelial neoplasia[31]. These observations have potentially interesting pathogenic correlates, since they would suggest a role of OCs in one of the later stages of the process of cervical carcinogenesis.

LIVER CANCER

Several epidemiological studies have suggested a positive association between OC use and liver cancer in developed countries, where the prevalence of hepatitis B is low, while no clear evidence of association has been reported in developing countries, where hepatitis B is endemic[3,4,32]. Thus, it appears that, in developing countries, where the prevalence of hepatitis B (the most important etiological factor for liver cancer) is very high and liver cancer incidence is correspondingly elevated, OC use is not a major risk factor. Conversely, in developed countries, where the prevalence of hepatitis B and the incidence of liver cancer are low, case–control studies indicate that OC use is a risk factor.

CUTANEOUS MALIGNANT MELANOMA

An increased risk of cutaneous malignant melanoma in ever users of OCs was suggested in the 1970s[33]. However, subsequent research did not confirm these suggestions. In particular, two cohort studies conducted in Great Britain (the Royal College of General Practitioners' Oral Contraception Study and the Oxford/Family Planning Association Contraceptive Study) found a relative risk of 0.9 for ever use and no trend with increasing duration of use, although a

Table 2 Estimates of the incidence of and mortality from unsafe abortions (World Health Organization Position Paper, International Conference on Population and Development 1994, Cairo)

Region	*Unsafe abortions (millions)*	*Deaths from unsafe abortions*
World	20.5	67 000
Africa	3.3	21 000
Asia	10.3	39 000
Latin America	4.2	5 500
USSR (former)	2.1	500
Europe	0.26	200

non-significant relative risk of 1.8 for a duration of use longer than 10 years emerged in the first study[5,6].

CONCLUSIONS

The main clinical role of oral contraceptives is, of course, contraception, and the first public health impact is reduction of unplanned pregnancies, and hence of maternal mortality due to induced abortions or delivery, particularly in developing countries (Table 2). However, in developed countries, the impact of oral contraceptives on cardiovascular diseases and carcinogenesis is a major issue in clinical practice and research.

In an effort to summarize the main evidence from the more recent research, we can conclude that:

(1) Oral contraceptives lower the risk of endometrial and ovarian cancer, and the protection seems to persist in the long term; and

(2) There is no association with skin melanoma and breast cancer risk, although there is a moderately increased risk among *current* users for breast cancer.

These results have important implications for making an informed choice about contraception. In contrast, information leaflets about oral contraceptives include a particularly detailed, but in several aspects, critical list of contraindications and side-effects. These include idiopathic jaundice, herpes gestations, unspecified liver disease, metrorrhagia, disorder of lipid metabolism, thromboembolic disorders, Dubin–Johnson syndrome, Rotor syndrome, thrombophlebitis, deteriorating otosclerosis, sickle cell anemia and pruritis, but do not generally indicate the main evidence about carcinogenesis. These confusing indications may decrease compliance, and also lack any general clear and quantitative indication[34], causing confusion and leading to withdrawal from oral contraceptive use by some women who have no real contraindications.

REFERENCES

1. Crosignani PG, La Vecchia C. Hormonal contraception. In Dooley MM, Brincat MP, eds. *Understanding Common Disorders in Reproductive Endocrinology*. Chichester: John Wiley, 1994; 123–43
2. Rivera R. Oral contraceptives: the last decade. In Van Look PFA, Pérez Palacios G, eds. *Contraceptive Research and Development 1984 to 1994*. Oxford, UK: Oxford University Press; 23–27
3. La Vecchia C, Franceschi S, Bruzzi P, Parazzini F, Boyle P. The relationship between oral contraceptive use, cancer and vascular disease. *Drug Safety* 1990; 5: 436–46
4. La Vecchia C, Tavani A, Franceschi S, Parazzini F. Oral contraceptives and cancer. A review of the evidence. *Drug Safety* 1996; 14: 260–72
5. RCGP (Royal College of General Practitioners). *Oral contraceptives and health: an interim report from the Oral Contraception Study of the Royal College of General Practitioners.* London: Pitman Medical, 1974
6. Vessey MP, Doll R, Peto R, Johnson B, Wiggins PA. Long-term follow-up study of women using different methods of contraception: an interim report. *J Biosoc Sci* 1976; 8: 373–427
7. Slone D, Shapiro S, Kaufman DW, Rosenberg L, Miettinen OS, *et al.* Risk of myocardial infarction in relation to current and discontinued use of oral contraceptives. *N Engl J Med* 1981; 305: 420–4
8. Stampfer MJ, Willet WC, Colditz GA, Speizer FE, Hennekens CH. A prospective study of past use of oral contraceptive agents and risk of cardiovascular diseases. *N Engl J Med* 1988; 319: 1313–17
9. Jick H, Dinan B, Rothman KJ. Oral contraceptives and non-fatal myocardial infarction. *J Am Med Assoc* 1978; 239:1403–6
10. Mann JI, Inman WHW, Thorogood M. Oral contraceptive use in older women and fatal myocardial infarction. *Br Med J* 1976; 2: 445–7
11. Shapiro S, Slone D, Rosenberg L, Kaufman DW, Stolley PD, *et al.* Oral contraceptive use in relation to myocardial infarction. *Lancet* 1979; 1: 743–7
12. Vessey MP, Doll R. Investigation of relation between use of oral contraceptives and thromboembolic disease. *Br Med J* 1968; 2: 199–205
13. Stadel BV. Oral contraceptives and cardiovascular disease. *N Engl J Med* 1981; 305: 612–18, 672–7
14. Rosenberg L, Bégaud B, Bergman U, Brown B, Buist AS, Cramer D, Daling J, Grimes D, Kemper F, Mills A. What are the risks of third-generation oral contraceptives? Are third-generation oral contraceptives safe? *Hum Reprod* 1996; 11: 687–93
15. Prentice RL, Thomas DB. On the epidemiology of oral contraceptives and disease. *Adv Cancer Res* 1987; 49: 285–401
16. Olsson H. Oral contraceptives and breast cancer: a review. *Acta Oncol* 1989; 28: 849–63

17. La Vecchia C. Oral contraceptives and breast cancer. *Breast* 1992; 2: 76–81
18. Thomas DB. Oral contraceptives and breast cancer. *J Natl Cancer Inst* 1993; 85: 359–63
19. Schlesselmann JJ. Net effect of oral contraceptive use on the risk of cancer in women in the United States. *Obstet Gynecol* 1995; 85: 793–801
20. La Vecchia C, Parazzini F, Negri E, *et al.* Risks and benefits of oral contraceptives in Italy. In Andreoli M, Shields M, eds. *Highlights in Molecular and Clinical Endocrinology*, Ares-Serono Symposium 1994, May 22–24, Rome. Rome: Ares-Serono 1994; 327–36
21. Malone KE, Daling JR, Weiss NS. Oral contraceptives in relation to breast cancer. *Epidemiol Rev* 1993; 15: 80–97
22. Thomas DB, Noonan EA and the WHO Collaborative Study of Neoplasia and Steroid Contraceptives. Risk of breast cancer in relation to use of combined oral contraceptives near the age of menopause. *Cancer Causes Control* 1991; 2: 389–94
23. White E, Malone KE, Weiss NS, *et al.* Breast cancer among young US women in relation to oral contraceptive use. *J Natl Cancer Inst* 1994; 86: 505–14
24. Stanford JL, Brinton LA, Berman ML, *et al.* Oral contraceptives and endometrial cancer: do the other risk factors modify the association? *Int J Cancer* 1993; 54: 243–8
25. Voigt LF, Deng Q, Weiss NS. Recency, duration and progestin content of oral contraceptives in relation to the incidence of endometrial cancer (Washington, USA). *Cancer Causes Control* 1994; 5: 227–33
26. Rosenblatt KA, Thomas DB and the WHO Collaborative Study of Neoplasia and Steroid Contraceptives. Hormonal content of combined oral contraceptives in relation to the reduced risk of endometrial carcinoma. *Int J Cancer* 1991; 49: 870–4
27. Franceschi S, Parazzini F, Negri E, *et al.* Pooled analysis of three European case–control studies of epithelial ovarian cancer. III. Oral contraceptive use. *Int J Cancer* 1991; 49: 61–5
28. Parazzini F, Franceschi S, La Vecchia C, *et al.* The epidemiology of ovarian cancer. *Gynecol Oncol* 1991; 43: 9–23
29. Gwinn ML, Lee NC, Rhodes PH. Pregnancy, breast feeding and oral contraceptives and the risk of epithelial ovarian cancer. *J Clin Epidemiol* 1990; 43: 559–68
30. Rosenblatt KA, Thomas DB, Noonan EA, WHO Collaborative Study of Neoplasia and Steroid Contraceptives. High dose combined oral contraceptives: protection against epithelial cancer and the length of protective effect. *Eur J Cancer* 1992; 28A: 1872–6
31. Parazzini F, La Vecchia C, Negri E, Fedele L, Franceschi S, Gallotta L. Risk factors for cervical intraepithelial neoplasia. *Cancer* 1992; 69: 2276–82
32. WHO Collaborative Study of Neoplasia and Steroid Contraceptives. Combined oral contraceptives and liver cancer. *Int J Cancer* 1989; 43: 254–9
33. Beral V, Ramcharan S, Faris R. Malignant melanoma and oral contraceptive use among women in California. *Br J Cancer* 1977; 36: 804–9
34. Fioretti F, La Vecchia C, Tavani A, Parazzini F. Package inserts of oral contraceptives in Italy. *Pharmacoepidemiol Drug Safety* 1996; 5: 226–32

This paper has been reproduced from *Eur J Contracept Reprod Health Care* 1997; 2: 117–21

3 Biochemical aspects of hormonal contraception: effects on bone metabolism

A. Volpe, A. Amram, A. Cagnacci and C. Battaglia

INTRODUCTION

Osteoporosis is a major health-care problem leading to the increased incidence of vertebral, radial and hip fractures in the aging population. The magnitude of the problem is likely to increase as the proportion of elderly people increases. Both trabecular and cortical bone mineral content reduction occurs physiologically during the premenopausal period[1] and, overall, at the time of menopause. It is related to the fall of plasma estrogen levels[2–4]. *In vitro* studies have demonstrated that estrogens can act directly on osteoblasts by a receptor-mediated mechanism and modulate skeletal mineralization and remodelling[5,6].

The measurement of bone mineral density (BMD) can be predictive of future fracture risk. Several studies have examined the relationship between bone density and oral contraceptives (OCs). From the bulk of published reports it emerges that there is no consensus on whether OCs have a real protective effect on bone metabolism[7]. The different results can be explained by different techniques and different sites for measuring bone density, different OCs used, small number of subjects studied and trials not adequately controlled.

Our previous study[8] showed that, in premenopausal women (aged 40–45 years) with regular menstrual cycles, treated with OCs over a period of 24 months, the bone mineral density and biochemical markers of bone metabolism were unchanged.

The aim of the present study was to investigate in perimenopausal women the effect of an oral contraceptive on bone density and biochemical markers of bone metabolism.

MATERIALS AND METHODS

The study protocol was approved by the local Ethics Review Committee. Perimenopausal patients (n = 17) (aged 46–53 years), who experienced oligomenorrhea (cycle length ≥ 35 days) in the 3–6 months before the study, entered the study after informed consent was obtained. The patients were randomly assigned to Group I ($n = 8$), who received OCs containing 0.02 μg of ethinylestradiol (EE) and 0.15 μg of desogestrel (DOG) for 36 months, and Group II ($n = 9$) who received a placebo.

The inclusion criteria were normal thyroid, renal and adrenal function as assessed by clinical, hormonal and biochemical evaluations. None of the subjects had any pathological conditions influencing calcium metabolism and none received hormones or other medical treatments known to interfere with bone metabolism in the 6 months before observation. Furthermore, no therapies known to affect calcium metabolism were allowed during the study. All subjects were studied prior to initiation of therapy and every 6 months up to the 36th cycle of treatment, for the evaluation of bone mineral density (BMD), plasma osteocalcin, alkaline phosphatase and urinary hydroxyproline.

The bone density (mg/cm^2) of lumbar vertebrae L2–L4 was measured with the woman in the supine position, with her legs elevated to minimize lordosis, using dual energy X-ray absorptiometry (Lunar DPX; Lunar Corp., Madison, WI). Factors that may influence BMD were adjusted for age, body mass, physical activity, calcium intake and total duration of breastfeeding.

Fasting urinary excretion of hydroxyproline, a biochemical marker of bone resorption, was measured by a spectrophotometric method[9]. Serum alkaline phosphatase, a biochemical marker of bone formation was measured, enzymatically according to the Scandinavian recommendations[10]. Plasma osteocalcin, another parameter of bone formation, was measured in duplicate by radioimmunoassay using commercially available kits (Osteocalcin kit; Technogenetics, Trezzano sul Naviglio, Italy).

Statistical analysis

All the results were reported as the mean ± standard error (SE). Statistical analysis of the results was performed using the Student's t-test for unpaired data. The possible correlation between the observed data was studied by a simple linear regression analysis. A probability value < 0.05 was considered to be statistically significant.

RESULTS

In the treated group, a slight but non-significant bone mass improvement was observed during the entire period of OC therapy (36 months), whereas a continued and progressive bone loss was observed in the control group. After 3 years, the difference in BMD between the two groups was found to be significant (Figure 1). In OC-treated women, the pattern of urinary excretion of hydroxyproline (OHP) showed a progressive decrease from the baseline values (Figure 2a). This result correlated inversely with the vertebral bone density ($r = -0.6420$; $p < 0.05$).

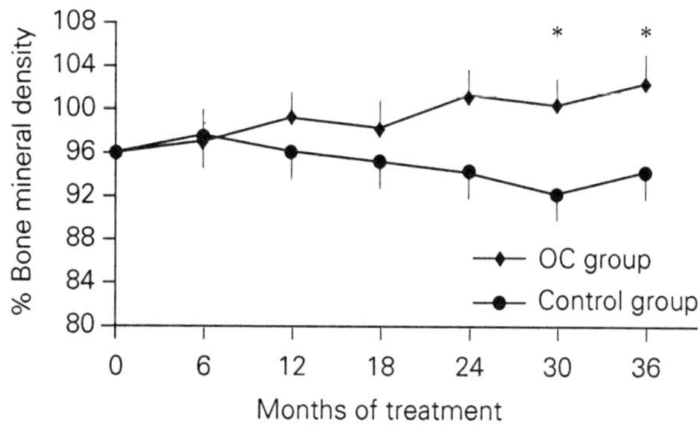

Figure 1 Bone mineral density in perimenopausal women. *, $p < 0.05$

Serum alkaline phosphatase (AP) significantly decreased from the 30th month of therapy until the end of the study (Figure 2b). Serum osteocalcin levels were also significantly decreased at the end of the therapy (Figure 2c).

DISCUSSION

The present study showed that, during 36 months of therapy, there is a modest increase in the spinal BMD among perimenopausal women treated with OCs, whereas a continuous and progressive bone loss was observed in the control group. The positive effect of OCs on BMD seems to be confirmed by continuous and progressive reduction of catabolic bone biochemical markers. Furthermore, the present study confirms previous observations in the literature. Goldsmith and colleagues[11] showed that peripheral bone mass was higher in premenopausal women who were taking oral contraceptives. Lindsay and colleagues[12] found, in 57 premenopausal women, a 1% increase in vertebral BMD for each year of exposure to OCs. Stevenson[13] showed a significant increase in bone density in postmenopausal women who previously used OCs. Gambacciani and co-workers[14] evaluated bone density and metabolism in a longitudinal 2-year follow-up study conducted in healthy, normally menstruating perimenopausal women, perimenopausal oligomenorrheic women, and age-matched oligomenorrheic women using OCs. He showed that there were no significant modifications in hormonal levels, biochemical markers of bone turnover and vertebral density in normal women. However, a significant increase in bone turnover associated with a decreased bone mass density in oligomenorrheic, hypoestrogenic and untreated patients was observed. On the other hand, Lindsay and colleagues[12] found no change in bone density in postmenopausal women who had previously used OCs and Rodin and co-workers[15], in a study involving 102 women, failed to find any significant difference in BMD between current OC users and never users. The discrepancy in findings may be attributed to differences in study design (cross-sectional study in which there is limited information on the past

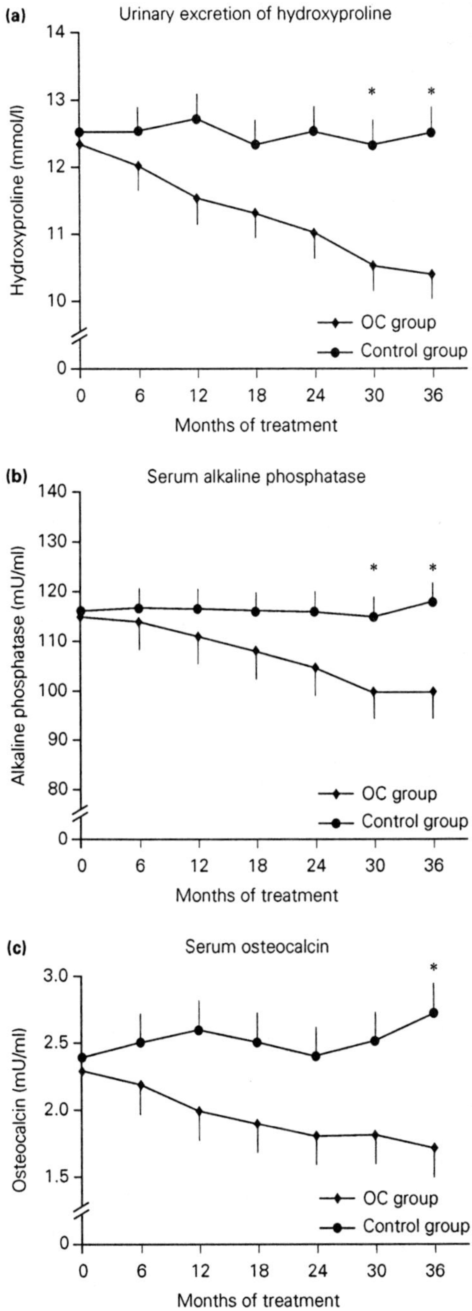

Figure 2 Biochemical markers of bone metabolism in perimenopausal women. *, $p < 0.05$; OC, oral contraceptive

exercise, diet, body weight and other lifestyle factors), small samples of women, and no complete information on the type of OCs used in the past by the women. The relationship between the ovarian function and bone turnover suggests that, during the perimenopausal transition, the decreased production in ovarian estradiol induces an activation of bone turnover that in turn causes a BMD decrease.

Our data confirm that OC therapy has a positive effect on bone density in perimenopausal women, suggesting that a long period of OC therapy is able to inhibit the activation of bone turnover. Furthermore, it seems to have a metabolic action on bone remodelling, and to induce the maintenance of BMD. The positive effect appears to be significant after 30 months of OC therapy, as supported by a significant reduction of biochemical markers of bone turnover.

CONCLUSIONS

Our findings support the previously observed associations between osteoporosis and the positive effect of oral contraceptive therapy. Moreover, the study confirmed that a long period of oral contraceptive therapy can be beneficial to inhibiting bone resorption and seems to be able to prevent the progressive decrease of bone loss in the perimenopausal age. Since controversial data are reported in the literature, we think
that they can be ascribed to many different factors: racial and hereditary factors, hormonal status, diet, smoking and physical activity. The effect of oral contraceptive therapy on bone mineral density still needs to be completely clarified. Further prospective random and extensive studies would be needed to substantiate these findings.

REFERENCES

1. Louis O, Devroey P, Kalender W, Osteaux M. Bone loss in young hypoestrogenic women due to primary ovarian failure: spinal quantitative computed tomography. *Fertil Steril* 1989; 52: 227–31
2. Lloyd T, Buchanan JR, Ursino GR, Myers C, Woodward G, Halbert DR. Long-term oral contraceptive use does not affect trabecular bone density. *Am J Obstet Gynecol* 1989; 160: 402–4
3. Stevenson JC, Lees B, Devenport M, Cust MP, Ganger KF. Determinant of bone density in normal women: risk factors for future osteoporosis? *Br Med J* 1989; 298: 924–8
4. Biller BMK, Coughlin JF, Saxe V, Schoenfeld D, Spratt DI, Klibanski A. Osteopenia in women with hypothalamic amenorrhea: a prospective study. *Obstet Gynecol* 1991; 78: 996–1001
5. Komm BS, Terpening CM, Benz DJ. Estrogen binding receptors mRNA, and biologic response in osteoblast-like osteosarcoma cells. *Science* 1988; 241: 81–4
6. Erikson EF, Colvard DS, Berg NJ. Evidence of estrogen receptors in normal human osteoblast-like cells. *Science* 1988; 241: 84–6

7. Stephen L, Corson MD. Oral contraceptives for the prevention of osteoporosis. *J Reprod Med* 1988; 38: 1015–20
8. Volpe A. The effect of the pill on bone metabolism. *Proceedings of the 3rd Congress of the ESC*, Athens 1994; 78–80
9. Newman RE, Logan MA. The determination of hydroxyproline. *J Biol Chem* 1950; 84: 299–303
10. Christiansen C, Riis BJ. 17β-Estradiol and continuous norethisterone: a unique treatment for established osteoporosis in elderly women. *J Clin Endocrinol Metab* 1990; 71: 836–41
11. Goldsmith NF, Johnston JO. Bone mineral effects of oral contraceptive, pregnancy and lactation. *J Bone Joint Surg* 1975; 57A: 657
12. Lindsay R, Tohme J, Kanders B. The effects of oral contraceptive use on vertebral bone mass in pre- and postmenopausal women. *Contraception* 1986; 34: 333–40
13. Stevenson JC. Pathogenesis, prevention and treatment of osteoporosis. *Obstet Gynecol* 1990; 75: 36S–41S
14. Gambacciani M, Spinetti A, Taponeco F. Longitudinal evaluation of perimenopausal vertebral bone loss: effects of a low-dose oral contraceptive preparation on bone mineral density and metabolism. *Obstet Gynecol* 1994; 83: 392–6
15. Rodin A, Chapman M, Fogelman I. Bone density in users of combined oral contraception. *Br J Fam Plann* 1991; 16: 125

This paper has been reproduced from *Eur J Contracept Reprod Health Care* 1997; 2: 123–6

4 Effects of sex steroid hormones on the neuroendocrine system

A.R. Genazzani, A. Lucchesi, M. Stomati, S. Catarsi, A.D. Genazzani, M. Criscuolo and F. Petraglia

INTRODUCTION

Estrogen and progesterone are the most important ovarian steroid hormones regulating female fertility, and have a profound effect on the central nervous system[1]. Pituitary and hypothalamic hormone release, thermoregulatory and cardiocirculatory activities and behavior and mood changes are targets of sex steroids in the brain. Recent studies have revealed that a correlation exists between sex steroid hormones and changes in brain neurotransmitters and neuropeptides: sex steroids exert their influence on synthesis and release of norepinephrine, dopamine, serotonin, gonadotropin releasing hormone (GnRH), corticotropin releasing factor (CRF) and β-endorphin[2].

Because inhibition of ovulation is the main objective of oral contraception, suppression of follicle-stimulating hormone (FSH) levels is of prime importance. Oral contraceptives inhibit folliculogenesis and ovulation by blocking the activity of the hypothalamus–pituitary–gonadal axis, in particular by suppressing the release of gonadotropins. This inhibitory effect seems to be due to the action of both estrogens and progestins on both hypothalamus and pituitary. Oral hormonal contraceptives exert their feedback effects at either the pituitary or the hypothalamic level, or both[3,4]. Oral contraceptives inhibit folliculogenesis and ovulation by acting on FSH secretion: FSH levels and the FSH response to an exogenous GnRH challenge, in fact, are uniformly depressed in oral contraceptive users. Progestins administered alone do not affect FSH levels, and the observed reduction in FSH output is attributed to a negative feedback effect of estrogen at the pituitary level. In addition to the negative feedback of estrogens, the decreased number of luteinizing hormone (LH) pulses and, by inference, of GnRH pulses, which occurs uniformly during oral contraceptive use, may contribute to the reduction in FSH release during oral contraceptive administration[3,5].

EFFECTS OF SEX STEROID HORMONES ON GnRH

Progesterone is a potent hormone which exerts its action mainly on the female reproductive tract, but also on a series of other functions, such as lipid metabolism and smooth muscle contractility. Therefore, the use of progesterone or progestins for chronic treatments (oral contraception or postmenopausal hormone replacement therapy) may cause several possible central actions and a series of side-effects[2,6]. Experimental studies conducted in female rats have shown that treatment with progesterone and norethisterone enanthate significantly increased the hypothalamic GnRH concentrations, whereas desogestrel and medroxyprogesterone acetate did not change hypothalamic GnRH or pituitary and plasma LH; progesterone and norethisterone enanthate concomitantly decrease pituitary LH and increase circulating LH. These data show a stimulatory action of progesterone on LH secretion, indicating that progesterone and norethisterone enanthate act on the hypothalamus-pituitary axis[7]. In fact, progesterone or norethisterone enanthate administered with estradiol benzoate significantly increase the hypothalamic GnRH content, reversing the negative effect of estradiol benzoate[1]. Therefore, these two steroid compounds have a positive stimulatory action on neuronal GnRH production. All gestagens reduced the increase of LH content induced by estradiol benzoate at the pituitary level (Figure 1); this means that an antagonistic effect of progesterone on estrogen-induced changes of the hypothalamus–pituitary–gonadal axis exists[1]. The negative feedback of estradiol benzoate on plasma LH is associated with a reduction of hypothalamic GnRH content and pituitary LH release (see Figure 1). The decreased estradiol benzoate-induced LH storage, caused by synthetic gestagens, may be due either to reduced LH synthesis or to changes in LH secretion.

Clinical studies have shown that progesterone exerts a positive effect on LH secretion in women if they have been pretreated with estradiol, and a negative effect when progesterone and estradiol administration start at the same time. These results have also been demonstrated in women using oral contraceptives[3,5,8]. Furthermore, because pituitary sensitivity is not compromised, and stimulation with GnRH results in a normal LH response of the pituitary, the reduction of LH pulse frequency in oral contraceptive users is probably caused by a gestagen-induced slowing of the hypothalamic pulse generator[3,9]. Elevated circulating inhibin levels may also play a role in determining the restriction of FSH release at pituitary level.

These results show that progesterone and progestins have a marked effect on hypothalamic and pituitary hormone secretion, and that they modulate estrogen-induced effects.

EFFECTS OF SEX STEROID HORMONES ON OPIOID PEPTIDES

Several studies have shown an important role of endogenous opioid peptides in the control of reproductive function. Whereas estrogens do not alter plasma β-endorphin levels, an important effect of progesterone on the opioidergic regulation of LH secretion has been shown: in fact, progesterone has been demonstrated to decrease hypothalamic and pituitary β-endorphin concentrations that, in turn, stimulate LH secretion, acting on the pulsatile release of GnRH from the mediobasal

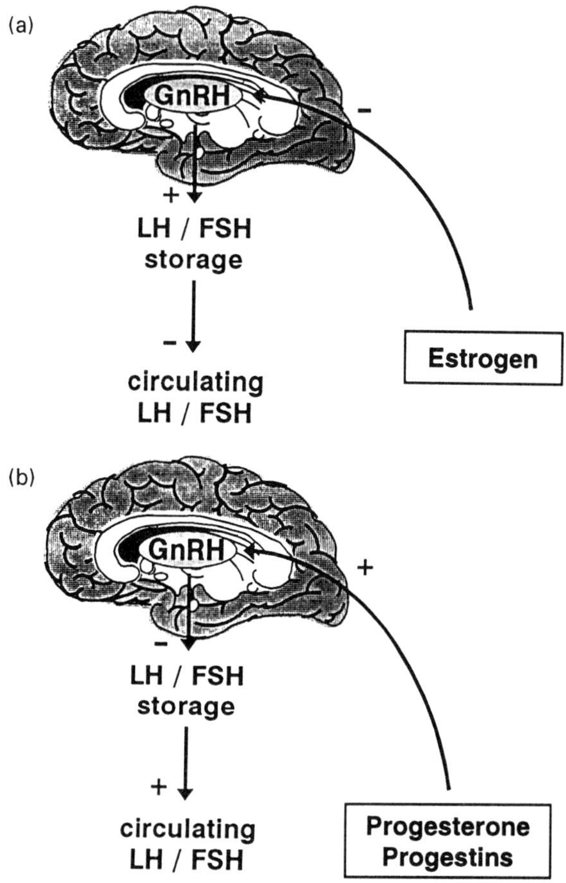

Figure 1 Effects of (a) estrogen and (b) progesterone and progestins on gonadotropin releasing hormone (GnRH). LH, luteinizing hormone; FSH, follicle stimulating hormone

hypothalamus (Figure 2)[10,11]. Because pituitary corticotropes are the major sources of plasma β-endorphin, this peptide has been proposed as part of the hypothalamus–pituitary–adrenal axis. Therefore, CRF increases and glucocorticoids decrease plasma β-endorphin, and circadian changes of plasma β-endorphin are similar to those of hypothalamus–pituitary–adrenal axis hormones[12]. Furthermore, plasma β-endorphin levels change during the menstrual cycle, and the increased β-endorphin plasma levels during the periovulatory days seem to be related to ovulatory function, suggesting a central activity modulated by gonadal steroids. In particular, a possible cause of plasma β-endorphin changes during the periovulatory phase seems to be the typical midcycle increase of plasma estradiol levels. The close correlation between ovulation and the midcycle plasma β-endorphin peak suggests an ovarian origin for this peak[13]. This is further supported by the evidence

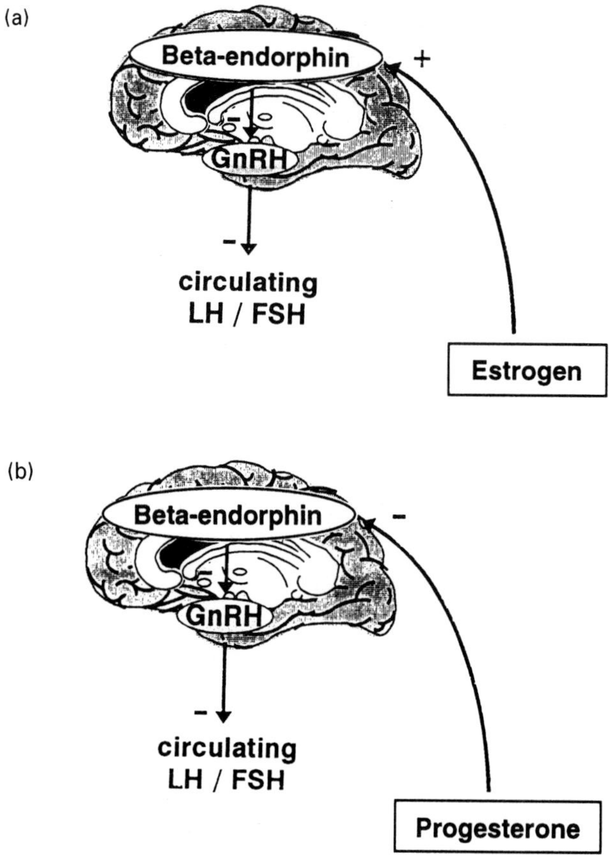

Figure 2 Effects of (a) estrogen and (b) progesterone on opioid peptides. GnRH, gonadotropin releasing hormone; LH, luteinizing hormone; FSH, follicle stimulating hormone

that oral contraceptives inhibit the periovulatory increase of β-endorphin plasma levels. In normal conditions, during the menstrual cycle, gonadal steroids change over time with a pattern that may not be mimicked by oral contraceptives. Therefore, the gonadal steroids may play an important role in determining the midcycle plasma β-endorphin peak. Therefore, the inhibition of ovulation by oral contraceptives is associated with a lack of both LH and β-endorphin surges, suggesting a relationship between the midcycle surges of these two hormones[11].

In female rats, the administration of estradiol benzoate increases hypothalamic β-endorphin concentrations (Figure 2)[14], modulating circadian changes[15]. Progesterone and synthetic progestins exert a similar effect. Among the progestins, while desogestrel increases pituitary β-endorphin, norethisterone acetate stimulates the hypothalamic pool[16], whereas norgestimate, a new potent progestin, shows an action at both pituitary and hypothalamic level. The different mechanism of action of norgestimate when associated with estrogens suggests a synergism with estradiol benzoate in increasing β-endorphin. Furthermore, the action of norgestimate, at pituitary and brain level, suggests that this progestin may act on β-endorphin-related neuroendocrine functions[2].

In the rat, receptor sites for progesterone have been demonstrated at the pituitary, hypothalamic and extra-hypothalamic levels. In several cases the distribution of progesterone receptors overlaps with that of estrogen binding sites, resulting in estrogen inducibility[2]. β-Endorphin exerts its actions through μ-type receptors and inhibits GnRH and LH release[17]. In fact, it has been observed that, in the whole brain of the female rat, the number of opioid receptors of the μ-type fluctuates during the phases of the estrous cycle. This may explain the different magnitude of the effects of opioid agonists and antagonists on gonadotropin release in the different phases of the ovulatory cycle[17]. During proestrus, in coincidence with the initiation of the LH surge, a progressive decrease in the number of hypothalamic μ-receptors has been demonstrated. In fact, it is possible that this decrease in the number of hypothalamic μ-receptors might be indicative of a decreased opiatergic tone, and that this might cause the release of GnRH. However, it is not well known why the number of hypothalamic μ-receptors declines during this phase of the estrous cycle, but it might be related to the increase in serum estradiol and progesterone levels occurring during proestrus. Indeed, an increase in the number of μ-receptors has been observed in the hippocampus and thalamus: this might be indicative of an estrogen-mediated increase in the opiatergic inhibitory tone, which occurs in these areas. Furthermore, the hippocampus has been demonstrated to be a target for estrogens: it might exert an inhibitory influence on gonadotropin release[17].

Thus, the opioidergic pathway may play an important role in reproductive function, as well as in sexual behavior, mediating the inhibition of the hypothalamus–pituitary–ovarian axis induced by oral contraceptives[2].

EFFECTS OF SEX STEROID HORMONES ON ADRENOCORTICOTROPIC HORMONE

Stress has been demonstrated to inhibit reproductive function: this effect is due to a decrease in gonadotropin secretion, as well as an inhibition of sexual behavior. Sex steroids, in turn, have been demonstrated to have an influence on hypothalamic–pituitary–adrenal function and activity. Estrogens are potent modulators of the pituitary–adrenal axis: basal levels of adrenocorticotropic hormone (ACTH) and corticosteroids increase at the time of proestrus in female rats, and toward the end of the follicular phase in women, when estrogen plasma levels are elevated (Figure 3)[18,19].

The effect of estrogens on pituitary–adrenal axis responsiveness in humans has been investigated. Activation of the hypothalamic–pituitary–adrenal axis is a

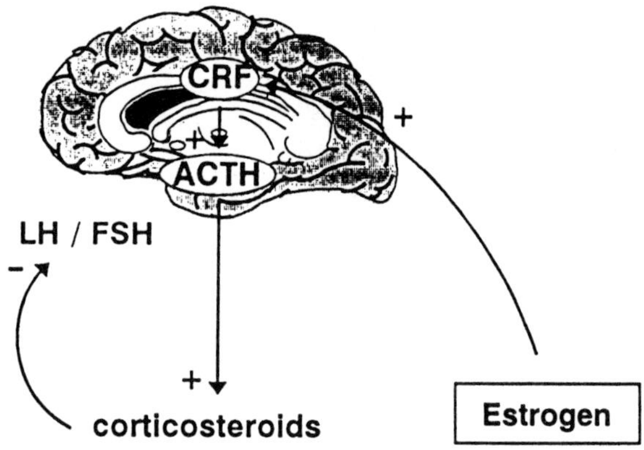

Figure 3 Effect of estrogen on adrenocorticotropic hormone (ACTH). CRF, corticotropic releasing factor; LH, luteinizing hormone; FSH, follicle stimulating hormone

characteristic physiological response to stress, and estrogens may affect endocrine response to stress. The stimulatory effect of estrogen on ACTH responses to stress seems to be transient; in fact, the enhanced ACTH responses to stress have been shown 24 h, but not 48 h, after estrogen administration[18]. A sex difference exists in both circulating corticosterone and in the corticosterone response to stress, with females having higher levels than males. This sex difference in ACTH and corticosterone levels during stress is abolished by ovariectomy. Other studies have shown that ovariectomy reduces basal corticosterone levels, while indeed estradiol administration increases them[20]. This is consistent with studies showing that basal and stress responsive corticosterone levels are highest during proestrus, when estrogen levels are highest[21].

Previous studies have classified two types of receptors for corticosterone: type I and type II, which are the products of the mineralocorticoid receptor gene and the glucocorticoid receptor gene, respectively. Chronic estrogen administration might cause a loss of glucocorticoid receptor ability to autoregulate, and this suggests that estrogen might cause a functional impairment of the glucocorticoid receptor. These data suggest that hyperactivation of the hypothalamic–pituitary–adrenal axis after stress in estrogen-treated rats might be due to impaired glucocorticoid receptor-mediated negative feedback[20,21].

EFFECTS OF SEX STEROID HORMONES ON CATECHOLAMINES

An increase in central noradrenergic and dopaminergic pathways following progesterone treatment has been demonstrated (Figures 4 and 5). Estradiol also regulates central catecholamine systems, which are a major modulator of the hypothalamic–pituitary–adrenal axis.

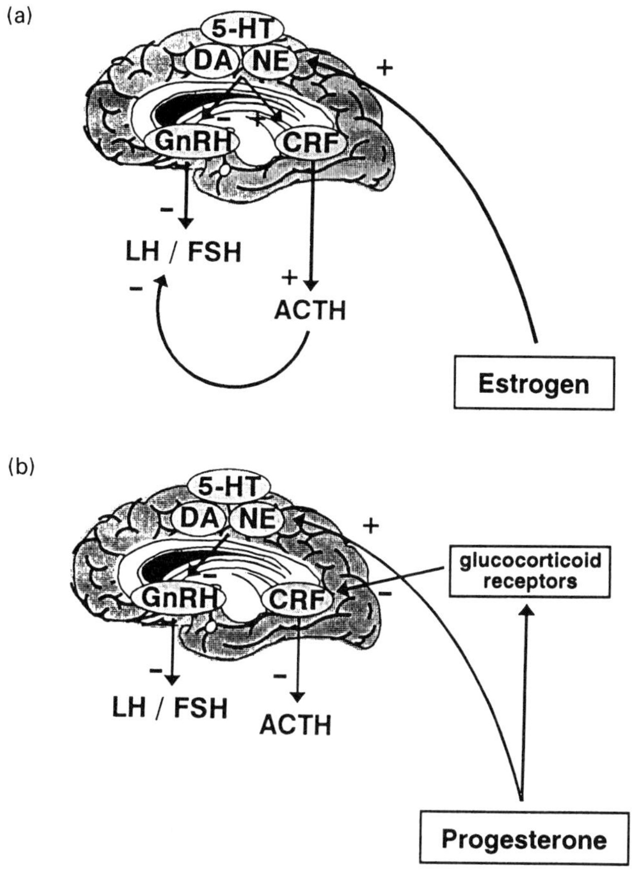

Figure 4 Effects of (a) estrogen and (b) progesterone on catecholamines. LH, luteinizing hormone; FSH, follicle stimulating hormone; GnRH, gonadotropin releasing hormone; ACTH, adrenocorticotropic hormone; CRF, corticotropic releasing factor; 5-HT, serotonin; DA, dopamine; NE, norepinephrine

During early proestrus, estradiol increases the norepinephrine and dopamine turnover rates at hypothalamic level, that mediate CRF activity during basal and stress conditions. The effects of catecholamines on CRF synthesis and release are dose dependent: in fact, intracerebroventricular low-dose administration of norepinephrine increases CRF release (at α_1-adrenergic receptors), while high-dose administration inhibits CRF release (at β-adrenergic receptors)[22].

In women with hypothalamic amenorrhea, who are estrogen deficient, elevated basal cortisol secretion as well as elevated responses to CRF have been demonstrated[23].

Estradiol appears to up-regulate α_1-adrenergic and down-regulate β-adrenergic receptors. Thus, it is possible that during early proestrus, when

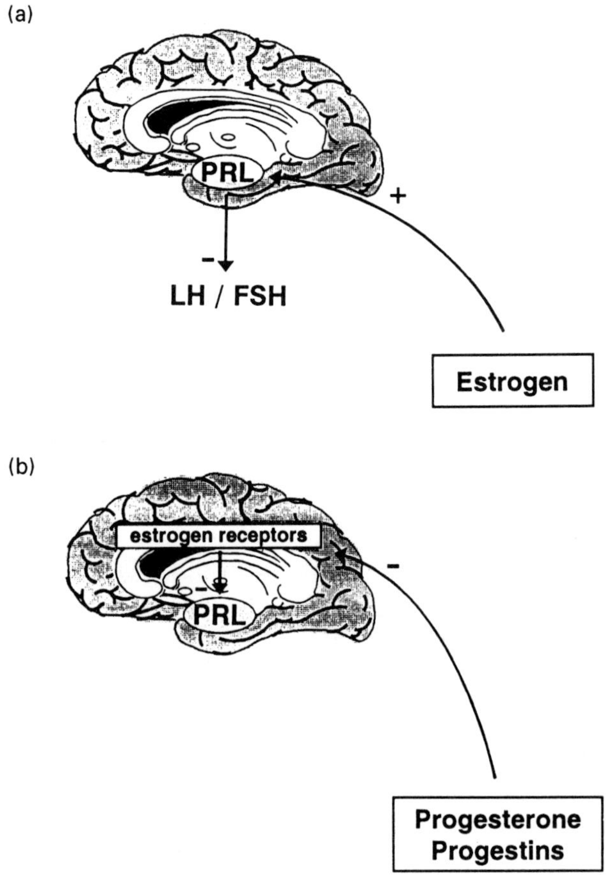

Figure 5 Effects of (a) estrogen and (b) progesterone and progestins on prolactin (PRL). LH, luteinizing hormone; FSH, follicle stimulating hormone

norepinephrine levels are rising, CRF release is increased as a function of increased α_1-adrenergic and decreased β-adrenergic receptor density, leading to an enhancement of ACTH synthesis (Figure 4). In fact, α_1-adrenergic receptors are stimulatory, while β-adrenergic receptors are inhibitory. Progesterone, indeed, seems to limit enhanced ACTH responses occurring during early proestrus. This hormone has been shown to inhibit hypothalamic CRF and pituitary ACTH production during stress in estrus, perhaps because of its affinity for the glucocorticoid receptor (Figure 4)[24].

Central serotonin and catecholamine systems seem to be implicated in mediating feedback mechanisms occurring during stress (Figure 4). Hypothalamic serotonin content varies throughout the estrous cycle, and estradiol has been demonstrated to cause an acute biphasic up- and down-regulation of serotonin receptors – an early decrease in serotonin receptor concentration is followed by a delayed increase[25]. Furthermore, serotonin receptors are co-expressed in many brain regions with the glucocorticoid receptors[18,26]. This suggests that estradiol can influence glucocorticoid feedback via its affects on serotonin transmission[18].

EFFECTS OF SEX STEROID HORMONES ON PROLACTIN

Significant changes in circulating prolactin levels during the menstrual cycle have been shown. In fact, during the late follicular phase, there is a progressive increase in serum prolactin levels, reaching a maximum value concomitantly with the LH peak. Subsequently, serum prolactin levels remain significantly higher during the luteal phase than during the early follicular phase[27]. However, the variations in prolactin are of moderate amplitude when compared with those reported for LH[28–30].

Observations that a high rate of patients with prolactinoma had previously used estrogen-containing oral contraceptives, and that prolactinomas developed in laboratory animals after estrogen administration, suggested a possible relationship between the use of estrogen and prolactin secretion[31,32]. A midcycle and luteal phase hyperprolactinemia has also been documented during ovulation induction with human gonadotropins in amenorrheic women[30]. It has been demonstrated that estrogens are important physiological stimulators of prolactin secretion both in humans[30,33] and in rats[1]. This regulation may at least partly be exerted at the pituitary level, by stimulating prolactin synthesis (Figure 5). Furthermore, some reports have shown that treatment with estradiol benzoate significantly increases the pituitary concentration of prolactin in ovariectomized rats. Hyperprolactinemia has been shown to disturb follicular maturation and corpus luteum function in women[34]. Administration of progesterone or progestins did not induce significant changes in pituitary or plasma prolactin[33], but reversed the estradiol benzoate-induced increase, by decreasing the number of available receptor sites (Figure 5). On the other hand, progesterone treatment does not alter the binding affinity of the estradiol receptor, but acts through a reduction in the availability of cytoplasmic estrogen receptors[1]. Therefore, progesterone could interfere with the action of estradiol on prolactin secretion by decreasing the availability of estrogen receptor, either by reducing its synthesis or by preventing the re-utilization of existing receptor after nuclear accumulation. This effect of progesterone is not dependent on its binding to the estrogen receptor, and the mechanism of action of progesterone is thus different from that of the antiestrogens, which bind to the cytoplasmic estrogen receptor[35].

CONCLUSIONS

In conclusion, the various progestins show different effects on hypothalamic gonadotropin releasing hormone and on pituitary luteinizing hormone and prolactin, but all modulate in the same manner the estrogen-induced effect on these structures. These data support the concept that when progestins are used alone or in association with ethinylestradiol for contraception, they have different effects on pituitary and hypothalamic cells[1].

REFERENCES

1. Genazzani AR, Petraglia F, Silferi M *et al.* Progestins modulate the action of estrogen on gonadotropin-releasing hormone, luteinizing hormone and prolactin in the rat. *Gynecol Obstet Invest* 1990; 29: 197–202
2. Genazzani AR, Petraglia F, Cleva M *et al.* Norgestimate increases pituitary and hypothalamic concentrations of immunoreactive beta-endorphin. *Contraception* 1990; 40: 605–13
3. Hemrika DJ, Slaats EH, Schoemaker J. The response of the pituitary–ovarian axis to pulsatile administration of gonadotropin-releasing hormone in long-term oral contraceptive users. *Am J Obstet Gynecol* 1994; 170: 462–8
4. Mishell DR, Kletzky OA, Brenner PF. The effect of contraceptive steroids on hypothalamic–pituitary–function. *Am J Obstet Gynecol* 1977; 128: 60–6
5. Labrie F, Lagacé L, Drouin J *et al.* Direct and differential effects of sex steroids at the anterior pituitary level on LH and FSH secretion. In Klopper A, Lerner AB, van der Molen HJ, Sciarra, J.J. eds. *Research on Steroids.* London: Academic Press, 1979; Vol 8: 207
6. Diczfalusy E. Mode of action of contraceptive drugs. *Obstet Gynecol* 1968; 100: 136–46
7. Mann DR, Barraclough CA. Role of estrogen and progesterone in facilitatng LH release in 4-day cyclic rats. *Endocrinology* 1973; 93: 694–7
8. Goodman RL. The sites of action of ovarian steroids in the regulation of LH secretion. *Neuroendocrinology* 1981; 32: 57–61
9. Mais V, Cetel NS, Muse KN, Quigley ME, Reid RL, Yen SSC. Hormonal dynamics during luteal–follicular transition. *J Clin Endocrinol Metab* 1987; 64: 1109–14
10. Shoupe D, Montz FJ, Lobo RA. The effects of estrogen and progestin on endogenous opioid activity in oophorectomized women. *J Clin Endocrinol Metab* 1985; 60: 178–83
11. Comitini G, Petraglia F, Fachinetti F *et al.* Effect of oral contraceptives or dexamethasone on plasma beta-endorphin during the menstrual cycle. *Fertil Steril* 1989; 51: 46–50
12. Petraglia F, Facchinetti F, Parrini D *et al.* Simultaneous circadian variations of plasma ACTH, β-lipotropin, β-endorphin and cortisol. *Horm Res* 1983; 17: 147–52
13. Petraglia F, Segre A, Facchinetti F *et al.* β-Endorphin and met-enkephalin in peritoneal and ovarian follicular fluids of fertile and postmenopausal women. *Fertil Steril* 1985; 44: 615–21
14. Petraglia F, Penalva A, Locatelli V *et al.* Effects of gonadectomy and gonadal steroids replacement on pituitary and plasma B-EP levels in the rat. *Endocrinology* 1982; 111: 1224–9
15. Genazzani AR, Trentini GP, Petraglia F *et al.* Estrogens modulate the circadian rhythm of hypothalamic beta-endorphin contents in female rats. *Neuroendocrinology* 1990; 52: 221–4

16. Genazzani AR, Petraglia F, Bergamaschi M *et al.* Progesterone and progestins modulate β-endorphin concentrations in the hypothalamus and in the pituitary of castrated female rats. *Gynecol Endocrinol* 1987; 1: 61–9
17. Piva F, Limonta P, Dondi D *et al.* Effects of steroids on the brain opioid system. *J Steroid Biochem Molec Biol* 1995; 53: 343–8
18. Viau V, Meaney MJ. Variations in the hypothalamus–pituitary–adrenal response to stress during the estrous cycle in the rat. *Endocrinology* 1991; 129: 2503–11
19. Carey MP, Deterd CH, de Koning J *et al.* The influence of ovarian steroids on hypothalamic–pituitary–adrenal regulation in the female rat. *J Endocrinol* 1995; 144: 311–21
20. Redei E, Li L, Halasz I *et al.* Fast glucocorticoid feedback inhibition of ACTH secretion in the ovariectomized rat: effect of chronic estrogen and progesterone. *Neuroendocrinology* 1994; 60: 113–23
21. Burgess LH, Handa RJ. Chronic estrogen-induced alterations in adrenocorticotropin and corticosterone secretion, and glucocorticoid receptor-mediated functions in female rats. *Endocrinology* 1992; 131: 1261–9
22. Plotsky PM, Cunningham ET, Widwaier EP. Catecholaminergic modulation of corticotropin-releasing factor and adrenocorticotropin secretion. *Endocr Rev* 1989; 10: 437–58
23. Biller BMK, Federoff HJ, Koenig JI *et al.* Abnormal cortisol secretion and responses to corticotropin-releasing hormone in women with hypothalamic amenorrhea. *J Clin Endocrinol Metab* 1990; 70: 311–17
24. Sarrieau A, Rostene W, Antakly T *et al.* Modulation of glucocorticoid binding capacity in selected brain regions and pituitary of adrenectomized rats by various steroids. *Soc Neurosci Abstr* 1987; 13: 725 (Abstr 201.8)
25. Biegon A, McEwen BS. Modulation bv estradiol of serotonin$_1$ receptors in brain. *J Neurosci* 1982; 2: 199–205
26. Wise PM, Rance N, Barraclough CA. Effects of estradiol and progesterone on catecholamine turnover rates in a discrete hypothalamic region in ovariectomized rats. *Endocrinology* 1981; 108: 2186–93
27. Djahanbakhch O, McNeilly AS, Warner PM *et al.* Changes in plasma levels of prolactin, in relation to those of FSH, oestradiol, androstenedione and progesterone around the preovulatory surge of LH in women. *Clin Endocrinol* 1984; 20: 463–72
28. Vekemans M, Delvoye P, L'Hermite M *et al.* Serum prolactin levels during the menstrual cycle. *J Clin Endocrinol Metab* 1977; 44: 989–93
29. McNeilly AS, Chard T. Circulating levels of prolactin during the menstrual cycle. *Clin Endocrinol* 1974; 3: 105–12
30. Messinis IE, Templeton A. Changes in serum prolactin levels during the follicular phase and the endogenous luteinizing hormone surge of cycles hyperstimulated with follicle stimulating hormone. *Clin Endocrinol* 1988; 28: 243–51
31. Badawy SZA, Rebscher F, Khon L *et al.* Progesterone suppression of estrogen-stimulated prolactin secretion and estrogen receptor levels in rat pituitary cells. *Endocrinology* 1979; 104: 429–32
32. Bevan J, Sussman J, Roberts A *et al.* Development of an invasive macroprolactinoma: a possible consequence of prolonged oestrogen replacement. *Br J Obstet Gynaecol* 1989; 96: 1440
33. Ehara Y, Siler TM, Yen SSC. Effects of large doses of estrogen on prolactin and growth hormone release. *Am J Obstet Gynecol* 1976; 125: 455–8

34. Kauppila A, Leinonen P, Vihko R *et al.* Metoclo-pramide-induced hyperprolactinemia impairs ovarian follicle maturation and corpus luteum function in women. *J Clin Endocrinol Metab* 1982; 54: 955–60
35. Haug E. Progesterone suppression of estrogen-stimulated prolactin secretion and estrogen receptor levels in rat pituitary cells. *Endocrinology* 1979; 104: 429–32

This paper has been reproduced from *Eur J Contracept Reprod Health Care* 1997; 2: 63–9

5 Long-term experience of a levonorgestrel-releasing intrauterine system

V. Odlind

INTRODUCTION

The initial purpose for the development of intrauterine hormone administration was to decrease the risk of expulsion of intrauterine devices (IUDs) by administering uterine-relaxing hormones into the uterine cavity. This theory proved wrong as the expulsion rate of the progesterone-releasing system did not differ from that of other IUDs, but it was found that intrauterine progesterone significantly reduced menstrual blood loss[1]. In order to distinguish the steroid-releasing intrauterine methods from inert or copper IUDs, which have a very different mechanism of action, the former devices are usually referred to as intrauterine systems (IUSs). The levonorgestrel-releasing IUS (LNG-IUS), which is the most extensively tested and most widely used IUS, has the frame of a Nova T on which a silastic capsule has been attached to the vertical arm, releasing 20 μg per 24 h from a total load of 52 mg of levonorgestrel. The LNG-IUS was developed during the late 1970s and the 1980s, and it was first marketed in Finland in 1990 and in Sweden in 1992. It is currently being introduced on to the market in several European countries. There are still limited numbers of large studies relating to the use of the LNG-IUS, particularly long-term follow-up studies, and studies of the LNG-IUS in women with various medical conditions.

MECHANISM OF ACTION

The LNG-IUS exerts its contraceptive effect by a strong progestational influence on the cervical mucus, which becomes thick and impermeable to sperm, and on the endometrium which becomes thin and inactive, which is believed to be the main mechanism of contraceptive action[2]. In addition to that, the LNG-IUS probably causes a foreign-body reaction, similar to that of copper IUDs. Because the levonorgestrel release is low, ovulation is not normally inhibited[3]. However, minor effects on ovulatory function have been reported with the LNG-IUS[4].

EFFICACY AND SIDE-EFFECTS

Use of the LNG-IUS has been shown to result in a significantly lower pregnancy rate than with use of the Nova T during 5 years in one randomized study[5]. In another study with a duration of 7 years, the pregnancy rate of the LNG-IUS was slightly, but not significantly, lower than that of the TCu380[6]. Thus, the LNG-IUS is one of the most effective contraceptive methods available (Table 1).

The most common side-effects resulting in discontinuation of use are bleeding pattern disturbances and hormonal side-effects, i.e. breast tension, mood changes and acne. These side-effects are mostly reported in the beginning of treatment and the rate is low, probably as a result of the low steroidal dose[5].

BLEEDING PATTERN WITH USE OF LEVONORGESTREL-RELEASING INTRAUTERINE SYSTEM

After insertion of the LNG-IUS, there is often a period of frequent, irregular bleeding or spotting during the initial 2–3 months. During this time the number of bleeding/spotting days is usually increased, but the volume of blood lost is reduced as compared to the woman's normal menstruation[7,8]. With prolonged use, the menstrual blood loss is dramatically reduced and many women develop amenorrhea or report extremely scanty regular bleeds[5]. This profound change in menstrual pattern is the result of the strong progestational effect exerted on the endometrium, which becomes very thin[2]. Few women develop amenorrhea during the first months of use but at the end of the first year around 20% of LNG-IUS users have amenorrhea or extremely scanty bleeding[5]. There is no difference in ovulatory function between those women using the LNG-IUS who do, and those who do not, experience amenorrhea[3,9]. The amenorrhea is uterine, i.e. the women usually remain ovulatory throughout LNG-IUS use. With long-term LNG-IUS use, increasingly more women develop amenorrhea, and at the end of 5 years around 50% report amenorrhea, the remaining women reporting short irregular or regular episodes of spotting[5]. Almost no woman reports menstrual-like bleeding after 5 years. When a new LNG-IUS is inserted immediately upon removal of the old one, there is usually very little bleeding disturbance, and most women continue to have exactly the bleeding pattern that they have experienced during the latter phase of the first segment of LNG-IUS use. Women with regular but heavy menses (idiopathic menorrhagia) and no apparent abnormalities at pelvic examination may be recommended use of the LNG-IUS, since it will considerably reduce menstrual blood loss[10].

ECTOPIC PREGNANCY

The relative risk of ectopic pregnancy in users of hormone-releasing IUSs is higher than that in users of copper-releasing IUDs. However, the risk of ectopic pregnancy is strongly related to the total risk of pregnancy associated with the

Table 1 Reasons and cumulative discontinuation rates for levonorgestrel-releasing intrauterine system (LNG-IUS) and other IUDs: results from two randomized comparative long-term studies

Device	*Pregnancy*	*Expulsion*	*Bleeding/pain*	*Reference*
60 months				Andersson *et al.*[5]
Nova T	4.2	5.5	20.4	
LNG-IUS	0.3	4.9	15.1	
84 months				Sivin *et al.*[6]
TCu 380Ag	1.4	7.4	23.3	
LNG-IUS	1.1	11.8	15.4	

IUD. Thus, the progesterone-releasing IUS (Progestasert) has been associated with a higher ectopic rate than copper IUDs[11]. Progesterone is a much less potent hormone than levonorgestrel, but, when levonorgestrel was administered into the uterine cavity in an extreme microdose, levonorgestrel was also less in preventing ectopic pregnancy. An IUS releasing only 2 μg/24 h of levonorgestrel resulted in a significantly higher risk of pregnancy and an almost seven-fold risk of ectopic pregnancy as compared with two different copper IUDs with around 200 mm^2 copper area[12].

In a European multicenter trial, including 5615 woman-years of LNG-IUS use and 2776 woman-years of Nova T use, Andersson and colleagues[5] reported an ectopic pregnancy rate of 0.2 per 1000 woman-years of use of the LNG-IUS and 2.5 per 1000 woman-years with the Nova T. In another large multicenter study of the LNG-IUS and the TCu380, both IUDs were shown to be highly effective with few pregnancies, and there were no ectopics reported for the LNG-IUS after 5 years and around 3000 woman-years of observation for each device[13]. In a multicenter study in India, the LNG-IUS was compared with three different copper-releasing IUDs for 36 months. There were no pregnancies at all with the LNG-IUS during 10 500 woman-months of observation[14]. In a report by Allonen[8], all data from randomized comparisons between the LNG-IUS and various copper IUDs were pooled and the ectopic rate for the LNG-IUS was calculated to be 0.2 per 1000 woman-years, compared with 0.9 per 1000 woman-years for copper IUDs in the same studies. Thus, the LNG-IUS is associated with a highly protective effect against ectopic pregnancy, both compared with other IUDs and compared with non-contraceptors (Table 2).

LEVONORGESTREL-RELEASING IUS AND PELVIC INFLAMMATORY DISEASE

Several large epidemiological studies have looked at the association between IUD use and pelvic inflammatory disease (PID), and generally come to the

Table 2 Rate of ectopic pregnancy during first 2 years of randomized trials of non-medicated IUDs, copper-releasing IUDs with copper area of < 200 mm^2, copper-releasing IUDs with copper area of > 200 mm^2, and during 5 years of LNG-IUS use. From reference 15

Type of device	*Women-years of use*	*Pregnancies per 1000 woman-years*	*Ectopic pregnancies (%)*	*Ectopics per 1000 woman-years*
Non-medicated	4600	19.0	4.6	0.87
Cu < 200 mm^2	21 000	20.8	3.6	0.75
Cu > 200 mm^2	39 200	7.3	3.2	0.23
LNG-IUS	5615	0.9	20.0	0.20

conclusion that the risk of PID is related to sexual behavior and the risk of sexually transmitted disease (STD) rather than to IUD type. Because of its progestational effects on the cervical mucus, it has been suggested that the LNG-IUS may protect against PID.The European multicenter study showed a lower risk of PID in LNG-IUS users as compared with users of Nova T, which, because of low numbers, did not become statistically significant until 3 years of accumulated use[5,16].When the data were analyzed according to age of the women, the difference was most pronounced in women below 25 years.All the women in the study were considered at low risk for PID at inclusion in the study. Although these data suggested a protective effective of the LNG-IUS against PID, more studies, particularly in groups at some known risk of PID, need to be performed before such an association is proven.

CANCER

No study has addressed an association between LNG-IUS use and malignancy or premalignant conditions. No difference was found in the European multicenter study in the incidence of atypical cervical smears between users of LNG-IUS and users of Nova T[5]. Two studies have reported successful treatment of endometrial hyperplasia or precancerous lesions in the endometrium with the LNG-IUS, but the clinical significance of these findings is still unclear and further studies are needed[17,18].

LEVONORGESTREL-RELEASING IUS IN COMPARISON WITH OTHER INTRAUTERINE DEVICES

The mechanism of action of the LNG-IUS is very different from that of a copper IUD, resulting in a pattern of scanty bleeding. For this reason, women with heavy menses could be recommended the LNG-IUS although they would be discouraged from using a copper IUD which results in a very different bleeding pattern[7,10]. Amenorrhea during use of LNG-IUS has to be interpreted differently than during use of a copper-releasing IUD.

LEVONORGESTREL-RELEASING IUS IN COMPARISON WITH OTHER PROGESTOGEN-ONLY METHODS

The LNG-IUS is a progestogen-only contraceptive method, and could therefore, metabolically, be compared with progestogen-only pills, Norplant and progestogen-only injectables. The release rate of 20 μg/24 h of levonorgestrel makes the progestogen load lower than any other progestogen-only method, about two-thirds or less of the daily dose of a progestogen-only oral pill (levonorgestrel 30 μg/24 h) and Norplant (levonorgestrel 30–60 μg/24 h). Therefore, some of the systemic hormonal effects of the LNG-IUS are less pronounced than those of the levonorgestrel-containing progestogen-only pill or Norplant, although few comparative studies exist.

ELIGIBILITY FOR THE LEVONORGESTREL-RELEASING IUS

Whereas most healthy parous women are eligible for LNG-IUS as well as IUD use, neither of these methods is the first choice in young, nulliparous women. However, if there is no apparent increased risk of STD (i.e. the woman is in a monogamous, stable relationship) the LNG-IUS may be a possible method also for nulliparous women, for example to be inserted after an abortion[19]. The LNG-IUS has been studied in breast-feeding women, and the effects on milk composition, milk yield, duration of breast feeding and growth and development of the breast-fed infants did not differ in comparison with a group of women using the Nova T[20,21].

For women suffering from heavy menstrual periods and dysmenorrhea, the LNG-IUS is highly recommended, because of its potential to reduce menstrual blood loss. However, women who have vaginal bleeding irregularities must be properly evaluated before LNG-IUS insertion.

Women who have had an ectopic pregnancy in the past may be recommended use of an LNG-IUS, which is protective against ectopic pregnancy as discussed above.

INSERTION ROUTINES

The LNG-IUS can be inserted at any time during the menstrual cycle when it is reasonable to believe that the woman is not pregnant. Insertion can be done immediately postabortion in the first trimester, if no infection is suspected. However, insertion of a LNG-IUS is usually recommended to be postponed until 6 weeks postpartum, although there are no studies to support this. Before insertion it is important that prospective users of the LNG-IUS are carefully informed about the mechanism of action of the LNG-IUS, and especially counselled about the profound change in bleeding pattern that can be expected. It is recommended that the woman be asked to keep a bleeding diary.

LEVONOGESTREL-RELEASING IUS USE IN THE LATER REPRODUCTIVE YEARS AND BEYOND

After 5 years the LNG-IUS can be replaced by a new system, if the woman so requests. The limited experience as yet from second and third segments of LNG-IUS use suggests that the pregnancy rate remains extremely low, side-effects few and the bleeding pattern scanty and unchanged throughout. Thus, the LNG-IUS seems to be a particularly suitable method for women who have completed child-bearing and who are approaching an age when heavy and/or irregular menses become more prevalent: the premenopausal years. There are already a few studies suggesting that the LNG-IUS or similar intrauterine levonorgestrel-releasing systems may be successfully used throughout the climacteric period and into the menopause as an addition to estrogen replacement therapy[22–24].

REFERENCES

1. Bergkvist A, Rybo G. Treatment of menorrhagia with intrauterine release of progesterone. *Br J Obstet Gynaecol* 1983; 90: 255–8
2. Nilsson CG, Luukkainen T, Arko H. Endometrial morphology of women using a d-norgestrel-releasing intrauterine device. *Fertil Steril* 1978; 29: 397–401
3. Nilsson CG, Lähteenmäki P, Luukkainen T. Patterns of ovulation and bleeding with a low levonorgestrel-releasing intrauterine device. *Contraception* 1980; 21: 155–64
4. Barbosa I, Bakos O, Odlind V, *et al.* Ovarian function during use of a levonorgestrel releasing IUD. *Contraception* 1990; 42: 247–59
5. Andersson K, Odlind V, Rybo G. Levonorgestrel-releasing and copper-releasing (Nova T) IUDs during five years of use. *Contraception* 1994; 49: 56–72
6. Sivin I, Stern J, Coutinho E, *et al.* Prolonged intrauterine contraception: a seven-year randomized study of the levonorgestrel 20 mcg/day (LNG 20) and the copper T380Ag IUDs. *Contraception* 1991; 44: 473–80
7. Nilsson CG. Comparative quantitation of menstrual blood loss with a D-norgestrel-releasing IUD and a Nova-T-Copper device. *Contraception* 1977; 15: 379–87
8. Allonen H. The levonorgestrel IUD. In Bardin CW, Mishell DR Jr, eds. *Proceedings from the 4th International Conference on IUDs*. Newton, MA, USA: Butterworth Heinemann, 1994; 284–92
9. Nilsson CG, Lähteenmäki P, Luukkainen T. Ovarian function in amenorrhoeic and menstruating users of levonorgestrel-releasing intrauterine device. *Fertil Steril* 1984; 41: 52–4
10. Andersson K, Rybo G. Levonorgestrel-releasing intrauterine device in the treatment of menorrhagia. *Br J Obstet Gynaecol* 1987; 97: 690–4

11. Alza Corporation. Progestasert intrauterine progesterone contraceptive system. Alza Product Information, 1986
12. World Health Organization Task Force on Intrauterine Devices for Fertility Regulation. Microdose intrauterine levonorgestrel for contraception. *Contraception* 1987; 35: 363–79
13. Sivin I, El Mahgoub S, McCarthy T, *et al.* Long-term contraception with the levonorgestrel 20 mcg/day (LNg 20) and the CopperT380Ag intrauterine devices: a five-year randomized study. *Contraception* 1990; 42: 361–78
14. Indian Council of Medical Research Task Force on IUD. Randomized clinical trial with intrauterine devices (levonorgestrel intrauterine device (LNG), CuT380Ag, CuT220C and CuT200B). A 36-month study. *Contraception* 1989; 39: 37–52
15. Sivin I. Dose- and age-dependent ectopic pregnancy risks with intrauterine contraception. *Obstet Gynecol* 1991; 78: 291–8
16. Toivonen J, Luukkainen T, Allonen H. Protective effect of intrauterine release of levonorgestrel on pelvic infection. Three years comparative experience of levonorgestrel- and copper-releasing intrauterine devices. *Obstet Gynecol* 1991; 77: 261–4
17. Perino A, Quartararo P, Catinella E, *et al.* Treatment of endometrial hyperplasia with levonorgestrel releasing intrauterine devices. *Acta Fertil Eur* 1987; 18: 137–40
18. Scarselli G, Tantini C, Colafranceschi M, *et al.* Levonorgestrel-Nova-T and precancerous lesions of the endometrium. *Eur J Gynaecol Oncol* 1988; 9: 284–6
19. Heikkilä M, Lähteenmäki P, Luukkainen T. Immediate postabortal insertion of a levonorgestrel-releasing IUD. *Contraception* 1982; 26: 245–59
20. Heikkilä M, Luukkainen T. Duration of breast-feeding and development of children after insertion of a levonorgestrel-releasing intrauterine contraceptive device. *Contraception* 1982; 25: 279–92
21. Heikkilä M. Puerperal insertion of a copper-releasing and a levonorgestrel-releasing intrauterine contraceptive device. *Contraception* 1982; 25: 561–72
22. Andersson K, Mattson LÅ, Rybo G, *et al.* Intrauterine release of levonorgestrel – a new way of adding progestogen in hormone replacement therapy. *Obstet Gynecol* 1992; 79: 963–7
23. Suhonen SP, Holmström T, Allonen H, *et al.* Intrauterine and subdermal progestin administration in postmenopausal hormone replacement therapy. *Fertil Steril* 1995; 63: 336–42
24. Wollter-Svensson LO, Stadberg E, Odlind V, *et al.* Intrauterine administration of levonorgestrel 5 and 10 μg/ 24 hours in perimenopausal hormone replacement therapy. A randomized clinical study during one year. *Acta Obstet Gynecol Scand* 1996; in press

This paper has been reproduced from *Eur J Contracept Reprod Health Care* 1996; 1: 319–23

6 Hormonal postcoital contraception

A.A. Kubba

INTRODUCTION

The recognition that not every sexual act was pre-planned, let alone protected, led to the development of postcoital contraception. Postcoital (emergency) methods of contraception are suitable and highly effective only in emergencies. An emergency arises when a contraceptive accident, such as condom breakage, or unprotected sexual intercourse takes place. Unwelcome spermatozoa may then gain access to the ovum and result in an 'accidental pregnancy'. Postcoital contraception aims to intercept this union of egg and sperm and/or prevent the implantation of the fertilized egg. Hormonal postcoital contraception has to be applied during a critical time window of 72 h from the unprotected exposure.

In the 1960s, Haspels introduced high-dose, estrogen-only emergency contraception in Europe[1] and Yuzpe introduced the combined estrogen/progestogen method in North America in the 1970s[2]. Over the past 30 years, several reports and studies have demonstrated the safety and efficacy of hormonal (as well as intrauterine) postcoital contraceptives. A recent review of the literature on efficacy[3] leads to the conclusion that the Yuzpe method is of even higher efficacy than that so far acknowledged.

COMBINED HORMONAL POSTCOITAL CONTRACEPTION

The so-called Yuzpe method consists of two doses, each of 100 μg ethinylestradiol and 1000 μg norgestrel (equivalent to 500 μg levonorgestrel). Each dose can be made up with two tablets of a 50 μg/500 μg ethinylestradiol/norgestrel pill. In the UK, a preparation is marketed for sole use as a postcoital contraceptive under the name Schering PC4. In Germany, the same preparation is known as Tetragynon®.

The first dose of the combined method should be taken within 72 h from the unprotected exposure, followed by the second dose 12 h later. When bioavailability of the steroids is thought to be reduced, such as in women taking liver enzyme-inducing drugs, the dose should be increased to three tablets initially followed by three tablets 12 h later[4].

MODE OF ACTION

The effect of postcoital hormones is multi-focal. In the author's view, the most consistent action is on the endometrium, effected by changes in endometrial receptors and enzymes. This renders the endometrium unsuitable for implantation. The steroids also disrupt ovarian activity; ovulation may be delayed if the treatment is given before ovulation and, if the treatment is given after ovulation, luteolysis may occur. In addition, there are also potential effects on tubal motility.

There is no evidence (clinical or theoretical) that postcoital contraception exhibits an abortifacient effect.

INDICATIONS

Unprotected intercourse

The non-use of contraception is an obvious indication for emergency contraception. Included in this category are failed coitus interruptus, ejaculation on the external genitalia or miscalculation of the rhythm method of periodic abstinence.

Contraceptive 'accidents'

Contraceptive 'accidents' include condom rupture, displacement, misuse, or incorrect placement of a diaphragm, expulsion or removal of an intrauterine device (especially in mid-cycle) and missed pills.

Sexual assault

Sexual assault is an extremely important indication for emergency contraception. The latter method is an important component of any relief-aid operation in areas of conflict where violence against women is anticipated. Women experiencing sexual assault may also require long-term emotional support.

Recent use of suspected teratogens

Suspected teratogens include drugs such as cytotoxic drugs or live vaccines such as yellow fever.

EFFICACY OF HORMONAL POSTCOITAL CONTRACEPTION

The probability of conception varies on different days of the menstrual cycle, depending on the proximity of the time of exposure to ovulation. Sperm survival of up to 6 days has to be taken into account. With these considerations in mind, the probability of conception in mid-cycle is between 20 and 30%.

The failure risk of the Yuzpe treatment can be regarded in two ways. When calculated as a percentage of those treated per cycle, the failure rate varies from under 1% to as high as 5%. A recent review of the efficacy literature[3] points to factors that confound this failure risk. The author's assessment of the literature leads to the belief that the Yuzpe method has a failure rate of under 1%, as long as the conditions for its use are not violated by omitting to consider an earlier episode of unprotected intercourse before the index event or because of unprotected intercourse taking place after the treatment has been given.

The second, and more appropriate, way of expressing the efficacy of the Yuzpe method is to use the true effectiveness rate defined as the number of pregnancies prevented by the use of the method and calculated from the ratio of the observed to expected pregnancies. The effectiveness rate of the Yuzpe method is at least 75% and could be as high as 80%.

SIDE-EFFECTS OF HORMONAL POSTCOITAL CONTRACEPTION

The main side-effect of the Yuzpe method is nausea, which occurs in up to 50% of cases[5]. The role of antiemetics in reducing nausea and vomiting, thereby enhancing the efficacy of the method, needs further study. Vomiting occurs in 20% of cases. If a patient vomits either dose within 2 h of ingestion, a repeat dose should be considered or an intrauterine device inserted. Headaches, dizziness and breast tenderness have all been reported as side-effects, but causation is not established.

CONTRAINDICATIONS

Table 1 lists the small number of contraindications that apply to hormonal postcoital contraception. Most are relative.

REPEATED USE OF HORMONAL POSTCOITAL CONTRACEPTION

There is no limit to the number of times the emergency method can be used. The dosage of steroids in the Yuzpe treatment is equivalent to no more than seven pills of a low-dose combined pill preparation. Therefore, even if the method is used three times in a cycle, the dose is no greater than the total dose of one packet of combined pills. Women who resort to emergency hormonal methods as alternatives to using an effective planned method of birth control should be warned that the risk of pregnancy when hormonal postcoital contraception is used repeatedly is much higher than the risk of the method when used in emergencies only.

Table 1 Contraindications for hormonal postcoital contraception

Condition	*Degree of contraindication*
Suspected pregnancy	absolute contraindication
Past history of thromboembolism	relative contraindication
Migraine at presentation in a woman with previous history of migraine with aura	absolute contraindication

MANAGEMENT OF FAILED HORMONAL POSTCOITAL CONTRACEPTION

A woman who presents with an accidental pregnancy following the failure of hormonal postcoital contraception should be counselled along the same lines applying to any other unintended pregnancy. In addition, the following points need to be emphasized:

(1) Data so far do not point to an adverse effect of hormonal postcoital contraception on a continuing pregnancy[6]. However, the clinical experience is based on a relatively small number of pregnancies that have continued to term.

(2) Failed emergency contraception is not an indication for a termination of pregnancy.

(3) A normal pregnancy outcome cannot be guaranteed.

PROGESTOGEN-ONLY EMERGENCY CONTRACEPTION

Levonorgestrel has been widely used as an emergency contraceptive. There are a number of ongoing studies to investigate this method further. Levonorgestrel at a dose of 0.75 mg is marketed as an emergency contraceptive in several Eastern European countries. Ho and Kwan[7] reported the use of two doses, each of 0.75 mg levonorgestrel, taken 12 h apart and initiated within 48 h of intercourse. Efficacy was equivalent to the Yuzpe method. When progestogen-only emergency contraception is considered, the patient should be made aware of the limited experience with such regimens.

THE FUTURE

Anti-progestins may prove to be the most effective and most convenient forms of emergency contraceptives. Mifepristone[8] has been used as a single dose of 600 mg taken within 72 h of unprotected intercourse, and has proved to be highly acceptable and efficacious.

REFERENCES

1. Haspels AA. Postcoital oestrogen in large doses. *IPPF Med Bull* 1972; 6: 2
2. Yuzpe AA, Thurlow HJ, Ramzy I, Leyshon JI. Postcoital contraception – a pilot study. *J Reprod Med* 1974; 13: 53–8
3. Trussell J, Ellertson C, Stewart F. The effectiveness of the Yuzpe regimen of emergency contraception. *Fam Plann Perspect* 1996; 28: 58-64
4. Kubba AA. Emergency contraception guidelines for doctors. Faculty of Family Planning and Reproductive Health Care, London 1993
5. Yuzpe AA, Percival Smith R, Rademaker AW. A multicenter clinical investigation employing ethinylestradiol combined with dl-norgestrel as a postcoital contraceptive agent. *Fertil Steril* 1982; 37: 508–13
6. Cardy GC. Outcome of pregnancies after failed hormonal postcoital contraception – an interim report. *Br J Fam Plann* 1995; 21: 112–15
7. Ho PC, Kwan MSW. A prospective randomised comparison of levonorgestrel with the Yuzpe regimen in post-coital contraception. *Hum Reprod* 1993; 8: 389–92
8. Webb AMC, Russell J, Elstein M. Comparison of Yuzpe regimen, Danazol and Mifepristone (RU 486) in oral postcoital contraception. *Br Med J* 1992; 305: 927–31

This paper has been reproduced from *Eur J Contracept Reprod Health Care* 1997; 2: 101–4

7 Gestagens, danazol and antiprogestogen in emergency contraception

A.M.C. Webb

INTRODUCTION

Emergency contraception has been attempted throughout history but it was not until the 1960s that hormones were used. Initially, estrogens in varied doses were utilized, and in the 1970s Albert Yuzpe described the method which has become the most widely known, using two doses of ethinylestradiol and levonorgestrel[1]. Although its effectiveness has been demonstrated, this method still has a true failure rate of around 25%[2] and causes not insignificant nausea, vomiting and cycle disturbance. The search for a method which is more effective, or has fewer side-effects, or preferably both, has continued. This paper describes work using progestogen alone, danazol and the antiprogestogen, mifepristone.

PROGESTOGENS

Various trials have been carried out using a variety of progestogens, but they are either non-comparative or are too small to prove the effectiveness of the method. Despite this, a levonorgestrel-only method has been commercially available in some countries for a number of years, under the trade name of Postinor. The World Health Organization concluded that, as a repeated method, progestogens alone caused too much cycle disturbance to be acceptable[3]. As an occasional method, they did not feel there was enough evidence and so conducted a trial comparing levonorgestrel 0.75 mg, repeated after 12 h, with the standard Yuzpe regimen[4]. The study was randomized and both treatments were started within 48 h of unprotected intercourse. The study included 834 women and the pregnancy rates in both groups were found to be very similar, with 2.6% in the Yuzpe group and 2.4% in the levonorgestrel group being pregnant (excluding the women who had further acts of intercourse during the same cycle). The incidences of nausea and vomiting were much lower in the levonorgestrel group (16.1% and 2.7%, respectively) than in the Yuzpe group (46.5% and 22.5%, respectively). The World Health Organization have proceeded to carry out a further, larger study in 22 centers, comparing the same methods but over a longer period of 72 h in order to try to substantiate these findings. The target

Table 1 Number of pregnancies expected and observed in women receiving the Yuzpe regimen, danazol and mifepristone; 95% confidence intervals shown in parentheses

	Yuzpe regimen (n = 191)	*Danazol* (n = 193)	*Mifepristone* (n = 195)
Expected pregnancies	11.290	11.735	11.690
Observed pregnancies	5	9	0
Pregnancy rate (%)	2.62 (0.86–6.00)	4.66 (2.15–8.67)	0
Standardized ratio	0.433 (0.144–1.030)	0.767 (0.351–1.460)	0 (0–0.316)

was to recruit 2200 subjects by the end of 1996. If this study confirms the original findings, it will expand the choice of methods without reducing efficacy.

DANAZOL

Initial results suggested that danazol, a potent antigonadotropin, and progestogen, which also has a direct effect on the ovary, might be as effective as the Yuzpe regimen but with considerably fewer side-effects[5]. Unfortunately, when a randomized trial was carried out, using 600 mg, repeated after 12 h, and started within 72 h of unprotected intercourse, in comparison with the Yuzpe regimen, no clinical effect was noted and the number of pregnancies observed was virtually the same as those that were predicted had no treatment been given (Table 1)[6]. As other methods are available, danazol cannot be recommended as a method of emergency contraception[7].

MIFEPRISTONE

Mifepristone has a strong antiprogestogenic effect and has been demonstrated to be a potent abortifacient. Due to its actions, it was thought to be a good candidate for use in emergency contraception. Two randomized trials were carried out in the UK, with World Health Organization support, comparing the Yuzpe regimen to one 600 mg dose of mifepristone, given within 72 h of intercourse.

The first trial randomly allocated women to receive either the Yuzpe regimen, danazol, as described earlier, or mifepristone[6]. A total of 616 women were recruited, all between 16 and 45 years. Of the 191 women receiving the Yuzpe regimen, five became pregnant, which gave a pregnancy rate of 2.62%, and of the 195 receiving mifepristone, none became pregnant (Table 1). The women receiving mifepristone also had lower rates of nausea and vomiting (Table 2), although they were more likely to experience significant delay in the next period, with only 19% bleeding before they expected and 39% bleeding later than they expected (Table 3).

Table 2 Side-effects experienced in the first 4 days following treatment with the Yuzpe regimen and mifepristone

Side-effects	*Percentage of women receiving Yuzpe regimen*	*Percentage of women receiving mifepristone*
Nausea		
None	30	63
Mild	26	22
Moderate	25	11
Severe	19	3
Vomiting		
None	78	97
Mild	9	2
Moderate	7	1
Severe	6	0

Table 3 Timing of menstruation after taking emergency contraception relative to expected date of next period

Timing of menstruation (relative to expected date of next period)	*Percentage of women receiving Yuzpe regimen*	*Percentage of women receiving mifepristone*
> −7 days	23	5
−7 to −4 days	16	14
−3 to +3 days	51	37
+4 to +7 days	5	13
> +7 days	2	26
Bled twice	3	5

The second study showed similar results to the first trial, with no pregnancies in the mifepristone group, and a pregnancy rate of 1% (95% confidence interval 0.3–3.5) in the Yuzpe regimen group. Side-effects in the mifepristone group were also greatly reduced[8].

The work with mifepristone as an abortifacient suggested that much lower doses than the initially used 600 mg would be just as effective[9]. The World Health Organization, therefore, has funded a further multicenter study to confirm the previous findings, to investigate whether lower doses of 50 mg and 10 mg are as effective as the initial dose, and whether the timing of the treatment can be extended to 120 h without compromising efficacy. This study included 1717 women from 11 centers across the world, and the results should be available in the near future. A further comparative study looking at the Yuzpe regimen vs. mifepristone is currently being carried out in China.

CONCLUSIONS

The World Health Organization studies have gone a long way in expanding the choice of effective methods of emergency contraception. If the further studies confirm the effectiveness of progestogens alone, there should be little problem in making this alternative available. Although treatment with mifepristone is more politically sensitive, if a dose can be found that, although ineffectual as an abortifacient, still works postcoitally and does not cause significant cycle disturbance, some of the objections to its more widespread use may disappear, even in countries where access to abortion is limited.

REFERENCES

1. Yuzpe AA, Smith RP, Rademaker AW. A multicenter clinical investigation employing ethinylestradiol combined with dl-norgestrel as a postcoital contraceptive agent. *Fertil Steril* 1982; 37: 508–13
2. Trussel J, Stewart F. The effectiveness of postcoital hormonal contraception. *Fam Plann Perspect* 1992; 24: 262–4
3. Task Force on Post-ovulatory Methods for Fertility Regulation, WHO. Postcoital contraception with levonorgestrel during the peri-ovulatory phase of the menstrual cycle. *Contraception* 1987; 36: 275–86
4. Ho PC, Kwan MSW. A prospective randomized comparison of levonorgestrel with the Yuzpe regimen in post-coital contraception. *Hum Reprod* 1993; 8: 389–92
5. Zuliani G, Colombo UF, Molla R. Hormonal postcoital contraception with an ethinylestradiol–norgestrel combination and two danazol regimens. *Eur J Obstet Gynecol Reprod Biol* 1990; 37: 253–60
6. Webb AMC, Russel J, Elstein M. Comparison of Yuzpe regime, danazol and mifepristone in oral postcoital contraception. *Br Med J* 1992: 305: 927–31
7. Von Hertzen H, Van Look PFA. Alternative methods of emergency contraception. *Fertil Control Rev* 1995; 4: 22–5
8. Glasier A, Thong KJ, Dewar M, Mackie M, Baird D. Mifepristone (RU486) compared with high-dose estrogen and progestogen for emergency postcoital contraception. *N Engl J Med* 1992; 327: 1041–4
9. Van Look PFA, von Hertzen H. Clinical uses of antiprogestogens. *Hum Reprod Update* 1995; 1: 19–34

This paper has been reproduced from *Eur J Contracept Reprod Health Care* 1997; 2: 127–9

8 Rhythm methods and devices

G. Freundl

INTRODUCTION

It is the aim of rhythm methods to identify the fertile time in the cycle, so that couples can choose to abstain from sexual intercourse if they wish to avoid a pregnancy or continue sexual activity if they wish to conceive[1].

There are certain requirements for these methods of fertility control. They should be:

(1) Effective;

(2) Without adverse side-effects (secure);

(3) Easy to use;

(4) Ethically acceptable;

(5) Cheap;

(6) Independent of educational status (available for everybody);

(7) Accepted by the partner.

The scientific evaluation of methods of fertility control requires analysis of each of these aspects. All existing methods of contraception fail to meet all of these criteria. Indeed, no medical scientist who is aware of the problems in these areas related to current contraception technology can readily envisage any universal remedy for the control of fertility. This chapter focuses on rhythm methods.

HISTORY

The attempt to regulate fertility by using abstinence during the cycle is not new (Figure 1). In ancient times, attempts had been made to investigate the length of the fertile phase. It is interesting to note where various authors located the fertile phases. Susruta, in about 1000 BC, located the fertile phase in the first 12 days of the cycle. Charata, in 900 BC, extended this phase to 16 days. Aristotle reduced this to only 5 days. Soranus of Ephesus, the Greek gynecologist, believed that conception was most likely to occur immediately after menstruation, when

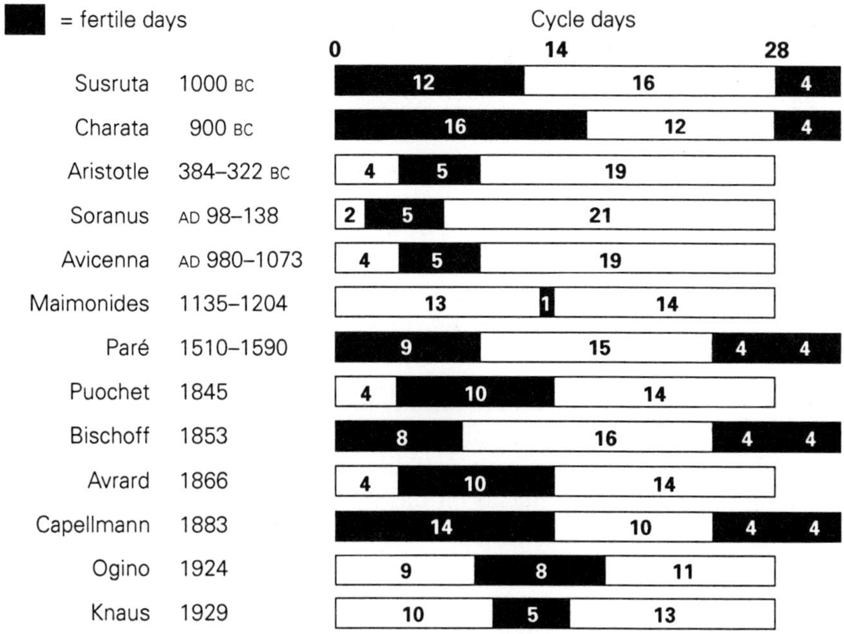

Figure 1 Assumed position and length of the fertile period in a woman's cycle in various centuries. Black, fertile time

the womb had been 'scrubbed clean' ready for the male seed to attach itself to the wall of the womb. He recommended, therefore, that the couple should abstain from intercourse before, during the last days of and shortly after menstruation, if pregnancy was to be avoided – advice which, if followed, greatly increases the likelihood of conception, as the couple will have intercourse on the most fertile days. It is very interesting that only one author, Maimonides, in the late 11th century, located the fertile phase in the middle of the cycle. However, he gave only 1 day as the length of the phase. Interestingly, he followed exactly the Jewish beer purity regulations, which are cited in the Bible, chapter 15, verses 19 and 28: 'If a woman has her bloodflow, she has to be regarded as unclean. When the bloodflow stops, she has to count 7 days and then she will be clean.' This physiological misconception of equating menstruation with fertility persisted through the 19th century and, in fact, was not corrected until the 1930s.

In the 1930s, two physicians, Ogino of Japan[2] and Knaus of Austria[3], independently confirmed that the time of ovulation or peak fertility usually occurred 14 days before the next menses. Ogino and Knaus had given new impulse to cycle research. However, the effectiveness of the so-called calendar method is rather low. Therefore, it again cannot be recommended by physicians and gynecologists.

Temperature method

The temperature method for detection of the fertile and infertile phases using the basal body temperature is a very accurate method. The first descriptions of the change of temperature before the menses came from the English physician Squire, in 1867 and the French physician Rabuteau in 1870. The Americans Mary Jacobi and John Goodman (1877) developed their so-called 'wave theory of menstruation'. The German internist Hansen, in 1913, published very carefully registered temperature charts.

The first correct interpretation of the cause of the hyperthermic phase of the cycle was given in 1926 by the Dutch gynecologist Henry van de Velde. He wrote: 'I am quite sure, that the temperature rise does not precede the beginning function of the corpus luteum but temperature rise is caused by the function of the corpus luteum'.

The first to develop a method of family planning from the cyclic changes of the basal body temperature was the German Catholic priest Wilhelm Hillebrand in 1935. The Belgian gynecologist Ferrien wrote in 1947 that the postmenstrual infertile period starts 48 h after the beginning of the hyperthermic phase of the cycle. The German gynecologist Döring suggested in 1950[4] to determine by taking basal body temperature not only at the beginning of the postovulatory infertile time but also the end of the postmenstrual infertile time.

In 1966, a scientific group of the World Health Organization (WHO) published the following rule: 'a significant temperature rise is characterized by rising of the temperature within 48 hours or less. The temperatures of 3 consecutive days have to be at least 0.2 °C higher than the temperatures at the preceding 6 days.'

Cervical mucus method

Changes in cervical mucus secretion were published prior to observations concerning the temperature: in 1837 by the French gynecologist Donne and in 1847 by the French physician Pouchet. In 1855, Tyler Smith gave a wonderful description of the cervical mucus behavior during the cycle. Marion Sims, in 1868, compared the qualities of cervical mucus with egg white. Clift, a Briton, called this phenomenon 'spinnbarkeit' for the first time in 1946. Shettles recommended for the first time, in 1949, mucus observation for family planning.

In 1973, the Australian neurologist John Billings developed the so-called pure 'cervical mucus observation method = ovulation method'[5].

Symptothermal method

The American gynecologist Keefe has stressed, since 1949, the advantages of the combination of temperature and mucus observation.

The Austrian physician Josef Rötzer was the great promoter of the symptothermal method in Europe[6]. In a similar way, the Polish priest Jan Mucharski promoted the 'double-check method of family planning' in the USA. In 1973, Thyma published his work about the fertile and infertile days of married life, recommending the double-check method.

All the methods described above became known as natural family planning (NFP), and they rely on observations of cervical mucus, temperature or a combination of these physiological signals to determine the fertile and infertile phases of the cycle.

Natural methods of family planning rely on the following biological conditions:

(1) Periodicity of fertility and infertility;

(2) The ovum can only be fertilized during 12–18 h after release (limited life span of the ovum);

(3) The life of sperm is longer and more susceptible to variation and can reach 3–5 days when cervical mucus is present;

(4) There is only one ovulation per cycle;

(5) The fertile days can be determined by the woman herself by self-observation of signs and symptoms of her body.

PRESENT SITUATION

Periodic abstinence techniques include:

(1) The basal body temperature method (Döring, Marshall);

(2) The cervical mucus or ovulation method (Billings);

(3) The symptothermal method (Rötzer, Thyma).

(4) The calendar method = rhythm method (Ogino, Knaus);

Basal body temperature method

Definition

The basal body temperature (BBT) method is based on the increase in body temperature that occurs shortly after ovulation, associated with secretion of progesterone by the corpus luteum.

After ovulation, the body temperature rises 0.2–0.4 °C or 0.4–0.8 °F, and remains high until the next menstruation. The couple are advised to refrain from sexual intercourse between the first day of menstruation and the third consecutive day of elevated temperature. (This method does not reveal anything about the potential fertility of the days preceding ovulation.)

Table 1 Effectiveness temperature method

Author	Year	Cycles (n)	Women (n)	Pearl-Index theoretical	Pearl-Index practical
Döring[7]	1967	11 352	307	0.1	0.8
Marshall[8]	1968	4749	321	1.2	6.6
Vollmann[9]	1975	31 570	656	0	0.26

Pearl-Index theoretical, theoretical method effectiveness; Pearl-Index practical, method effectiveness following practical use

Indications

The BBT method may be found convenient by couples who have decided to use periodic abstinence and if the woman is willing to abstain from sexual intercourse for long periods of time, and has irregular menstrual cycles, so that the calendar method cannot be used.

Effectiveness

The effectiveness of the temperature method given as the Pearl Index (number of unwanted pregnancies per 100 women using the method for 1 year) is located within the range 0.26–6.6 (Table 1).The theoretical failure rate lies at about 1.0 and the practical failure rate between 2.5 and 6.6.

Cervical mucus (Billings) method

Definition

The cervical mucus method is based on the recognition and interpretation of cyclic changes in the cervical mucus that occur in response to the changing estrogen levels.

During a menstrual cycle, a woman may experience different sensations at the opening of the vagina and changes in the characteristics of the cervical mucus. Couples practicing this technique can have sexual intercourse during both pre- and postovulatory phases as it is possible to identify the infertile phase in both parts of the cycle by monitoring the mucus pattern.

Effectiveness

For the effectiveness of the cervical mucus method (Table 2), in prospective studies, a theoretical Pearl index between 1.2 and 2.9, and a practical Pearl index between 15.5 and 34.9 was found.

Table 2 Effectiveness ovulation method

Author	*Year*	*Cycles (n)*	*Women (n)*	*Pearl-Index theoretical*	*Pearl-Index practical*
Ball (Aust)[10]	1976	1626	122	2.9	15.5
Klaus (USA)[11]	1979	12 282	—	1.2	19.3
Wade (USA)[12]	1981	3232	573	—	34.9
WHO[13]	1981	10 215	869	2.0	20.6

Pearl-Index theoretical, theoretical method effectiveness; Pearl-Index practical, method effectiveness following practical use; WHO, World Health Organization

It is interesting to note that there are great differences between nations. In El Salvador, the practical effectiveness is about 30 and in the Philippines it is 16.5.

Modified mucus method

A modified mucus method is being used in some programs. The rules of the method are less conservative than the original mucus method. It differs from the original method with regard to the following points:

(1) The modified mucus method allows sexual intercourse in the first month of use, while the original method does not.

(2) In women who have regular cycles, the modified mucus method allows sexual intercourse on preovulatory days when thick mucus is present, contrary to the original method.

(3) Sexual intercourse is permitted on the third day after the peak mucus day in contrast to the fourth day in the original method.

Symptothermal method

Definition

The symptothermal method combines two or more indicators of fertility, especially cervical mucus changes, the calendar method and the BBT method, thus increasing the accuracy with which a woman can determine the different phases of her cycle. The days of required abstinence can be kept to a minimum, combined with a high efficiency rate.

Factors influencing use of symptothermal method

All factors affecting BBT and mucus pattern can also influence the efficiency of the symptothermal method. However, the combination of two (double-check)

Table 3 Effectiveness symptothermal method

Author	*Year*	*Cycles (n)*	*Women (n)*	*Pearl-Index theoretical*	*Pearl-Index practical*
Rice (multinat.)[14]	1977	14 416	723	0.75	7.16
Wade (USA)[12]	1981	3399	590	0	16.6
Europe[15]	1996	21 277	1372	—	2.5
Germany[16]	1997	14 870	758	0.63	2.2

Pearl-Index theoretical, theoretical method effectiveness; Pearl-Index practical, method effectiveness following practical use

or more indicators of fertility ensures the greatest possible accuracy and helps to override the margin of human error inherent in the interpretation of all indicators of fertility.

Effectiveness

With regard to the effectiveness of the symptothermal method (Table 3), Rice reported, in a multinational study, a theoretical Pearl index of 0.75 and a practical Pearl index of 7.16[14].

Wade published results in 1981 with a theoretical Pearl index of 0 and a practical Pearl index of 16.6[12]. In spring 1997, we evaluated the results of our prospective use-effectiveness of NFP with a total of 14870 cycles in 758 women, and achieved a use-effectiveness of 2.2%, which is a fairly reasonable result[16,17]. It is also interesting to note that great international variations were found in the Rice study, i.e. use-effectiveness of 18.05 in Columbia and 4.85 in the United States according to the actuarial method (or Kaplan–Meier method).

Calendar or rhythm method

Definition

The calendar or rhythm method, reportedly, is the most widely used of all periodic abstinence techniques. Properly used, it involves numerical calculations based on previous menstrual cycles to estimate the fertile period.

Effectiveness

Reports about the effectiveness of the rhythm method differ greatly (Table 4): the theoretical Pearl index is said to be 3.3 and the practical Pearl index lies between 5.9 and 47. There are great variations between locations and countries (Table 5).

Table 4 Effectiveness calendar method

Author	*Year*	*Cycles (n)*	*Women (n)*	*Pearl-Index theoretical*	*Pearl-Index practical*
Tietze[18]	1951	7267	409	—	14.4
Dunn[19]	1956	4687	156	3.3	5.9
Jaramillo[20]	1968	3802	—	—	47

Pearl-Index theoretical, theoretical method effectiveness; Pearl-Index practical, method effectiveness following practical use

NEW TECHNOLOGIES

Today, there are methods of replacing the personal observations by various modern techniques, summarized below.

Electronic thermometers

Electronic thermometers such as 'Evatherm®' and 'Roland®' are technically able to measure temperature with an accuracy of ± 0.1 °C. This accuracy is sufficient for these thermometers to be used in NFP. The advantage is that the time of measurement is minimized in relation to that of mercury thermometers.

Temperature computers

At the present time, the most advanced thermometers are computer thermometers, whose programs use the rules of the temperature method (Babycomp®, Ladycomp® Bioself 110®, Cyclotest D®). We have tested these devices, and some of them were found to be of great help to the users. Points of

Table 5 Effectiveness ovulation method – national variations (World Health Organization 1981)[13]

Country	*Pearl-Index theoretical*	*Pearl-Index practical*
Ireland	3.4	16.3
New Zealand	6.3	28.6
India	0.5	17.5
Philippines	0.7	16.5
El Salvador	0.0	30.6
Total	2.0	20.6

Pearl-Index theoretical, theoretical method effectiveness; Pearl-Index practical, method effectiveness following practical use reference for these tests were: ovulation detected by ultrasound, luteinizing hormone (LH) level in urine and the symptothermal method[21].

Babycomp, or *Ladycomp* is a computer which is programmed according to the rules of the temperature method.

To date, we have tested 20 women over 204 cycles. The age of the women ranged between 18 and 45 years and they mostly had a cycle length of 25–35 days. In conclusion, we found that Babycomp, on the whole, safely determined the beginning as well as the end of the fertile phase. However, it does not minimize but, on the contrary, extends the length of the fertile phase. In a retrospective efficacy study, Bachhofer (1997)[22] has evaluated 633 women using this design, finding a 12-months' rate of 5.3% (actuarial method). However, Babycomp is suitable for women who do not want to record their temperature every morning. The only problem of the design is the current high price.

The *Bioself* is a computer that uses the rules of the calendar method. Using these rules, it cannot be more effective than the calendar method itself. However, some women like this apparatus as it is very handy and easy to read[23].

Cyclotest D came onto the market just as we started testing, so there are only a few results available. However, this computer has been updated so that at the present time we are testing a new version, which offers the possibility to feed information relating to peak day of the mucus or the LH peak to the program. Testing is going well but, to date, we have not evaluated the results.

Electrical resistance gauges

We have tested electrical resistance gauges such as the Cue®, the ovulation controller or the dist-4.

The Cue fertility monitor measures the salivary and vaginal fluid resistance. We have checked 45 cycles of 8 women using the Cue fertility monitor, and found that the Cue peak occurred 7 ± 1.6 days prior to the first BBT rise[24]. The vaginal low occurred 1.6 ± 0.2 days prior to the first higher reading, and the vaginal rise 0.6 ± 1.9 days prior to BBT +1. From the standard deviations reported, it can be seen that there was not much difference between individual values.

In summary we found that it is possible to use the Cue peak to predict ovulation. In each normal and well-defined cycle, the Cue peak precedes the fertile phase of the cycle. We are still trying to find a better algorithm than the current one to evaluate comparison of the single reading of each day with the day of ovulation and with those of biphasic and monophasic cycles.

Volumemeters

There are, furthermore, self-tests available for measurement of body fluids. With plastic vaginal aspirators such as Rovumeter® and Ovutrac® it is possible to measure the varying volumes of the cervicovaginal fluid[25,26].

Hormonal computers

At the present time, field trials on the effectiveness of a system called Persona®, performed in Britain, Germany and Ireland, have been evaluated. A total of 710 women were admitted to the multicenter trial and followed for 7209 cycles. The calculated pregnancy rate was 2.2% (4.2–8.3). The method effectiveness of the system used with abstinence on red (fertile) days was calculated to be 94%[27]. The hand-held monitor and disposable urine test sticks measured changes in the urine levels of estrioglucuronide and luteinizing hormone and stored the information over six cycles for calculation of green (non-fertile) and red days in the cycle. With this knowledge, the user may abstain from intercourse or use a barrier method of contraception in order to prevent conception.

We have also evaluated the Ramp test, which is a urinary test that detects the pregnandiol glucuronide rise in the urine after ovulation. It is a test that should be able to detect the postovulatory infertile phase, but did not come up to our expectations.

A successor has recently been put onto the market: the *Safeplan* test. This is easier to handle and of more reliable technique, but also has the disadvantage that it can only encompass the postovulatory infertile phase.

CURRENT CONTRACEPTIVE USE

A 1994 report of WHO records that, in developed regions, 70% of couples use contraceptive methods and fewer than 50% use modern methods with no change between 1983 and 1990.

In developing regions, around 50% use contraceptive methods and, between 1983 and 1990, the use of modern methods increased from 40 to 48%.

In Germany, the following figures are available according to the Health Foundation Study of 1992[28]. The contraceptive pill is the most used contraceptive method. It is a little more frequently used in the new than in the old countries. The intrauterine device (IUD) is used by about 13%, and periodic abstinence is used by between 7 and 8% of couples.

The WHO 1994 report shows a marked difference between developed and developing regions. Sterilization and IUDs are the major contraceptive methods in developing regions. The pill and barriers are the major methods used in developed regions. Barrier contraception has a much higher usage in developed regions: 22% versus 5% in developing regions. Rhythm methods are also more frequently used in developed regions: 11% versus 4%

Periodic abstinence methods are used throughout the world, more so in developed countries. Among contraceptive users, a range of 5–20% use NFP or rhythm methods. Barrier contraception combined with the calendar rhythm method is also very widely used. A reliable objective method of defining the fertile phase would greatly enhance acceptance of natural family planning and the use of barrier contraception.

CONCLUSION

It is one of the basic human rights of a couple to be able to determine the size of their family. The present author believes that natural family planning is one of the methods that can be used to reach this goal.

In this sense, knowledge of the most fertile, least fertile and infertile phases of the human menstrual cycle is important to enable women to decide whether they wish to conceive, use periodic abstinence for fertility regulation, or use coitus interruptus and/or barrier methods only in the fertile phase.

In 1972, a Task Force established by WHO looking into methods for the prediction and detection of ovulation decided that the major objective was to develop a simple do-it-yourself method for women to use for the purpose of fertility control[29]. Today, we are one step beyond this, so that some technical assistance is available for women to use at home to rate their own fertility pattern, and, if necessary, to supplement their own observations.

REFERENCES

1. Flynn AM. *A Manual of Natural Family Planning*. Hemel Hempstead, UK: Allen and Urwin, 1984
2. Ogino K. Über den konzeptionstermin des weibes und seine anwending in der praxis. *Zentralbl Gynäkol* 1932; 12: 721–32
3. Knaus H. Die periodische frucht- und unfruchtbarkeit des weibes. *Zentralbl Gynakol* 1933; 57: 1393–1408
4. Döring GK. Temperaturmessung als einfaches hilfsmittel zur zyklusanalyse. *Geburtshilfe Frauenheilkd* 1949; 9: 757
5. Billings EL, Billings JJ, Brown JB, Burger HG. Symptoms and hormonal changes accompanying ovulation. *Lancet* 1972; 1: 282–4
6. Roetzer J. Erweiterte basaltemperaturmessung und empfängnisregelung. *Arch Gynäkol* 1968; 206: 196–214
7. Döring GK. Über die Zuverlässigkeit der Temperaturmethode zur Empfängnisverhütung. *Dtsch Med Wochenschr* 1967; 92: 1055–61
8. Marshall J. A field trial of the basal body temperature method of regulating birth. *Lancet* 1968; 2: 8
9. Vollmann RF. How effective is rhythm? *Fam Plann Perspect* 1975; 7: 53
10. Ball M. A prospective field trial of the "Ovulation Method" of avoiding conception. *Eur J Obstet Gynecol Reprod Biol* 1976; 6: 63–6
11. Klaus H, Goebel M, Muraski B. Use-effectiveness and client satisfaction in six centres teaching the Billings ovulation method. *Contraception* 1979; 19: 613–29
12. Wade ME, McCarthy P, Braunstein GD. A randomized prospective study of the use-effectiveness of two methods of natural family planning. *Am J Obstet Gynecol* 1981; 141: 368–76
13. World Health Organization. A prospective multicenter trial of the ovulation method of natural family planning. II. The effectiveness phase. *Fertil Steril* 1981; 36: 591–8
14. Rice FJ, Lanctot CA. Fairfield international collaborative study on the symptothermal method. In NFP Research Workshop, Linden Hill Hotel 1979: Bethesda, Maryland

15. Freundl G. Prospective European multi-center study of natural family planning (1989–1992): interim results. The European Natural Family Planning Study Groups. *Adv Contracept* 1993; 9: 269–83
16. Frank-Herrmann P, Freundl G, Gnoth C, Godehardt E, Kunert J, Baur S. Sottong, U. Natural family planning with and without barrier method use in the fertile phase: efficacy in relation to sexual behavior: a German prospective long-term study. *Adv Contracept* 1997; 13: 179–89
17. Gnoth C, Frank-Herrmann P, Freundl G, Kunert J, Godehardt E. Sexual behavior of natural family planning users in Germany and its changes over time. *Adv Contracept* 1995; 11: 173–85
18. Tietze C. The clinical effectiveness of contraceptive methods. *Am J Obstet Gynecol* 1959; 78: 650–6
19. Dunn HP. The safe period. *Lancet* 1956; II: 441–2
20. Jarmillo-Gomez M. Rhythm: a hazardous contraceptive method. *Demography* 1968; 5: 433
21. Freundl G, Baur S, Bremme M, Döring GK, Frank-Herrmann P, Godehardt E, Kunert J. Temperaturcomputer zur bestimmung der fertilen zeit im zyklus der frau: Babycomp, Bioself 110, Cyclotest D. *Fertilität* 1992; 8: 66–76
22. Bachhofer D. *Der Miniaturcomputer Babycomp/Ladycomp in der natürlichen Familienplanung.* Dusseldorf: Medizinische Fakultät der Heinrich-Heine-Universität 1997; 1–83
23. Drouin J, Guilbert EE, Desauliners G. Contrceptive application of the Bioself fertility indicator. *Contraception* 1994; 50: 229–38
24. Freundl G, Bremme M, Frank-Herrmann P, Baur S, Godehardt E, Sottong U. The CUE fertility monitor compared to ultrasound and LH peak measurements for fertile time ovulation detection. *Adv Contracept* 1996; 12: 111–21
25. Flynn AM, McCarthy AM, Docker M, Royston JP. The temporal relationship between vaginal fluid volumes obtained with Rovumeter vaginal aspirator and the fertile phase of the cycle. *Hum Reprod* 1988; 32: 201–5
26. Barbato M, Pandolfi A, Guida M. A new diagnostic aid for natural family planning. *Adv Contracept* 1993; 9: 335–40
27. Bonnar J, Flynn A, Freundl G, Kirkman R, Royston P, Snowden R. Effectiveness of personal hormone monitoring for contraception. *Lancet* 1997; in press
28. Oddens BJ, Visser AP, Vemer HM, Everaerd WT. Contraceptive use and attitudes in reunified Germany. *Eur J Obstet Gynecol Reprod Biol* 1994; 57: 201–8
29. World Health Organization, Task Force on Methods for the Determination of the Fertile Period: Special Programme of Research Development and Research Training in Human Reproduction. Temporal relationship between ovulation and defined changes in the concentration of plasma estradiol-17-beta, luteinizing hormone, follicle stimulating hormone, and progesterone. I. Probit analysis. *Am J Obstet Gynecol* 1980; 138: 383–90

9 Postpartum contraception: the lactational amenorrhea method

M. Vekemans

INTRODUCTION

Breastfeeding still accounts for a significant proportion of all fertility reduction, the average birth interval being longer among populations that breastfeed than among populations that do not breastfeed[1]. However, for the individual, breastfeeding *per se* is not reliable for fertility suppression[2].

The lactational amenorrhea method (LAM)[3] is a tool for the individual woman to utilize breastfeeding physiology in order to help space her births.

PHYSIOLOGY

Infertility usually occurs for the first 50 days postpartum. Thereafter, suckling suppresses follicular development in 65% of lactating mothers, and, in most of the remaining, follicular development is incomplete[4]. The pattern differs between societies and between individuals, nutrition of the mothers possibly being one of the determinants (studies are still inconclusive). Therefore, it has been difficult to develop universal guidelines to recommend the use of natural postpartum infertility as a contraceptive method. LAM is a response to the difficulty of predicting the duration of the natural postpartum infertility period. It has proven to be highly efficient, as will be shown below.

Suckling induces a reduction in the pulsatile release of gonadotropin releasing hormone (GnRH) which almost suppresses luteinizing hormone (LH) and follicle stimulating hormone (FSH) secretions, which in turn increases the duration of the lactational amenorrhea. The mechanism seems to involve an intracerebral opioid pathway (local release of β-endorphin, inhibiting hypothalamic release of GnRH and suppressing dopamine secretion, thereby stimulating prolactin secretion). Prolactin maintains milk production, and thus encourages suckling, but has no major role in the lactational infertility[4,5]. Reduced suckling precipitates the return of ovulation.

Table 1 Cumulative probability of ovulation during lactational amenorrhea

	At 6 months	*At 12 months*
Ovulation	31%	67%
Ovulation + adequate luteal phase	14%	38%
Menses	19–67%	—

The cumulative probability of ovulation during lactational amenorrhea[5-9] varies. A few typical results are presented in Table 1.

In breastfeeding mothers, the first postpartum menstruation usually occurs before the first ovulation, if blood appears during the first 6 months postpartum[5]. In a study in Manila[6], for women menstruating before 6 months postpartum, the lag between anovular first menses and subsequent ovulation was 16 weeks (± 4.4 weeks standard deviation). This figure shows that the LAM criterion 'amenorrhea' is very conservative, which explains the very good protection offered.

The return of menstruation indicates ovarian hormonal activity. The later this occurs, the more ovulation occurs before the vaginal blood loss.

THE LACTATIONAL AMENORRHEA METHOD

LAM is based on three conditions which have to be respected simultaneously:

(1) The baby is under 6 months of age. Experiments with LAM-9 (the baby is under 9 months of age) and 'extended LAM' (the baby is over 9 months of age) are being conducted;

(2) The mother is still amenorrheic;

(3) The mother practices exclusive or quasi-exclusive breastfeeding (on demand, day and night).

The use of the questionnaire in Figure 1 is recommended to assess the suitability of the lactational amenorrhea method for nursing mothers[2,10].

During lactation, fecundity still remains impaired after menstruation resumes. However, menstruation is a more important indication of the return of fertility, as compared to the age of the baby, especially if breastfeeding remains quasi-exclusive (i.e. maternal milk constitutes the major part of the infant's food).

LAM is a way of both spacing births and supporting breastfeeding, and this method is also a means by which the user knows when a complementary

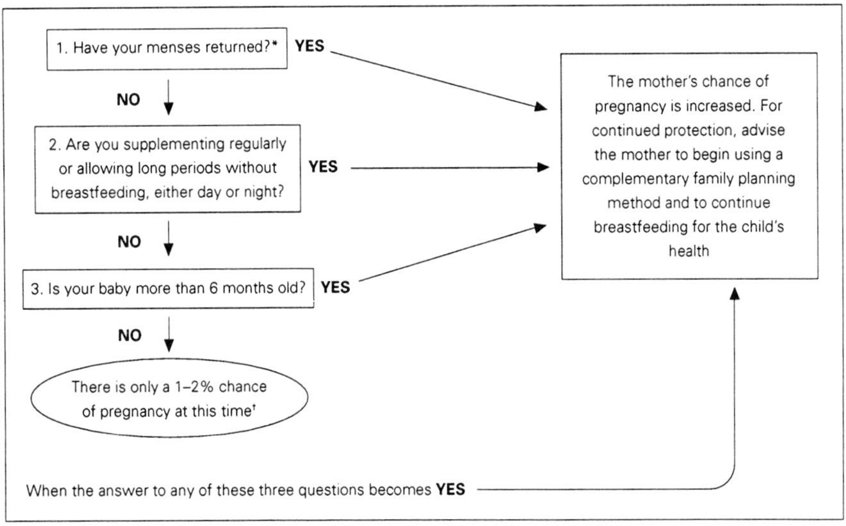

*Spotting that occurs during the first 56 days is not regarded as menses; †the mother may choose to use a complementary method of contraception at any time

Figure 1 Questionnaire to assess suitability of mothers for the lactational amenorrhea method

method of family planning must be started. Evidence exists that exclusive breastfeeding for the first 6 months has a positive impact on the nutrition of the infant, when mothers are properly nourished and socially supported. Their infants grow as well as, or better, than formula-fed infants[2]. Mothers should receive, or be spared through decreased workload, the excess calories needed to fully breastfeed. Feed the mothers and they will breastfeed the babies. In addition, a subsequent pregnancy does not obviate breastfeeding.

To succeed at breastfeeding, a number of rules must be followed:

(1) No supplements (except vitamins, or to taste, or exceptionally);

(2) Frequent sucklings (≥ 10/24 h; in total 100 min/24 h);

(3) Each breast stimulated each time;

(4) Offer the breasts soon after delivery, best within 1 h and always within 12–24 h;

(5) Night sucklings;

(6) If a supplement is exceptionally given, let the infant suckle first. Decreasing duration or number of sucklings increases the risk of ovulation before the first menstruation.

Health workers should help to improve breastfeeding practices. The appearance of the first tooth can be used as a signal for supplementing with other food, where, and when the 6 months' time span is difficult to assess[5].

LAM must be followed by another contraceptive method or periodic abstinence

Breastfeeding should be encouraged in maternity wards, and substitutes avoided as much as possible. Hospitals should refrain from offering the mothers milk powder, presents and leaflets from milk powder manufacturers. Cohabitation between mother and newborn must be allowed and organized from the beginning. The creation of a breastfeeding-LAM-family planning team would be very helpful in many hospitals and maternity wards in order to modernize their practices, i.e. promoting breastfeeding, LAM and contraception. Suppression of barriers and misconceptions surrounding breastfeeding is a priority in many settings.

Efficacy

LAM is at least 98% effective[11,12]. In one study[13] the pregnancy rate was 1.7%. In a multicentric prospective study (centers in Mexico, Thailand, Egypt, Pakistan, the Philippines, Canada and Australia)[14] strict LAM-6 (i.e. with quasi-exclusive breastfeeding of babies up to 6 months of age) resulted in a life table pregnancy rate of 0.7%. With food supplementation, the rate remained quite low (2.9%) although this figure can be considered too high for going over to the promotion of 'unstrict' LAM (i.e. when breastfeeding is supplemented).

In a Slovenian study[15], LAM was found to be very efficient until 32 weeks postpartum, even with partial breastfeeding.

In order to remain objective when studying the efficacy of LAM, the low pregnancy rates obtained with the method must be compared with figures obtained in a control population not trained in the method. The probability of pregnancy in early postpartum may also be low because intercourse is less frequent at that time. A study in Chile has shown a very small difference in pregnancy rates between the LAM group and the control group, 1% and 1.7% at 6 months, respectively. The main LAM promoters (i.e. The Institute for Reproductive Health, Georgetown University, Washington DC, USA) found that pregnancy rates in LAM users and control cohorts do not differ statistically at 6 and 12 months postpartum. The gain is rather in the field of family health (mother, infant, siblings, husband) through, for the infant, optimal breastfeeding, and of economic gain for the remainder of the family.

Acceptability

A study in Ecuador found that 31% of the women to whom LAM was presented accepted participation. Of them, 90% correctly understood the method after two visits and 75% expressed satisfaction.

Continuity

At 12 months postpartum, menstruation had returned in 87.5% of all the women in a multicentric study[14]. The authors noted high discontinuation rates, so they recommend use of LAM only to the time before beginning other contraceptive methods. In prospective studies, continuation rates are to be calculated using life table analysis. Two different curves have to be considered: first, the ongoing users (how many still use the method after *x* months?) and second, the complete cohort (how many changed to other methods?). Pregnancy rates must be presented for the two groups, and for a control group. It is not sufficient only to present failure rates in women strictly adhering to the LAM criteria. A table can be set up reporting the number of women contacted at the start and during months 1-6, the number of women using LAM (with number of pregnancies and number lost to follow-up), the number of women who changed from LAM to another contraceptive method (again with number of pregnancies and number of lost for follow-up) and the number of women who stopped using LAM without having recourse to an alternative method (with number of pregnancies and number of lost for follow-up). There is an urgent need for such investigations.

Double protection

Using modern contraceptives during the first 6 months in amenorrheic, lactating women is economically a waste, since the double protection (mean 26 weeks) offered is unnecessary[10]. The question is, is it necessary, or indeed recommended, to start contraception soon after delivery, where there is substantial lactational amenorrhea? Rather, LAM should be offered as a contraceptive method.

Indications

In the USA, the extent of combined pill use among lactators has declined since the early 1970s[16]. The introduction of LAM, followed by another method of contraception, appears to be an excellent proposal nowadays.

Arguments in favor of the use of the lactational amenorrhea method

Some women may perceive contraception and breastfeeding as incompatible[11]. LAM is very well adapted to such individuals, and gives time to discuss the necessary move to natural family planning or use of a modern method of contraception after LAM ceases to offer protection.

LAM is certainly suitable for couples who want to practice natural family planning since body signs of ovulation are difficult to detect during lactational amenorrhea. However, LAM should not be restricted for use to natural family planning amateurs, as some authors feel[11], but rather be proposed as an intermediary method of contraception before changing to a modern one.

LAM gives time to the couples to choose their long-term method of contraception, and is accepted by all religious authorities. It saves money for the families and is in harmony with the prevailing belief that lactation delays fertility and is thus easily understood and accepted. LAM decreases the unnecessary use of contraceptives. It also regulates the introduction of supplements and improves babies' health.

Sustained breastfeeding saves family resources which helps to provide proper nutrition for other family members. Money saved helps to feed and clothe the other children. This is important in very poor families and in developing countries. Formula milk is extremely expensive for poor family budgets.

LAM establishes links between the maternity and the family planning programs.

Arguments against the use of the lactational amenorrhea method

Unwanted pregnancies conceived while using LAM, although infrequent, result in very short, and thus high-risk, birth intervals. This has to be kept in mind whilst counselling couples: if the risk taken is considered unacceptable, a modern method of contraception can be recommended and started. Some authors use this as an argument against LAM promotion[11]. This seems unwise. They do not seem to balance the risks and benefits properly, and assume that not having recourse to LAM results in the use of modern contraceptives, which is certainly far from being automatic. Only when a long-lasting method, not involving the user, can be started (e.g. 6-monthly injections, implants, intrauterine device, sterilization) is LAM not the first choice, on an individual scale. On a public health scale, double protection prevents savings.

Malnutrition should not be an obstacle for the use of LAM. Intervention projects should focus on the nutrition of the mother.

Early introduction of supplements is not a contra-indication for LAM. On the contrary, practices can be improved through the program. Similarly, late introduction of supplements is not an obstacle. LAM teaches the right moment for introduction of supplements.

The introduction of LAM in a family planning program necessitates the training of staff in order to ensure that all staff understand the special family planning needs of lactating women and that all staff are able to support breastfeeding (including the physical and psychological aspects).

Constraints

The often-used message that additional food has to be introduced to an infant at 4 months of age is not compatible with LAM-6. UNICEF, other agencies and non-governmental organizations active in co-operation could change their message, and advise giving additional food from 4 to 6 months of age.

Working mothers imagine difficulties with LAM. Co-operation by employers can alleviate the problems (e.g. time allowed for breastfeeding, going home at noon, expressed milk given during the day by a helper). However, LAM does not necessarily need to extend to the full 6 months. In addition, cultural norms and attitudes towards breastfeeding change. It is worthwhile to try to promote LAM everywhere.

Another difficulty is that nowadays LAM training is not given in medical and paramedical schools.

Some of the constraints can be summarized as follows, using four categories.

Providers and health workers

Easily give artificial milk (formula). Often don't encourage breastfeeding;
Don't think LAM is effective;
Have to be trained;
Are overwhelmed with work;
Think LAM does not add any good to the prevalent situation;
Have to add LAM to childbirth education classes;
Have to discard all obstacles: a team's work;
Have to teach mothers how to breastfeed;
Have to teach the advantages of breastfeeding:
  ideal growth and development of children;
  decreases infectious diseases;
  decreases breast and ovarian cancer risks;
  increases birth intervals (developing countries);
  saves money;
Have to teach mothers about timing of supplement introduction;
Have to encourage 2 years (after 6 months partial) lactation.

Sociocultural aspects

Marketing of human milk substitutes is free;
Artificial lactation is considered 'normal';
Women's work needs adaptation;
Breastfeeding in public has to be right;
Pacifiers are not indicated.

Mothers and healthcare providers

Incorrect breastfeeding practices may occur;
Artificial lactation is attractive.

Teaching

Need for new modules;
Use of the new LAM knowledge;
Follow-up of newly trained service providers has to be organized.

Promotion of LAM in developing and developed countries

More and more authors admit that LAM is a valuable tool which may be used to space families and control fertility in developing countries[12], as lactation has contraceptive properties. However, prolonged lactation has to be protected by efficient contraception because (1) a new pregnancy often means abrupt weaning of the last child, accompanied by bad health risks and (2) the contraceptive effect of lactation statistically decreases with time.

In developing countries, breastfeeding is a universal practice: often more than 95% of mothers start lactation. Throughout the world, 95% of newborns are breastfed. In Rwanda, for instance, 82% of the mothers still exclusively breastfeed their babies for 6 months, and 22% for 12 months (although this is not recommended: supplements should be started at 6 months of age). In rural Tunisia, a study showed figures for lactation of 91% at 6 months postpartum and 67% at 12 months postpartum. In such countries, which are representative of many developing countries, LAM can be welcome. LAM improves lactation, increases the mean amenorrhea duration and, in a cohort, the number of women continuing with lactation. As a consequence, LAM saves lives.

LAM seems less likely to be accepted in developed countries, because of a series of objections. In most developed countries, postpartum women are advised to initiate artificial contraception soon, or at the latest, 6 weeks after delivery.

On the other hand, almost all medical authorities currently admit that it is necessary to promote breastfeeding for health reasons. LAM and breastfeeding are complementary and support each other. LAM can be safely and efficiently encouraged as both a family planning method and as a method supporting breastfeeding. LAM constitutes a strong link between the postpartum clinic and the family planning clinic, in so far as those two activities are not integrated. Reproductive healthcare clinics ideally offer both services, as do maternity wards.

In 1994, LAM trials were conducted in at least 12 countries. In the author's opinion, nowadays reproductive health programs should integrate LAM. Programmatic aspects for introduction of LAM include the following short and incomplete list to show the complexity of starting with a new activity:

(1) Needs evaluation;

(2) Current situation evaluation including attitudes of the population, healthcare providers and decision-makers;

(3) Identification of resource-persons;

(4) Training;

(5) Set objectives;

(6) Describe the action plan;

(7) Calculate budgets;

(8) Implement, evaluate, follow-up, learn lessons, etc. . .

One complete case of LAM use gives 0.25 couple-years protection.

The costs related to the implementation of the method could include training costs, counselling time, follow-up activities, modifications of record keeping systems and of computing programs, National Committee meetings and changes in national family planning guidelines.

CONCLUSIONS

Breastfeeding, in contrast to the lactational amenorrhea method (LAM), is not a family planning method. In developed and developing countries, women ideally should exclusively breastfeed their infants for the first 6 months postpartum and, providing they have not experienced menstruation, they do not need to use other contraception than LAM. They should, however, use another contraceptive after 6 months.

Optimal breastfeeding, which is supported by LAM, followed by the use of a complementary form of family planning, should be considered as essential components of nutritional planning and of family planning interventions, for both mothers and children. There is a need for integration of postpartum, breastfeeding and contraception activities, as breastfeeding and family planning are complementary.

REFERENCES

1. Howie PW. Breastfeeding: a natural method for child spacing. *Am J Obstet Gynecol* 1991; 165: 1990–1
2. Labbok MH. Breastfeeding and fertility regulation: the impact of sustained breastfeeding and the lactational amenorrhea method (LAM) on the nutrition of mothers and children. Occasional paper no. 6, 1993, Institute for Reproductive Health, Georgetown University, Washington DC, USA
3. Labbok MH, Pérez A, Valdés V, Sevilla F, *et al.* The lactational amenorrhea method: a postpartum introductory family planning method with policy and program implications. *Adv Contracept* 1994; 10: 93–109
4. McNeilly AS. Breastfeeding and fertility. In Gray R, Leridon H, Spira A, eds. *Biochemical and Demographic Determinants of Reproduction*. Oxford, UK: Clarendon Press, 1993; 391–412
5. Short RV. Lactational infertility in family planning. *Ann Med* 1993; 25: 175–80
6. Eslami SS, Gray RH, Apelo R, Ramos R. The reliability of menses to indicate the return of ovulation in breastfeeding women in Manila. *Stud Fam Plann* 1990; 21; 243–50

7. Pérez A, Labbok MH, Queenan JT. Clinical study of the lactational amenorrhea method for family planning. *Lancet* 1992; 339; 968–70
8. Diaz S, Rodriguez G, Marshall G, *et al.* Breastfeeding pattern and the duration of lactational amenorrhea in urban Chilean women. *Contraception* 1988; 38: 37–51
9. Diaz S, Rodriguez G, Peralta O, *et al.* Lactational amenorrhea and the recovery of ovulation and fertility in fully nursing Chilean women. *Contraception* 1988; 38: 53–67
10. Laukaran VH, Rutstein SO, Labbok MH, Ballard E. Contraceptive use during lactational amenorrhea: estimates of double coverage among postpartum women using DHSI and DHSII data. Paper presented at the *Annual Meeting of the Population Association of America*, Miami, FL, May 1994
11. Millman S. Promoting breastfeeding as birth control. *Health Transition Rev* 1993; 3: 101–6
12. Howie PW. Natural regulation of fertility. *Br Med Bull* 1993; 49: 182–99
13. Distler W. Kontrazeptive Wirkung des Stillens. *Deutsche Medizinische Wochenschrift* 1992; 117: 1221
14. Kennedy KI,Visness CM. Contraceptive efficacy of lactational amenorrhoea. *Lancet* 1992; 339: 227–30
15. Rojnik B, Kosmelj K, Andolsek-Jeras L. Initiation of contraception postpartum. *Contraception* 1995; 51: 75–81
16. Ford K, Labbok M. Contraceptive use during lactation in the United States: an update. *Am J Pub Health* 1987; 77: 79–81

This paper has been reproduced from *Eur J Contracept Reprod Health Care* 1997; 2: 105–11

10 Fertility awareness and natural family planning

C.M.M. Pyper

INTRODUCTION

This paper will offer an overview of the scientific understanding we have of the signs and symptoms of fertility and how the interpretation of these signs and symptoms can be of benefit to both clients and health professionals. Although information about natural family planning is requested by a small number of clients seeking family planning advice, many more clients benefit from information about fertility awareness. Information about fertility awareness helps to fulfil the broader definition of the services many family planning clinics offer. If couples have a better understanding of when a woman is fertile they are in a stronger position to makes informed decisions about how they wish to manage their reproductive health[1,2].

FERTILITY AWARENESS

Fertility awareness is far more than just basic reproductive anatomy and physiology. A definition of fertility awareness is that it involves understanding basic information about fertility and reproduction, being able to apply it to oneself, and being able to discuss it with a partner or with a health provider.

For a woman, fertility awareness includes the ability to identify the signs and symptoms of fertility during the menstrual cycle. For a man, fertility awareness includes understanding that he is fertile all the time and, therefore, recognizing his own reproductive potential. For the couple, fertility awareness includes the understanding of their combined fertility at different stages of their lives.

Fertility awareness is fundamental to understanding and making informed decisions about reproductive health throughout the life-cycle (Figure 1), for example, as part of school education, adolescents are encouraged to adopt a healthy lifestyle, especially in relation to their sexual health. Figure 1 shows that, as well as accurate knowledge about their reproductive health, it is essential that adolescents are given time to explore their attitudes and acquire communication skills, not only to make informed decisions about their sexual health but to be capable of keeping to the decisions they have made even when under pressure from their peers to do otherwise. Fertility awareness is important because it offers clear knowledge as a basis for understanding sexual health and an accurate language to enable individuals to communicate more easily.

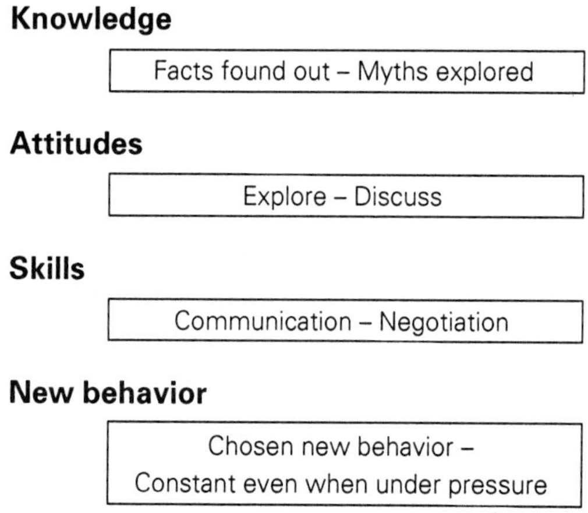

Figure 1 Understanding behavior change when addressing sexual health

Fertility awareness information is used to help couples to plan pregnancies as well as to avoid them. This can be helpful to couples having difficulty conceiving, both for the timing of intercourse or for the timing of some of the subfertility investigations.

Women who are fully breastfeeding value knowledge about reduced fertility[3–7]. A woman may use breastfeeding as a family spacing method, using the guidelines of the lactational amenorrhea method. If the baby is less than 6 months of age and the mother is fully or almost fully breastfeeding, providing menstruation has not returned, her chances of pregnancy are less than 2%. After childbirth, a woman who is fully breastfeeding learns that her fertility is likely to return when her baby is being weaned or after her baby is 6 months old. She will then need to consider an alternative method of family planning. Knowledge about fertility awareness enables her to monitor her return of fertility.

Women who understand fertility awareness during the years of the pre-menopause value being given clear information about their declining fertility. They value information about the signs and symptoms associated with the decreased levels of the hormones estrogen and progesterone. This helps them make a more informed decision about whether they wish to use hormone replacement therapy and the duration and timing of the therapy.

Fertility awareness information helps couples understand how sexually transmitted diseases may cause infertility in both women and men, especially if they are not treated early[8].

There are so many factors that influence a family planning decision. Figure 2 is very complicated, but so are many family planning decisions. Fertility awareness knowledge is a small but important part of the complex decision-making process. Decisions about when and whether to have a child, especially for those couples who are faced with an unplanned pregnancy, are often very complex. One

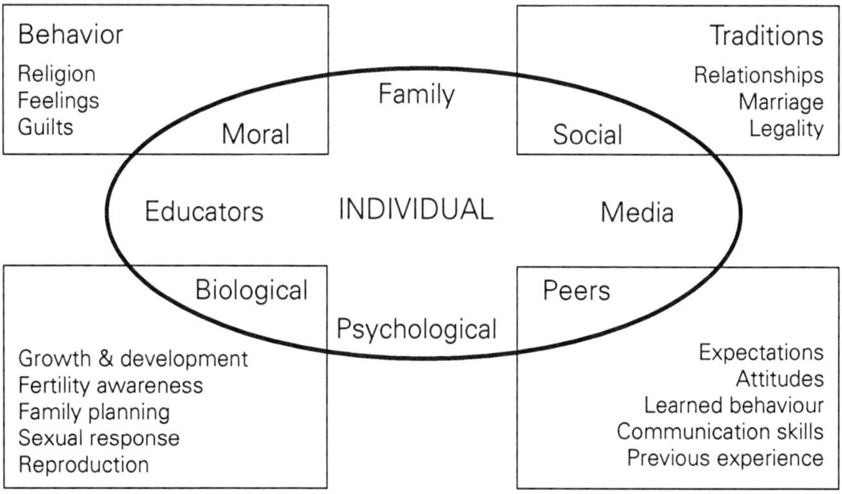

Figure 2 Influences on an individual making a reproductive health decision

factor that is frequently omitted is the knowledge that a woman's fertility gradually decreases once she is over 30 years old.

Fertility awareness information helps couples to make an informed decision when deciding which method of family planning they wish to use and can assist health professionals during family planning consultations to explain how each family planning method works, how the method will fail if not used correctly and how fertility returns when the method is discontinued.

Couples who choose only to use a barrier method during the fertile time are a group who do not readily identify themselves to family planning providers; these couples often do not have adequate information about fertility awareness. The use of diaphragms and contraceptive cream or foam make the recognition of the cervical mucus difficult, if not impossible, so it is not recommended that women should rely on interpreting cervical mucus. Some women choose to monitor the changes in the cervix. In some family planning clinics, the recommendation is made that barriers should be used from after menstruation until after the third high temperature is recorded on the chart.

NATURAL FAMILY PLANNING

Natural methods of family planning use fertility awareness to identify the fertile days of a woman's menstrual cycle. The essential features of natural family planning are:

(1) Observing the naturally occurring signs and symptoms of fertility;

(2) Abstaining from intercourse to avoid pregnancy when the signs and symptoms indicate the fertile time;

(3) If a couple wish to achieve a pregnancy, ensuring that they have intercourse during the fertile time.

The changes that occur in the cervical mucus, the basal body temperature and the cervix are all physiological and dependent on the changing levels of the hormones estrogen and progesterone. These changes indicate whether a woman is fertile or infertile. In order to understand the physiological basis of natural family planning, it is helpful to briefly review hormonal control of the menstrual cycle. Fertility in the menstrual cycle is controlled by a complex interplay of hormones. In a normal menstruating woman, the following events take place:

(1) Following menstruation, the hypothalamus in the brain releases gonadotropin releasing hormone which passes down to the pituitary gland.

(2) The pituitary gland responds to gonadotropin releasing hormone by secreting the two gonadotropin hormones, follicle stimulating hormone and a small amount of luteinizing hormone.

(3) Follicle stimulating hormone and luteinizing hormone stimulate the ovary and follicle to release the hormones estrogen and progesterone.

(4) Follicle stimulating hormone stimulates several follicles to develop. One of the follicles becomes the dominant follicle which grows and develops over 6 days, secreting increasing quantities of the hormone estrogen; the ovary also secretes estrogen. The estrogen level reaches a peak at the time the follicle has reached full maturity.

(5) The rising level of estrogen exerts a negative feedback on the hypothalamus which responds by producing a smaller amount of follicle stimulating hormone.

(6) The peak level of estrogen triggers the production of luteinizing hormone which helps to rupture the follicle releasing the ovum.

(7) Immediately following ovulation, the cells of the follicle are luteinized, forming a new endocrine structure, the corpus luteum, which produces progesterone.

To identify the fertile and infertile phase during each menstrual cycle, a knowledge of when ovulation takes place is not sufficient. The length of time during which the ovum can be fertilized after ovulation, and the life span of the sperm in the female genital tract before ovulation, must be known.

Research has shown that the life span of the ovum is only 12–24 h. Fertilization must take place during those few hours following ovulation if pregnancy is to occur. Research has shown that, occasionally, there is a second ovulation which may result in a twin pregnancy; this second ovulation will occur within 24 h of the first ovulation.

Research has shown that the life span of the sperm is variable and depends on environment. In the female genital tract, the survival of the sperm depends on the presence of cervical mucus that are produced from the secreting cells on the surface of the cervix. The fluid in the vagina, in the absence of cervical mucus, is acidic and the sperm will be rapidly destroyed. If fertile cervical mucus is present, sperm will live an average of 3 days, but it is possible for sperm to survive for 5 days or, rarely, even longer. Newly ejaculated sperm are not capable of fertilizing eggs. They must first undergo a series of changes that involve the release of enzymes from the sperm head. These changes need time and a mixture of cofactors. Some of these are provided by the cervical mucus[9].

METHODS OF NATURAL FAMILY PLANNING

Some methods of natural family planning depend on using only one of the indicators of fertility. Other methods of natural family planning are based on two or more indicators of fertility.

The single indicator methods are as follows:

(1) Observing cervical mucus (also known as the ovulation or Billings method);

(2) Recording basal body temperature;

(3) Palpating the cervix (this method is rarely used alone);

(4) Calculations based on cycle length (also known as the calendar method or rhythm method).

The hormones estrogen and progesterone cause other changes that women may recognize; these are called the minor indicators of fertility. Although they may be helpful in individual cases, they are not relied on to indicate the fertile time. It is also important that the women do not assume that some of these changes described are physiological, and they should check with a health professional if they are concerned. The changes women may notice include: mood changes, skin changes, breast changes, mid-cycle pain, back pain, abdominal heaviness and spotting of blood.

Single indicator methods

Observing cervical mucus

The cervical secretion indicator is based on the recognizable changes in the cervical secretions and sensation of dryness or moistness in the vulval area that occur during the menstrual cycle.

The cervical mucus is produced from the secreting cells in the mucosal lining of the cervix. The mucus consists of long strands of polymers of mucopolysaccharides. There are different types of mucus produced by the cervix during the menstrual cycle. The quantity and the consistency of cervical mucus

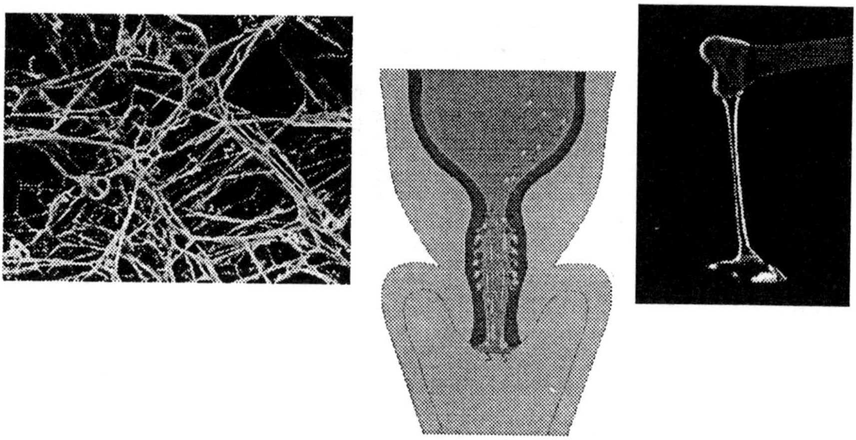

Figure 3 Illustration to show the effect of estrogen on cervical mucus. Illustrations were developed with support from the Institute for Reproductive Health, Georgetown University, Washington DC under the co-operative agreement DPE-3061-A-00-1029-00 with the Agency for International Development

are influenced by the hormones estrogen and progesterone. The different types of mucus either impede or encourage sperm motility, and this determines the state of fertility[10].

Early in the cycle, following menstruation, when the estrogen levels are low, the cervical mucus is small in quantity, white, thick and sticky. This thick sticky mucus forms a fibrillar network plugging the cervix, forming an effective barrier to sperm penetration. In addition, the secretions produced by cells lining the vagina are acidic, and sperm are rapidly destroyed. If the mucus is viewed using nuclear magnetic resonance, there are changes in the structure of the mucus during the cycle. The mucus is made up of filaments; in the following descriptions, they will be referred to as thin, medium or thick diameter. Using nuclear magnetic resonance, the structure of this mucus shows filaments of medium diameter forming a dense network.

The rising levels of estrogen alter the cervical mucus, which changes from being thick and sticky to become gradually clearer and more stretchy. This mucus has added nutrients to nourish the sperm and is alkaline in reaction. This fertile mucus flows into the vagina, neutralizing the acidity and creating an environment which enhances and prolongs the life of the sperm. This type of mucus is called fertile mucus. Using nuclear magnetic resonance, the structure of the mucus shows filaments of thick, medium and thin diameter. The filaments gradually stretch out forming a loose network which is easy for the sperm to swim through.

With the higher levels of estrogen, the cervical mucus becomes slippery, crystal clear and stretchy (Figure 3). There is a marked increase in this type of mucus due to an increased water content about 24 h before ovulation. The

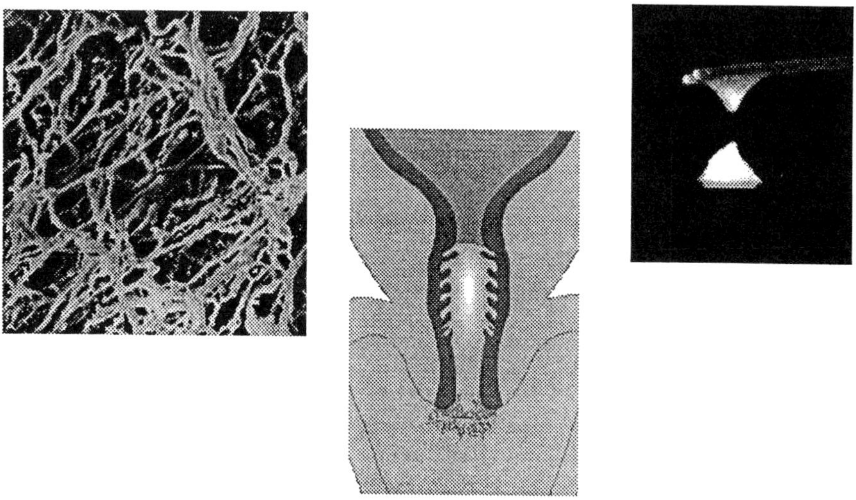

Figure 4 Illustration to show the effect of progesterone on cervical mucus. Illustrations were developed with support from the Institute for Reproductive Health, Georgetown University, Washington DC under the co-operative agreement DPE-3061-A-00-1029-00 with the Agency for International Development

sperm move easily in this fertile mucus. Some of the sperm swim to the uterus. Some sperm rest in crypts (which are small pockets in the mucosal lining in the cervix) before swimming up through the uterus. Using nuclear magnetic resonance, the structure of the mucus shows filaments of thick, medium and thin diameter. The filaments are more stretched out forming a loose network through which the sperm can swim easily.

After ovulation, under the influence of the hormone progesterone, the cervical mucus forms a thick sticky plug which is antagonistic to sperm penetration (Figure 4). The vaginal environment again becomes acidic, where any sperm are rapidly destroyed. Using nuclear magnetic resonance, the structure of the mucus shows filaments of thick, medium and thin diameter, forming a very dense network. Sperm are unable to swim through this thick, sticky cervical mucus.

Figure 5 shows that the ability of sperm to penetrate the cervical mucus increases with increased volume and decreased viscosity of cervical mucus. The fertile cervical mucus has certain properties that the non-fertile cervical mucus does not have. These properties are sometimes used to help identify fertile cervical mucus:

(1) The Spinnbarkeit test demonstrates the stretching ability of fertile mucus.

(2) The glass of water test involves putting the mucus in a glass of water. The fertile mucus will not dissolve in the water whereas most other vaginal secretions will.

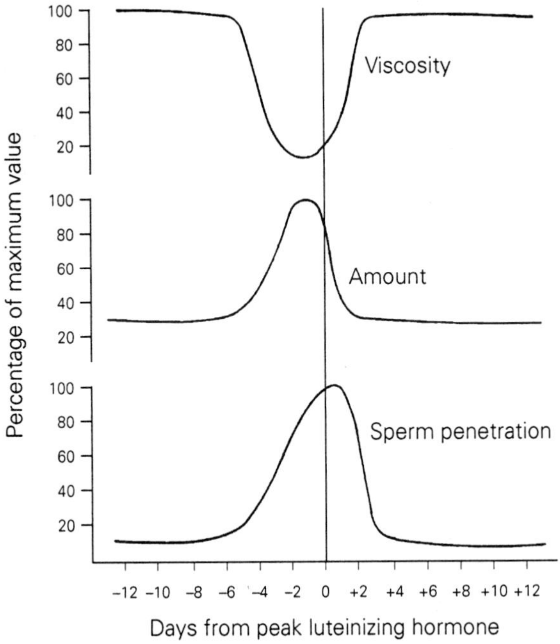

Figure 5 Effect of estrogen and progesterone on cervical secretions

(3) The Ferning test is demonstrated if samples of mucus are dried on a glass slide and observed under a microscope.

The mucus may be observed in three ways:

(1) By the feeling of dryness or moistness in the vulva area, especially at the entrance to the vagina;

(2) By the appearance of the mucus when wiping the vulva area with a tissue; it may be described in color as white or creamy, and whether it is opaque (cloudy) or clear;

(3) By touching the mucus to detect whether it is sticky or stretchy.

After having a menstrual period, a woman may notice a feeling of dryness in the vulva area; this indicates the absence of cervical mucus. The beginning of the fertile time is recognized by the appearance of cervical mucus or by a sensation of moistness at the entrance to the vagina. At first, there is only a small amount of mucus which is usually cloudy and sticky. Over the following few days, the mucus gradually gradually increases in the amount noticed and changes in appearance, gradually becoming transparent and stretchy. At this time, a woman will notice the maximum amount of moistness and lubrication at the vaginal entrance. The last day of this clear slippery mucus is known as the peak day which is only recognized on the following day because the cervical mucus has changed. After the peak day, the cervical secretions rapidly change to become thick and sticky or they may not be noticed at all. The fertile time continues for 3 days after the peak day.

Observation of cervical mucus for three menstrual cycles is normally required before a woman is confident in recognizing the cervical mucus changes. A couple using observation of cervical mucus to avoid pregnancy is taught to abstain from intercourse:

(1) When the woman is menstruating;

(2) On alternate days before the first signs of any cervical mucus;

(3) At the fertile time, beginning when the woman first observes cervical mucus.

The fertile time ends on the evening of the fourth day after the peak day.

Women are taught to record the signs of cervical mucus on a chart. Color codes are sometimes used to indicate the fertile and infertile times of the cycle. A symbol such as a column or triangle is marked on the chart as a sign for the peak day. Women are taught to record 3 days after the peak day. The day marked 3 is the last fertile day.

If couples are given proper instruction and follow the instructions correctly, the cervical mucus method has been estimated to have a failure rate of 3% (Table 1)[11]. This is only with perfect use, and other studies, such as the World Health Organization multicenter trial, 1980[11], have shown a higher failure rate if the method is used alone. Alfredo Perez carried out a study in Chile that illustrated the importance of the teaching. If women were taught by inexperienced teachers, their failure rate was far higher than when using experienced teachers.

Recording basal body temperature

The hormone progesterone causes a change in the basal body temperature:

(1) The basal body temperature is defined as the body temperature before rising and after resting for at least 3 hours.

(2) After menstruation, the basal body temperature stays at about the same level.

(3) The hormone progesterone increases the basal body temperature by about 0.2 °C (0.4 °F).

(4) The temperature rise occurs immediately after ovulation as the blood levels of progesterone increase.

(5) The higher temperature is maintained until the level of progesterone falls at menstruation.

A woman is taught to take her temperature on waking. The temperature may be taken orally, rectally or vaginally but, whichever route is used, it must be

Table 1 Effectiveness of single indicator: observation of cervical secretions

Study	*Method failure (%)*	*Overall failure (%)*	*Participants (n)*
WHO 1980	2.8	19.6	869
Perez[22]			
1981, inexperienced teachers		16.4	
1982, experienced teachers		2.6	

used consistently. Special mercury fertility thermometers or electronic digital thermometers and large-scale charts help to ensure accurate recordings of the small changes in basal body temperature. During the first part of the cycle, the temperature remains at the lower level but, after ovulation, a rise of at least 0.2 °C will be noted. This rise will be maintained until the beginning of the next menstrual period. The rule of 'three over six' is an aid to chart interpretation. A cross is drawn on the chart with three temperatures in the top right quadrant and the previous six in the bottom left quadrant. The higher temperatures must be at least 0.2 °C above the lower temperatures.

The fertile time ends after the third consecutive daily temperature has been recorded at the higher level.

The basal body temperature chart will not identify the beginning of the fertile time. Therefore, couples using this method alone as a method of family planning have to abstain from intercourse until after the fertile time.

Research into the chances of conception on each day of the menstrual cycle was carried out in 1969 by Barrett and Marshall[12] (Figure 6). They used the rise of basal body temperature to estimate the time of ovulation. In the study, they found that the chances of conception approximated to zero 6 days before the day of the temperature rise and 2 days after the day of the temperature rise.

Women in this study used a single indicator: the basal body temperature. Using the basal body temperature alone requires abstinence from intercourse until after the three high temperatures have been recorded. This method, therefore, requires abstinence for an average of about 16 days each cycle. The user failure rate was 6% compared with a method failure rate of 1% (Table 2). The overall failure compared with the method failure illustrates that this is only an effective method if used by highly motivated couples who can tolerate a long time of abstinence[13].

There have been several devices developed that combine an electronic thermometer with a small computer. The computer combines information about the basal body temperature recordings with a calculation based on the woman's cycle length. It calculates when a woman is likely to be fertile using the

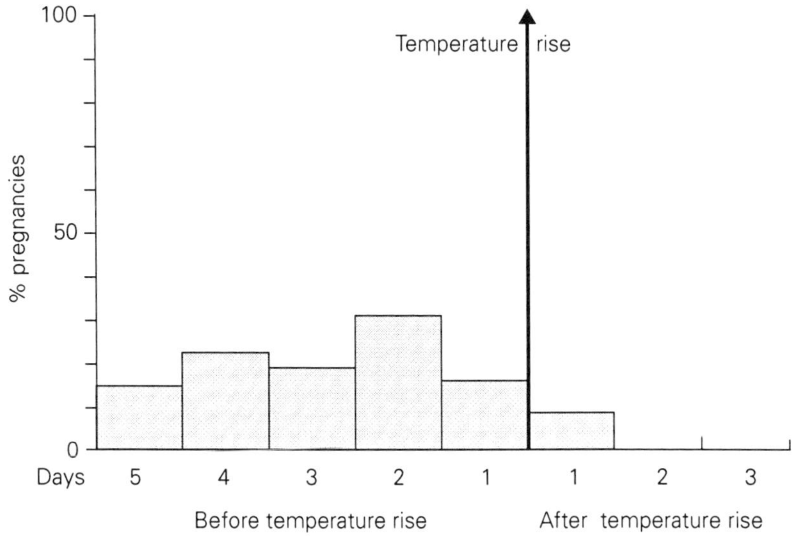

Figure 6 Chances of conception on given day of menstrual cycle using basal body temperature recordings. From reference 12

Table 2 Effectiveness of single indicator: basal body temperature alone. From reference 13

Study	*Method failure (%)*	*Overall failure (%)*	*Participants (n)*
Marshall, 1968	1	6.0	502

temperature rise. Colored lights indicate the likely fertile and infertile times. Examples of these types of devices are the Bioself® and Ladycomp®.

Palpating the cervix

Estrogen and progesterone cause subtle changes to take place in the muscle and connective tissue of the cervix. After menstruation, the level of the cervix is low in the vagina, the cervix is firm to the touch and the entrance to the cervix is closed. As estrogen levels rise, the level of the cervix rises higher in the vagina, the cervix softens and the entrance to the cervix opens slightly. After ovulation, as progesterone levels rise, the cervix returns to a lower position in the vagina, the cervix becomes firmer and the entrance becomes more closed.

Women can learn to become aware of the subtle changes in the cervix by gently palpating the cervix with the fingertip. A woman is taught to check her cervix at about the same time each day using the same position, for example with a leg raised or squatting. The three changes she feels for are:

(1) Whether the cervix is high or low in the vagina;

(2) Whether the cervix feels firm or soft to the touch;

(3) Whether the cervix is closed or slightly open.

A low, firm closed cervix indicates the infertile time. A high, soft open cervix indicates the fertile time.

It will take several months for a woman to be aware of these changes. The changes in the cervix may be recorded on the chart using a black dot low on the chart to represent the low, firm closed cervix and a circle higher on the chart to represent the high, soft open cervix.

Palpating the cervix is rarely used alone as a method of natural family planning, but the cervix changes are of particular value to women with long cycles, women during breastfeeding and women during the perimenopausal years.

This is an optional indicator of fertility and not all women wish to gently palpate their cervix.

Calculation based on cycle length

The calculation based on the length of the menstrual cycle needs the length of at least the previous six menstrual cycles. The lengths of the shortest and longest cycle are used in the calculation to identify the likely fertile time. The calendar calculation takes into account the life of the sperm and ovum.

The formula is: shortest cycle minus 19 = first fertile day; longest cycle minus 10 = last fertile day. To avoid conception, the couple is advised to abstain from sexual intercourse during this time.

This method gives an unnecessarily long period of abstinence, and is inefficient because the theory on which it is based is inaccurate. It is now known that the ovum can be fertilized only within a few hours of ovulation, and the viability of the sperm in the genital tract is variable and may be longer than 5 days.

Although the calendar method is not sufficiently reliable to be recommended, nevertheless, the information gained by recording the length of cycles and their variability is useful when used with another indicator.

Only a few reliable studies have been conducted on the effectiveness of the calendar method. The results are shown in Figure 7. It can be seen that the failure rate is less than 20%. This is a high failure rate and the method also requires a long period of abstinence. However, it is useful knowledge to couples who have no access to other methods of family planning. The far right column in Figure 7 shows the pregnancy rate for a couple using no contraception method.

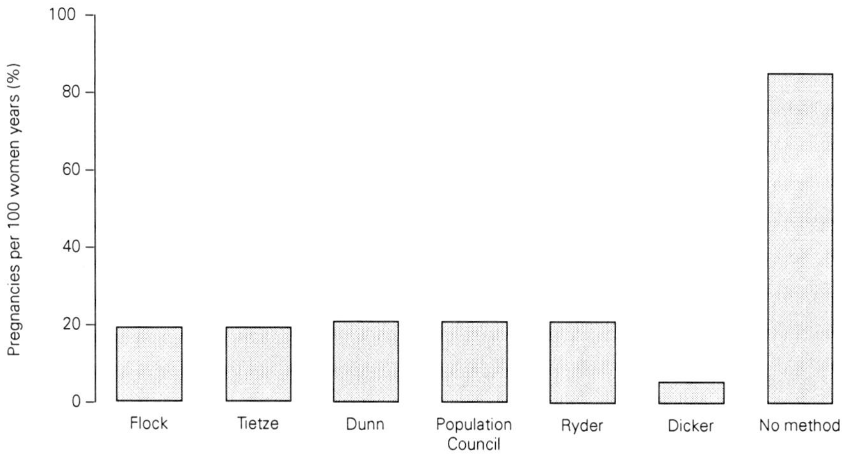

Figure 7 Effectiveness of single indicator: calculation based on cycle length

Natural family planning methods that combine indicators of fertility

Many women learn to use a combination of two or more of the following single indicators of fertility:

(1) Observing the cervical mucus;

(2) Recording basal body temperature;

(3) Palpating the cervix;

(4) Calculation based on cycle length.

In addition, some women may wish to record some of the minor indicators of fertility. In Figure 8, a woman has learnt to observe her cervical mucus and also to record her basal body temperature (Figure 9).

The beginning of the fertile time is recognized by the appearance of cervical mucus owing to the effects of estrogen.

The end of the fertile time is recognized by the effects of progesterone, showing that ovulation has taken place: first the rise in the basal body temperature and second the reduction and alteration of cervical mucus.

Double checking one symptom against another increases the reliability of the method.

Some women combine three or more of the indicators of fertility as shown in Figure 10. This is sometimes called the symptothermal method. The method combines observing the cervical mucus and recording the basal body temperature. If acceptable to the individual woman, she palpates her cervix and records the changes. She is also encouraged to use the calendar calculation to help identify the beginning of the fertile time. She also records other minor indicators of fertility such as ovulation pain and breast tenderness. She learns to record all the

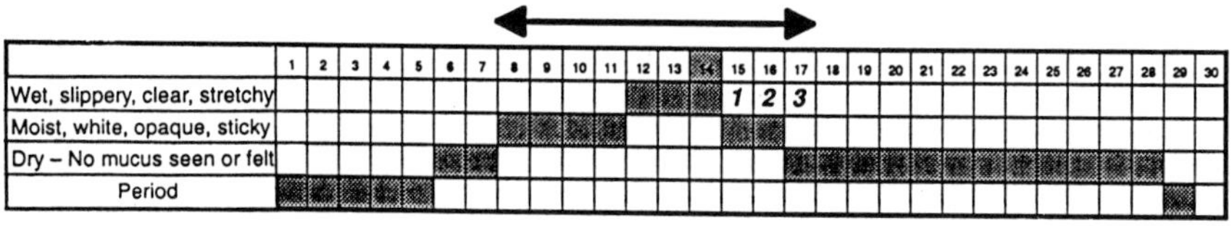

Figure 8 Recording changes in the cervical mucus on a chart. Produced in association with Jane Knight at Fertility UK

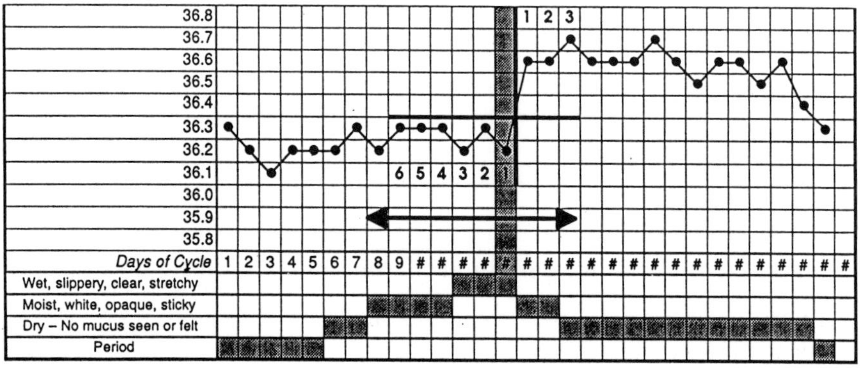

Figure 9 Combining the temperature indicator with the cervical mucus indicator. Produced in association with Jane Knight at Fertility UK

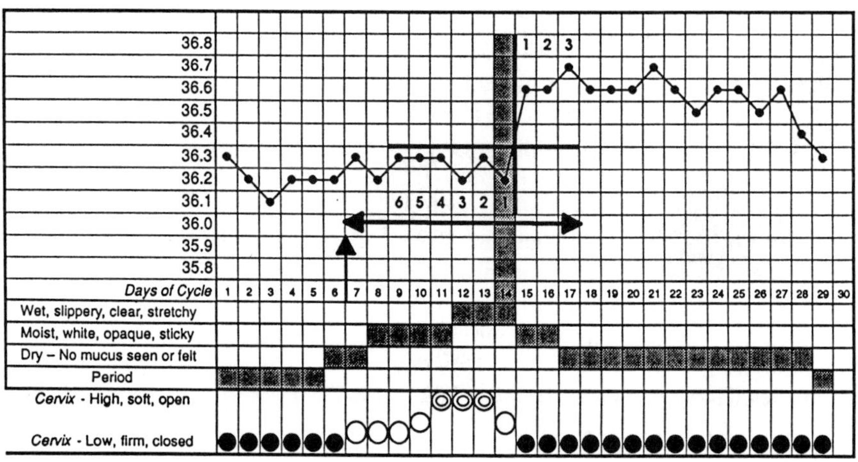

Figure 10 Chart showing four indicators of fertility recorded – the cervical mucus changes; the temperature changes; the cervix changes; and the calculation for the earliest fertile day marked by the upward arrow. Produced in association with Jane Knight at Fertility UK

Table 3 Effectiveness of using combination of indicators (symptothermal method). From references 14 and 15

Study	*Method failure (%)*	*Overall failure (%)*	*Participants (n)*
Marshall, 1982	0.3	3.9	108
Barbato, 1986	2.0	3.6	460
Freundl, 1987	1.0	2.6	387

observations on the same chart as shown. Checking several indicators increases the reliability of the method.

Table 3 gives results of three separate studies of women using a combination of the indicators[14,15]. The table shows that the failure rate using a combination of the indicators is less than that for most of the studies that use a single indicator.

In many settings, natural methods of family planning are taught on a one-to-one basis. In a primary health-care setting, this may be too costly and time-consuming. Therefore, a study was carried out in Oxford, UK to evaluate the cost-effectiveness of teaching fertility awareness and natural family planning in the National Health Service[16].

The study confirmed:

(1) The feasibility of a nurse teaching from a primary-care setting using a well structured course;

(2) That audio-visual materials reduced teaching time;

(3) That group teaching was feasible for some couples;

(4) That the failure rate was comparable with other natural family planning methods which combine several of the indicators of fertility and use experienced teachers;

(5) The educational value of teaching fertility awareness as part of reproductive health education;

(6) That the time-cost compared favorably with other family planning methods. Although it cost more in the first few months of nurses' time to teach natural family planning, once a couple understood the method, they no longer needed to attend the health clinic on a regular basis and the cost of charts and thermometers was very small. So, if the cost is adjusted over 10 years, then natural family planning becomes very cost effective.

RESEARCH INTO EFFECTIVENESS OF USER-DEPENDENT METHODS OF FAMILY PLANNING

Natural methods of family planning, as the contraceptive pill and barrier methods, are user-dependent methods. If natural methods of family planning are not used correctly, then intercourse is likely to occur at a time when pregnancy is more probable.

Figure 11 shows the average failure rates of natural family planning, oral contraceptives, male condoms and spermicides as reported by the Alan Guttmacher Institute. The top column shows the pregnancy rate for a couple using no contraception method. The first bar in each group shows the lower failure rates among those who are likely to use the methods correctly and consistently. The second bar in each group shows the relatively higher failure rates among those less likely to use the methods correctly or consistently. Some methods of natural family planning are more reliable than others. An average failure rate is used for Figure 11. The chart shows that natural methods of family planning are less effective than some of the other user-dependent methods.

The *advantages* of natural methods of family planning are:

(1) No chemical agents;

(2) No physical devices;

(3) No side-effects;

(4) Low cost;

(5) Not dependent on medical personnel after learning the method;

(6) Increased communication about fertility awareness and sexuality between a couple;

(7) The couple are both involved in the family planning method;

(8) They can use this knowledge to plan their family.

The *disadvantages* of natural methods of family planning are:

(1) Some couples never find abstinence easy and every teacher should be aware of this and counsel each couple;

(2) Do not protect against sexually transmitted diseases;

(3) Require several cycles to learn the method before it can be used with confidence;

(4) Cannot be used without the co-operation of the partner.

There is no ideal method of family planning. Many couples would like to have a non-invasive method which is reliable yet free from side-effects. Although natural methods of family planning are free from side-effects, their drawback is that they often require a long time of abstinence. If modern technology could allow the time of ovulation to be accurately predicted, then the method could become more reliable and the length of abstinence could be shortened. There are several groups of scientists around the world who are researching into methods

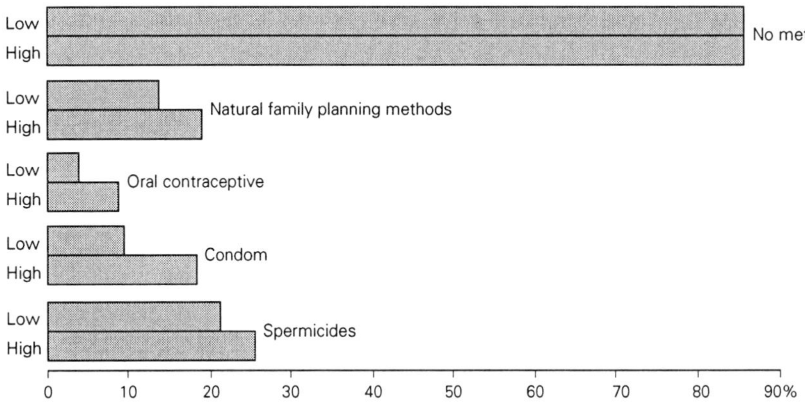

Figure 11 User-dependent family planning methods: percentage of women aged 15–44 years becoming pregnant in first year of use

to identify the fertile time. The research is mainly focused on the following hormones or their metabolites:

(1) Luteinizing hormone: high level just before ovulation;

(2) Urinary estradiol: raised levels at the outset of the fertile phase;

(3) Urinary pregnanediol: high level at the end of the fertile phase.

Research has confirmed that ovulation can be detected by hormone assays in plasma or urine[17] (Table 4). Rise in metabolites of estrogen may be used to indicate the probable start of the fertile phase. The maximum concentration of plasma estradiol is generally reached 1–2 days before ovulation.

It must be remembered that maturation of the follicle does not always end in ovulation; therefore, determination of the estrogen peak is less reliable in detecting ovulation than the rise in luteinizing hormone. The rise of luteinizing hormone occurs about 32 h before ovulation. The plasma concentration of progesterone

Table 4 Research into plasma hormone levels in relation to time of ovulation. From references 17–19

Hormone	*Onset of rise (h before ovulation)*	*Peak level (h before ovulation)*
Estradiol	83	24
Luteinizing hormone	32	16
Follicle stimulating hormone	21	15
Progesterone	8	(peak after ovulation)

begins to rise about 8 h before ovulation and the level rises rapidly following ovulation. This rise of progesterone is used clinically to confirm that ovulation has occurred.

Serial ultrasound studies of the ovaries during the menstrual cycle have confirmed the accuracy of the hormonal assays in pinpointing the likely time of ovulation[20]. Ultrasound gives the most accurate information on the time of ovulation. Using high resolution ultrasound scanners, the developing follicle is observed and measured. The diameter of the developing follicle has a wide range; it is impossible, therefore, to predict ovulation by a single measurement. Serial measurements are required by examination every day for several days prior to ovulation. Between one day and the next, the follicle will disappear, showing that ovulation has taken place. Ultrasound studies have also shown that the subjective signs such as temperature rise and cervical mucus changes are accurate in indicating the time of ovulation.

Research into the chances of conception on each day of the menstrual cycle was carried out in 1994 by Wilcox and colleagues[21]. They used hormone assays on daily urine collection to estimate the time of ovulation. Figure 12 shows that there were 6 days prior to ovulation during which, if a woman had intercourse, it was possible for her to conceive. The chances of conception fell to zero 24 h after ovulation.

Unipath have developed a personal system of family planning called Persona® which consists of a simple test using urine dip sticks combined with a computer for women to use in their own home. Together they identify the fertile time of the menstrual cycle by immune assay of the amount of luteinizing hormone and a metabolite of estrogen in a morning sample of urine. The computer monitors the changing levels of urinary metabolites and calculates the onset and end of the fertile phase. The device has colored lights that indicate the likely fertile and infertile times. The device has been researched in Europe. In September 1996 it was sold over the counter in the UK; it is also available in Italy and Ireland and will be available in the rest of Europe during 1997–1998. The results of the independent prospective clinical trial show a method failure rate of 6%; the data are due for publication later in the year. The potential use of devices such as Persona in the future, both as a method of family planning and as a teaching aid for helping women to learn about other aspects of fertility awareness, is very exciting.

CONCLUSIONS

It is well known that there is no ideal method of family planning but what is important is that new technologies will offer individuals and couples more choices of methods of family planning. A wide range of choice will meet the needs of more couples and, if a couple is satisfied with their method of family planning, they are more likely to use it consistently. The present author considers that all family planning health professionals should understand the scientific basis of

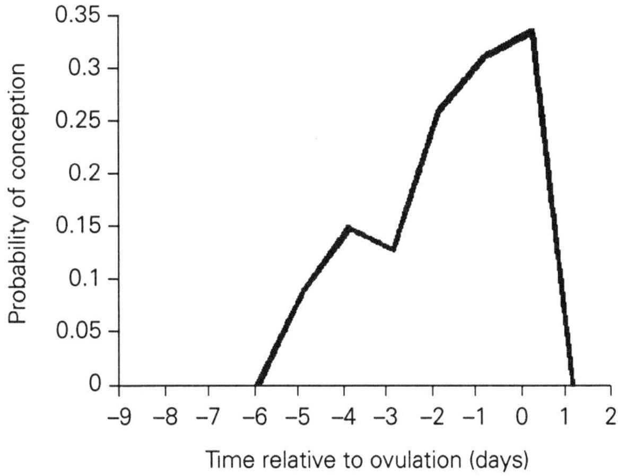

Figure 12 Chances of conception on given day of menstrual cycle using hormonal assays. From reference 21

family planning health professionals should understand the scientific basis of natural family planning, and that natural methods of family planning should be offered alongside other methods of family planning. In summary, the main objective has been to stress the importance of teaching individuals about fertility awareness so they are in a stronger position to make informed decisions about all aspects of their reproductive health and family planning.

ACKNOWLEDGEMENTS

I would especially like to thank especially Dr Victoria Jennings, Dr Elizabeth Clubb, Dr Anna Flynn, Jane Knight and Virginia Lamprecht for their support. I wrote this paper originally at the request of the Institute for Reproductive Health, and presented it in lecture form on their behalf at three reproductive health seminars in the Ukraine. Funding for the production of the slides was supported by the Institute for Reproductive Health, Georgetown University, Washington, DC under the co-operative agreement DPE–3061–A–00–1029–00 with the Agency for International Development. (The slides were also developed in Russian and recently translated into Ukranian.)

REFERENCES

1. Freely M, Pyper C. *Pandora's Clock 1994.* Cedar Press, 1994
2. Clubb EM, Knight J. *Fertility – Fertility Awareness and Natural Family Planning.* David & Charles, 1987
3. Howie P. Natural regulation of fertility. *Br Med Bull* 1993; 49: 182–99
4. Perez A, Labbok M, Queenan J. Clinical study of the lactational amenorrhoea method for family planning. *Lancet* 1992; 339: 968–70

5. Consensus Statement. Breast-feeding as a family planning method. *Lancet* 1988; 2: 1204–5
6. Gross B. *Breastfeeding and the return of fertility*. Report, Endocrine Unit, Department of Medicine, Westmead Centre, NSW, Australia, 1983
7. Vessey M, Smith A, Yeates D. Return of fertility after discontinuance of oral contraceptives – influence of age and parity. *Br J Fam Plann* 1986; III: 120–40
8. Aral S. Sexual behaviour as a risk factor sexually transmitted diseases. In Germain A, Holmes K, Piot P, *et al.*, eds. *Reproductive Tract Infections: Global Impact and Priorities for Women's Health*, Part III. New York: International Women's Health Coalition
9. Bromwich P. *Br J Sex Med* 1985; October: 124–5
10. Chretien FC, Cohen J. Human cervical mucus during the menstrual cycle and pregnancy in normal and pathological conditions. *J Reprod Med* 1975; 14: 192-6
11. World Health Organization. A prospective multicentre trial of the ovulation method of natural family planning: II. The effectiveness phase. *Fertil Steril* 1981; 36: 591–4
12. Barrett JC, Marshall J. The risk of conception on different days of the menstrual cycle. *Pop Stud* 1969; 23: 455–61
13. Marshall J. Thermal changes in the normal menstrual cycle. *Br Med J* 1963; 1: 102
14. Frank-Herrmann P, Freundl G, Baur, S. *et al.* Effectiveness and acceptability of the sympto-thermal method of natural family planning in Germany. *Am J Obstet Gynecol* 1991; 165: 2052–4
15. Barbato M, Bertolotti G. Natural methods of fertility control: a prospective study of 460 couples. Presented at *IV Congress of the International Federation for Family Life Promotion*, Serena, Canada, 1986; abstr.
16. Clubb EM, Pyper CM, Knight J. A pilot study on teaching natural family planning in general practice. In Proceedings of the Conference at Georgetown University, Washington, DC, 1991
17. Collins WP. The evolution of reference methods to monitor ovulation prediction. *Am J Obstet Gynecol* 1991; 165: 1994–6
18. Collins WP. Ovulation and the fertile period. *Med Forum* 1985; 17
19. World Health Organization Task Force. 1970
20. Flynn A, Docker M, Morris R, Lynch S, Royston J. The reliability of women's subjective assessment of the fertile period, relative to urinary gonadotrophins and follicular ultrasonic measurements during the menstrual cycle. In Bonnar J, Thompson W, Harrison RF, eds. *Research in Family Planning*. Lancaster, England: MTP Press, 1983; 3–11
21. Wilcox A, Weinberg M, Baird D. Timing of sexual intercourse in relation to ovulation. Effects on the probability of conception, survival of the pregnancy, and sex of the baby. *N Engl J Med* 1995; 333: 1517–21
22. Perez A, Labbok M, Barker D, Gray R. Use effectiveness of the ovulation method initiated during postpartum breastfeeding. *Contraception* 1998; 38: 499–508

This paper has been reproduced from *Eur J Contracept Reprod Health Care* 1997; 2: 131–46

11 Teaching natural contraception

F. Soler

INTRODUCTION

World Health Organization (WHO)

> *'Natural family planning (NFP) is a term used to describe methods of planning or preventing pregnancy based on observation of naturally occurring signs and symptoms of the fertile and infertile phases of the menstrual cycle. People who use NFP to avoid or delay pregnancy abstain from intercourse on potentially fertile days. Those wanting to achieve pregnancy use NFP to identify the fertile phase and hence maximise the probability of pregnancy'*[1].

The present author believes that NFP provides 'an alternative for those who, for any reason, cannot, or do not wish to use pharmacological or mechanical contraceptives'[1].

We must pay homage to the pioneers of modern NFP in the world: G. and R. Breault (Canada), Dr C.I. Lanctôt (USA), A. Cifuentes (Columbia), J. and E. Billings (Australia), R. and I. Ruiz, (Hong Kong) and particularly those from Europe: Dr T.H. Van de Velde (The Netherlands), R.F. Vollman (Switzerland), J.G.H. Holt (Austria), J. Marshall (England) and R. Palmer, G. Van der Stappen and C. Rendu (France).

BACKGROUND

Length of menstrual cycle

Menstruation is the normal periodic bleeding which results from the shedding of the lining of the uterus. The first day of menstruation is day 1 of the menstrual cycle and the last day of the cycle is the day before the next period.

Hormonal control of menstrual cycle

These cyclical changes in the womb directly depend on hormonal levels of ovarian activity and these, by a feedback process, depend on the follicle-stimulating hormone (FSH) and the luteinizing hormone (LH) released from the pituitary through the mediation of the gonadotropin-releasing hormone (GnRH) from the hypothalamus[2].

Natural signs of fertility and infertility

> *'Under estradiol dominance, the mucus becomes fluid and abundant: greatest release of mucus and maximal spinnbarkeit (an elastic-like quality to the mucus) will occur simultaneously with the estradiol peak, and hence signify follicular maturation. Under progesterone dominance, the cervical mucus becomes acidic and viscous (the uterine cavity becomes effectively sealed in preparation for embryo arrival and implantation)'*[2].

'A rise in basal body temperature occurs around the time of ovulation under the influence of progesterone'[3].

Phases of menstrual cycle

There are three phases of the normal ovulatory menstrual cycle: the relatively infertile phase, the fertile phase and the infertile phase. When the cycles vary, it is mainly the preovulatory phase that changes. The post-ovulatory or infertile phase remains fairly constant[3] (see Figure 1).

How long do gametes survive?

The ovum may survive in the reproductive system for about 12–24 h. On rare occasions in the same menstrual cycle, a second ovum is released within 24 h of the first. The spermatozoa may survive in the female reproductive system during the fertile phase for 3 days or longer. Survival beyond 5 days is unusual[3].

Planning intercourse

Men and women can plan and postpone intercourse. Every person has experience of sexual abstinence because of the changing circumstances of life[3]. Sexual appeal in humans is not only present and strong during the fertile phase[4], and psychological, physical or social reasons may interfere. The value system of both members of a couple and mutual understanding help to create optimum conditions for sex.

METHODOLOGY

Outline of anatomy and physiology of reproductive systems of men and women

Individually or in groups, it is first better to explain the male reproductive system, because sometimes it will be necessary to comment on the role of hormones, explain what a gland is and so on. The genital tract in men is responsible for the production and development of spermatozoa and the secretion of the male sex hormones, and serves for intercourse. The genital tract in women

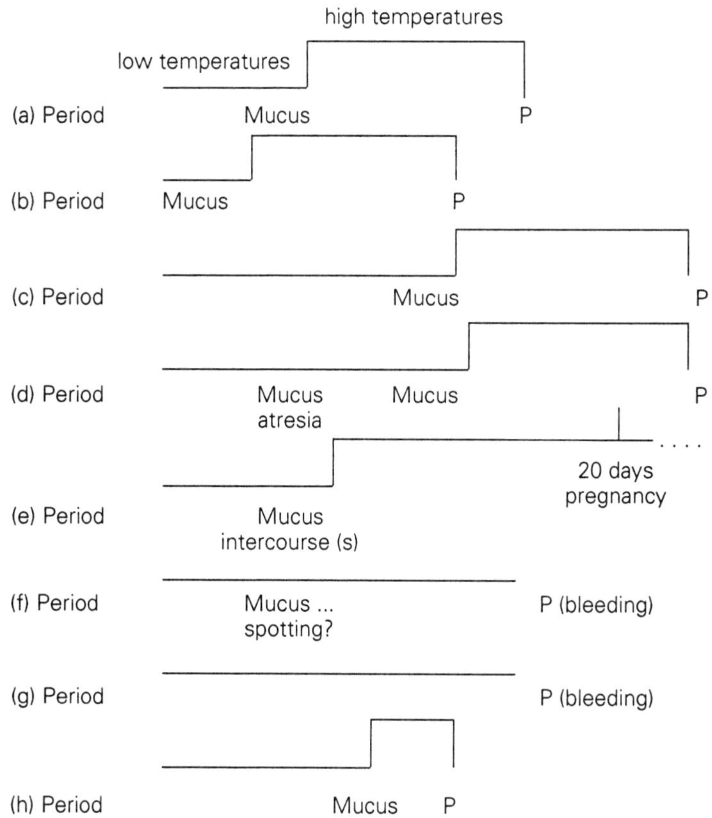

Figure 1 (a) A 'normal cycle'; (b) a short cycle; (c) a long cycle; (d) a long cycle with two phases of mucus, the first accompanying the atresia of the follicle; (e) 20 high days of temperature is a test of pregnancy; (f) an anovulatory cycle with mucus followed by either spotting or no spotting; (g) an anovulatory cycle without mucus; (h) a cycle with a deficient corpus luteum

serves similar functions (the development of the ovum and sex hormones, intercourse) and others such as pregnancy and breast-feeding. Consequently, it is necessary to explain the regulation of female hormones in more detail.

To remind (or to teach) people about the anatomy and physiology of the reproductive system of men, begins with description of the scrotum and its role in the thermal regulation of testes. These produce spermatozoa and the male sex hormones. A diagram of the internal anatomy of the male can show the bladder and the urethral sphincter and describe the function of the epididymus, the vas deferens, the seminal vesicle and the prostate gland. An accompanying diagram helps to explain changes in the penis during intercourse and the way spermatozoa enter the female reproductive system. Semen normally contains millions of spermatozoa. (If the penis is the starting point, some people may laugh or become embarrassed.) Finally, the relationship between the male sex hormones and the development of male sexual characteristics is explained[5].

Description of the female reproductive system begins with an external anatomical diagram of the female. Mention is made of the breasts and their functions and the vulva, with the labia majora, the labia minora, the clitoris, the urinary meatus and the hymen and the functions of each part. A front view is used to show the internal reproductive system with the vagina, the uterus, the Fallopian tubes and the ovaries, and a side view for the same parts between the urethra, the bladder, the pubic bone in front, and the rectum and the spine behind[6].

All women, with or without previous information about the physiology of the female reproductive system, know about the period. For this reason, the changes in the lining which covers the cavity of the uterus (the endometrium) are explained. The first day of the menstrual cycle is the day on which the menstrual flow starts, and the last day of the cycle is the day before the next menstrual flow begins. After the period, the endometrium develops and thickens, waiting for a fertilized ovum. If the woman does not become pregnant, 'the endometrium breaks up and is passed out of the body. This is menstruation'[7].

There are changes in the cervix between one period and another. After menstruation, it is closed, and progressively opens more and secretes the cervical mucus, which changes in quantity and quality from thick to thin and scanty to profuse, and disappears. It becomes sticky and acts as a 'plug' in the cervix until the following menstruation.

Why are there these changes in the endometrium and in the cervix? This process depends on changes in the ovaries. When menstruation begins, an immature ovum starts its development in a bag called a follicle and produces one hormone (estrogen), through which the bloodstream triggers the development of the endometrium, and the high level of estrogen triggers the secretion of cervical mucus. When the ovum is mature, the follicle expels it; the Fallopian tube regains it where fertilization is expected within no more than 24 h. Once fertilized, the Fallopian tube drives the egg to the endometrium. The empty follicle forms the corpus luteum, or yellow body, which starts to secrete another hormone called progesterone, responsible for the end of fluid mucus and preparation of the endometrium for a possible implantation of the egg, and which also causes a rise in the basal temperature and often breast tenderness and fullness. Two weeks after ovulation, the yellow body starts to disintegrate and stops producing progesterone and estrogen. A new menstrual cycle starts.

The ovaries are not independent and begin the maturation of the follicle answering to the FSH secreted by the pituitary gland. As the ovum continues to ripen, the estrogen level reaches a peak, and this triggers the pituitary gland to start releasing the LH which flows into the bloodstream and causes the rupture of the follicle.

The pituitary is not independent either, and these secretions of FSH and LH can be altered by stress, tiredness and so on.

The cervical mucus is favorable to the survival of the sperm, and the 'plug' in the cervix, after ovulation, stops sperm entering the uterus.

Combined fertility of men and women

The fertility of the couple starts with the lifespan of the spermatozoa in the fertile mucus (no more than 5 days) and ends with the lifespan of the ovum.

> *'The designated fertile phase was indeed fertile, as intercourse during this phase resulted in conception with increasing frequency the nearer to ovulation the intercourse occurred (there were two pregnancies for every three acts of intercourse on the peak day of the mucus sign)'*[8].

The study of Wilcox[9] has confirmed this hypothesis.

Observing and charting major signs of fertility and infertility

Cervical mucus

The following indicates:

> *'On each visit to the toilet, the woman, who can learn about mucus, WIPES across the lips that are the vaginal entrance, using a flat pad of tissue a few layers thick. As she does so, she easily notices if the vaginal entrance is 'dry', the tissue tends to catch, it will not glide. But when the vaginal entrance is 'slippery wet' (lubricated), the tissue glides easily. She then LOOKS at the tissue to see whether or not there is any mucous secretion adhering to the tissue (dampness from urine will simply absorb into the tissue). By folding and opening the pad of tissue, she TESTS it to see whether or not it is stretchable. She may obtain a sample by touching the lips at the vaginal entrance and to stretch it between her thumb and index finger. In order to avoid confusion, the beginner should take care not to place her fingers inside the vagina itself, which is always rather moist. The entire observation takes but a few seconds! . . . Each woman should learn for herself. As a beginner, she should do it before or after she urinates, or both ways for a while'*[10].

Some women find that mucus is particularly apparent after passing a stool and they use two tissues: one for the lips and the other for the rectum.

Women who complain of 'constant vaginal discharge' (seldom stretchable) should be aware that a continuous discharge is unlike the temporary mucous secretion of the fertile period, noticed as 'something that previously was not present'.

The peak day is the term applied to the last day when the mucus shows any of the signs of fertility: sensation of wetness/slipperiness (lubrication), and/or transparency and/or threadiness. The sensation of lubrication may last longer than the visible signs, in such a case it will determine the 'peak'[11]. Hormonal assays and ultrasonography studies have shown that ovulation occurs on the peak day or during the previous or following 3 days[12].

Active teaching

Active teaching is carried out using water, flour and raw egg-white and handtowels. Three glasses are needed: one contains water, another flour and the third, raw egg-white. The participants introduce their thumb and index finger into the water and develop a refined sensitivity. They experience a wet sensation (like the more fertile days). Afterwards, they dry their fingers and they introduce the same fingers into the raw egg-white. Out of the glass, their fingers glide easily (like the sensation produced by mucus, at the vulva, on the more fertile days). In the last exercise, they plunge their fingers in the water and then in the flour; they wipe their fingers and obtain a sticky paste like the less fertile mucus (with more water, the fluid paste can be compared with candidiasis).

To chart mucus, the World Health Organization designed a package for teachers of NFP and specifies for the cervical mucus method objectives[3] 'Recognise that a woman's own mucus pattern will be individual, cannot be predetermined and must be described in her own words' and[64] 'Recognise that a written description of all relevant observations throughout the day must be recorded on the chart along with the visual symbols being used. Describe the mucus with at least one sensation adjective, and one visual appearance adjective . . .' Then 'Explain that if both infertile-type and fertile-type mucus are recognised on the same day, only the fertile-type should be recorded. If bleeding and mucus of any type are observed on the same day, both are recorded'[3].

Spanish groups teach recording of sensation, color and elasticity. There are different charting methods according to the educational level of users, and the teaching groups. Some examples appear in Table 1. For illiterate people, very simple codes are prepared. For example, in the slums of Calcutta[13], X = period, O = moist discharge, a dot into O = thin, slippery and I = dry. For the Centre de Liaison des Equipes de Recherche (CLER)[14], with a very large experience in Francophone communities[15], keys are: — = without mucus, one black square = sticky mucus, two black squares = spinnbarkeit effect.

In his thesis, Lepault[16] presented the study of 757 charts of mucus (Billings method) from 116 women, and observed fewer unplanned pregnancies among the women who described only the sensation (with a single word), the number of unplanned pregnancies being 50% lower than among the women who described sensation and appearance. This confirms the wisdom of the Billings method that sensation is more important than appearance.

Biphasic pattern of basal body temperature

To measure and chart basal body temperature (BBT), the woman needs a normal clinical thermometer. Flynn[7] considers that 'it is better to use a special fertility

Table 1 How to chart the mucus symptoms. Color code used by the World Health Organization; *, Code of the slums of Calcutta; †, code of CLER; ‡, some Billings groups use marrow; **, Billings groups use yellow

	Description of the mucus			
Menstrual cycle events	*Sensation*	*Appearance*	*Abbreviation*	*Codes*
Period				red X* III†
Days of feeling dry	dry		d	green‡ I* —†
Days of not feeling dry	moist, sticky	white, yellow, scanty, thick, creamy, opaque	f	white** ○* ■†
	wet lubrication slippery	thin, profuse, watery, cloudy, raw egg-white, elastic, clear, reddish	F	white ⊙* ■■†
	Peak day	last day 'F'	X	
3 days after peak day	dry or moist		1 2 3	green‡ or white

thermometer, calibrated in tenths of a degree, and which only covers the range 35°C–39°C'. In Spain, fertility thermometers measure between 36 and 38°C; if a fever is suspected, these thermometers should not be used because a high temperature may break the mercury column. When the women uses a digital thermometer some charts are more difficult to interpret.

A special temperature chart has been designed for the purpose, because the ovulation-related temperature rise varies between 0.2 and occasionally 0.5°C.

The women takes her temperature on waking, before getting up in the morning. If she is working on night shifts, she will take her temperature after rest.

Temperature is taken as near as possible to the same time each day, and the woman will note the change if it is an hour or more earlier or later than usual.

She checks the internal temperature, rectally or vaginally, over 3 min. If she prefers to do it orally, she places the thermometer under her tongue, and closes her lips for 5 min. Clubb[17] specifies that 'oral temperatures can give satisfactory results if exact instructions are followed, but internal temperatures are more reliable'. Most digital thermometers emit a beeping sound after 45–60 s to signal that registration is complete. Some special fertility thermometers need 5 min (and more orally). For accuracy, whichever method has been chosen, it should be followed throughout the cycle.

The woman removes the thermometer, reads the temperature and records this reading on the chart by a dot in the centre of the appropriate square. If the mercury stops between two marks, WHO recommends recording the lower reading, whereas Flynn, Rötzer and others record the precise temperature, every 0.05°C (see Figure 2).

What disturbs BBT? Every event, such as a cold, a late night, drinking alcohol or any stressful situation should be noted on the chart to help interpretation. In Spain, Sunday lunch is very often a large meal eaten later in the afternoon than during the week. By contrast, the evening meal is light or non-existent. As a result, the BBT on Monday morning is lower than after a normal evening meal.

A disturbed night's sleep, such as getting up for children, can disturb the BBT; frequently, in this situation, an hour resting in bed before taking temperature is sufficient to optimize the temperature measurement. Other disturbances can be caused by changes in the environment, e.g. going away for holidays or the week-end.

Two thermometers can give different readings, one of 36.6°C and the other 36.8°C. For this reason the WHO chart for the symptothermal method states that 'If you change the thermometer, mark the day of the change on the chart'[3].

Usually, during the pre-ovulatory phase, the temperature taken 1 h later is 0.1 °C higher, and 2 h later is 0.2 °C higher but, during the following hours, the rate of rise decreases.

It is not necessary to chart the temperature every day. Some forgetfulness does not make interpretation of the chart more difficult. Six low temperatures and three high temperatures are necessary. During the first cycle, to chart the temperature for all the days of the cycle is recommended, but after three cycles, it is not necessary to chart after the third day of high temperature. An experienced woman charts temperatures when mucus starts or when she notices any change in the cervix, and stops observation when infertility is deduced.

Self-palpation of four changes in cervix during fertile phase

After a period, during which the cervix is low, and firm like the nose, it undergoes gradual changes as the level of estrogen increases before ovulation: it rises, opens, becomes softer, like the lips, and straightens out. Later, it lowers again and closes, becomes firmer and tilts rapidly due to progesterone release. If a woman wants to examine her cervix, she carefully washes her hands just before

SYMPTO-THERMAL CHART

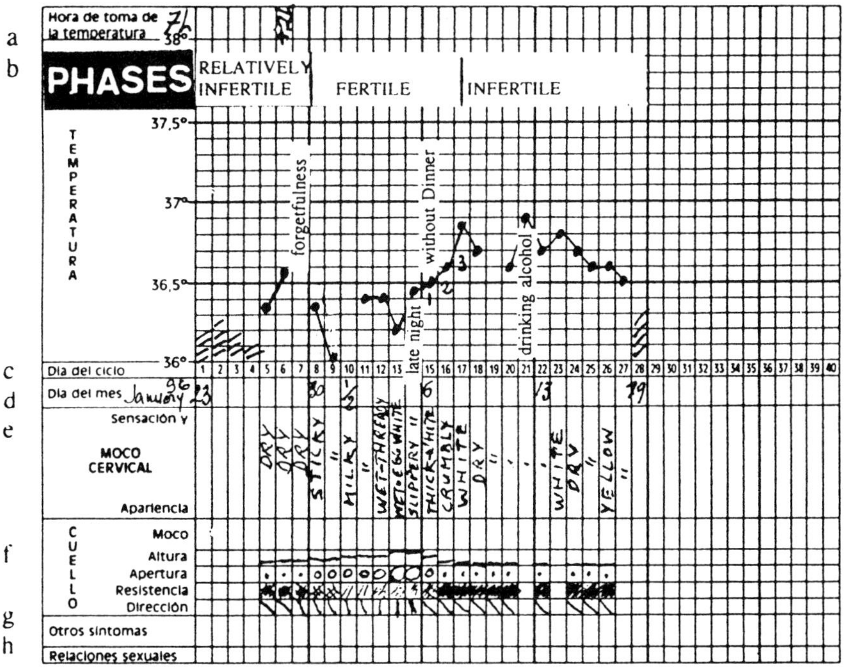

Figure 2 A typical sympto-thermal chart. (a) Time of taking temperature; (b) temperature; (c) day of the menstrual cycle; (d) day of month; (e) mucus: sensation and appearance; (f) cervix: mucus, level, opening, firmness, position; (g) other symptoms; (h) intercourse. Infertile days using Billings method: 5, 7 (or only 6) and 16–26; relatively infertile days (shortest cycle (26) minus 20 = 6): 1 to 6; infertile days: 16–26

introducing her index and middle fingers into the vagina. At the end of the vagina she touches the cervix (see Figure 3) with the tips of her fingers. Sometimes, it is necessary to press the abdomen with the other hand to force the uterus downwards. With two fingers, she can also 'milk' the cervix and collect the mucus[18].

Minor indicators of fertility

Ovulation pain, breast tenderness and so on

Pain may be in the side or mid-region of the abdomen, and be localized or diffuse, momentary or prolonged; this pain is related to the ovulatory period in general. Breast tenderness is frequent after ovulation, and is due to progesterone activity.

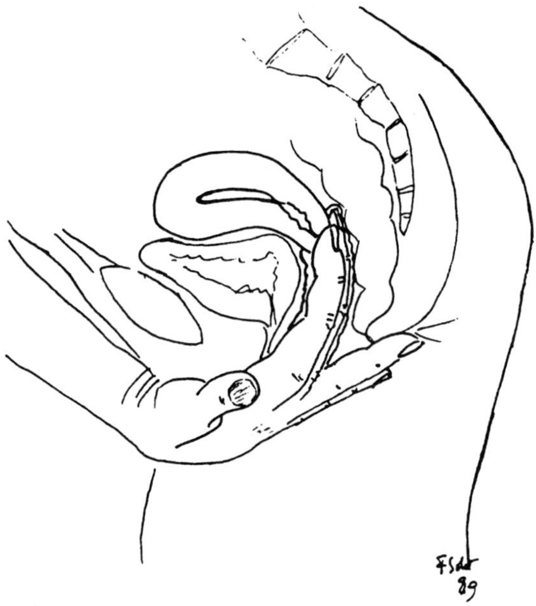

Figure 3 Self-examination of the cervix

Determining relatively infertile phase (in preovulatory phase) and infertile (post-ovulatory) phase by different methods of natural contraception

Billings method

During the first cycle, the couple abstain from intercourse for the entire cycle to enable the woman to distinguish the difference between mucus and sperm, and the woman, every night, charts the sensation given by the mucus at the vulva, and its appearance.

During menstruation, couples wishing to prevent conception should abstain from intercourse and all genital contact as if expecting a short cycle. 'Following menstruation there are usually several days when the woman notices no discharge at the vulva. These are the dry days. The couple may have intercourse at night'[15], (and, remembering recent observation of the mucus), 'but not the following day, to avoid confusing sperm with the beginning of mucus'.

At the first sign of mucus, the couple should regard itself as fertile (the mucus aids the survival of spermatozoa for 5 days) and abstain until the fourth day after the 'peak'. As of the fourth day after peak, the couple is free to have intercourse any time until the end of the cycle. However, observations continue to be made and noted because sometimes, by observation of mucus only, an atresia is not detected.

'The preovulatory and postovulatory days designed by the Billings method of NFP rules as infertile were indeed infertile as the pregnancies in this phase were 4 per 1000 acts of intercourse'[8].

Temperature method (to determine only infertile phase)

This method uses the WHO rules (Coverline) or the method of 'three over six'.

> *'To draw a Coverline: (1) omit the first four temperatures if taken on the first 4 days of the cycle; (2) take into account all the low phase readings unaffected by disturbance; (3) a minimum of six low temperatures is needed; (4) draw a Coverline 0.05 °C above the highest of these lower phase readings; (5) count three consecutive higher normal daily temperatures above this Coverline. The infertile phase begins on the morning on which the third consecutive higher daily normal daily temperature is recorded above the Coverline.*[3]*'*

The first chart of temperature determines infertile days.

Germanophone groups[19] and also Clubb[17] (England) consider only the last six low temperatures to be unaffected by disturbance. The third high temperature must be 0.2°C higher than the highest temperature of the six considered; if it is less than 0.2°C higher, a fourth day of high temperature checks infertility. CLER calculates the median of these six low temperatures and the high temperatures may be 0.3°C higher than this median and requires no more than 0.1°C between the first and the third high temperatures.

Symptothermal method

In this method, infertility starts on the third day after the peak of mucus and the third day of high temperature. Both sets of information must agree.

Determining relatively infertile phase (in preovulatory phase) by different methods of natural contraception

The last relatively infertile day can be determined by a calculation for the cycle–thermal method or the 'calculothermal' method: the shortest known cycle in the last six cycles minus 21; the shortest known cycle in the last year minus 20; or the earliest high temperature charted in the previous 12 cycles minus 8.

Both the Billings method and the mucothermal method rely on a sensation of dryness for determination of the last relatively infertile day.

A calculation together with the sensation of dryness (and without changes in the cervix) is used in the symptothermal method or multiple index method. (If mucus appears during one day calculated to be infertile, the fertile phase begins on this day, and although dryness exists over the calculated phase as relatively infertile, the potential fertile phase has begun.)

The fertile phase is between the relatively infertile phase and the infertile (postovulatory) phase.

Group and individual teaching

Young people and couples

For individual teaching, if the woman is a health worker or biologist, the explanation of the physiological basis of the methods is begun with the description of the effects of GnRH, and the changes in endometrium and the symptoms of fertility and infertility are discussed at the end. In other circumstances, the inverse order is better.

When young people receive information 'about the menstrual cycle of 28 days' and contraception, the lifespans of the ovum and spermatozoa are forgotten. Generally, books do not mention mucus characteristics, temperature changes or changes in the cervix. While there is an increasing tendency towards permissiveness and tolerance with regard to sexual relations, adolescents do not always appreciate the possibility of an unwanted pregnancy resulting from unprotected intercourse. They are interested in the 'subject' of sexuality rather than contraception. We need to teach adolescents in detail to observe these signs, so that they become aware of their own potential fertility, and use contraceptive methods[20].

After the physiology of men and women have been explained, the parts of a puzzle are given to each group of seven people (see Figure 4). One puts in the correct place the growing of the ovum and corpus luteum, another the changes to the endometrium, another the changes to the mucus, then temperature, etc., and all pieces of the puzzle fit together.

With a group of 26 or more, a performance is made of the menstrual cycle. One person, in a red pullover, pretends to be the first day of the cycle while others in white blouses are the days of mucus. Another possibility is to give each of them a colored paper cloak (red, green, white). A sitting-down circle is formed but after the 'days of mucus' the participants stand up (they are the 'high temperature level'). Afterwards a short cycle is portrayed, then a long cycle with late ovulation and another with an atresia and ovulation separated by dry days. If the group is small, each day of the cycle is represented by the head and raised hands of each participant. Some teachers help young women to chart and interpret the symptoms of the menstrual cycle.

Post-pill, breastfeeding and premenopause

After pill use, several months should elapse before return to normal charts. There are specific charts for breast-feeding and premenopause, and learning NFP in these periods of life needs more help from teachers.

Follow-up and help for first three cycles

Generally, help to interpret the first three charts (by phone at least) is enough to lead the woman or couple to autonomy; about 4 h during 3 months is required.

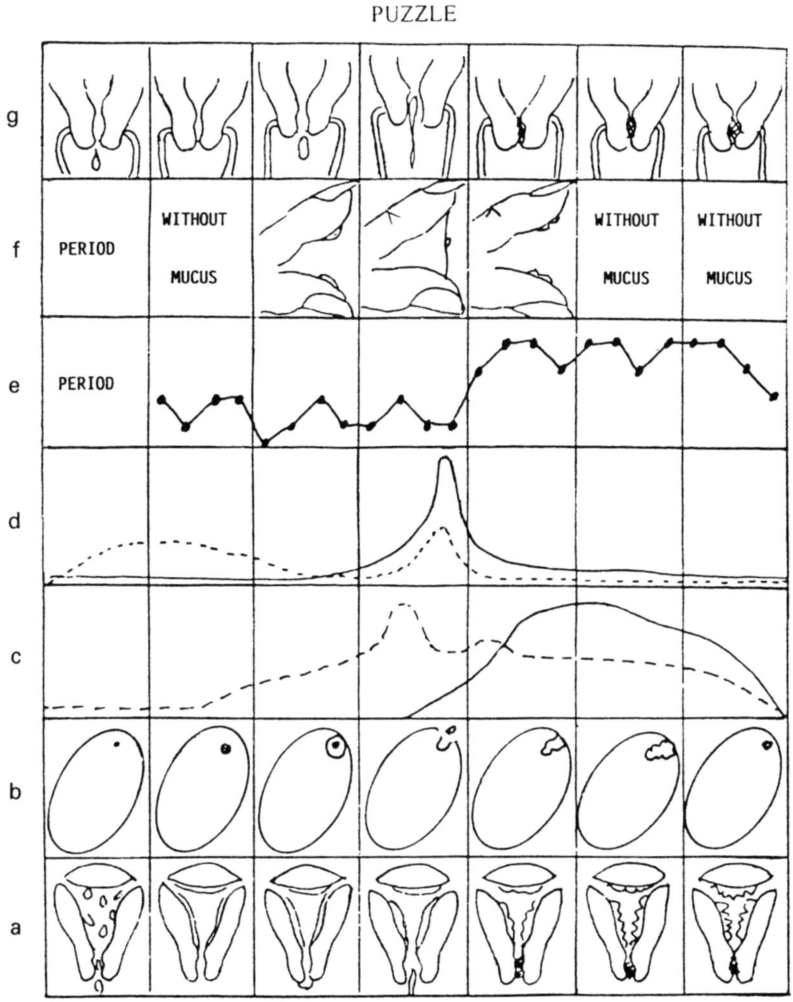

Figure 4 Puzzle used as a an aid to teaching natural contraception. (a) Destruction, reconstruction and transformation of the endometrium; (b) growth of the follicle, ovulation and the corpus luteum; (c) ovarian hormones; (d) hormones of the pituitary; (e) chart of temperature; (f) cervical mucus; (g) changes in the cervix

Who can teach natural contraception?

In the above-mentioned study from Calcutta[18], it is stated that 'If both (husband and wife) are unable to record the temperature, an educator helps them. These are women with education of about 6 years. They are trained regularly in weekly meetings by the specially trained sisters and the period of training is for 3 months. Soon a motived happy couple teaches other neighbors and thus the training becomes a continuous one.' In Western Europe, every country has one or more groups with a structured training for teachers of NFP. A mother using natural contraception can teach NFP to her daughter(s).

Who can use natural contraception?

Natural contraception can be used by every fertile woman or couple. An adolescent or a woman abstaining from intercourse can learn the natural signs of fertility and infertility to get to know their cyclical fertility and understand the changes in their body and mind. During the years of premenopause, observation of signs of fertility helps a woman to understand the longer cycles and other specific symptoms of this period of life.

Jennings has pointed out that 'It is interesting to note that, all over the world, women state that the principal reason for using natural contraception is fear of the side effects of other methods'[21].

> *'It is self evident that NFP will only work for couples who are prepared to co-operate . . . There are vast numbers of married couples around the world who are prepared to do so, and only a tiny proportion of these are aware that there are easily recognisable symptoms of ovulation'*[22].

Also, 'Some couples use NFP simply because they do not have access to other methods or because its use is consistent with their ethical or religious beliefs'[23].

> *'Klann and colleagues found that NFP-users did not differ much from the general population in Germany: they differed only in that they were much more willing to have further pregnancies and their attitude towards sexuality was positive and uninhibited. They described themselves more frequently as 'considerate, forbearing, rather trustful, having sophisticated moral opinions, and capable of dealing gently with others'. Women 'feel less subjectively helpless or dependent upon others'*[24].

'In Liberia a use- and cost-effectiveness study from 1983 to 1988 showed a total pregnancy rate of 4.3 (Pearl Index), in Zambia, the pregnancy rate was 8.9'. The symptothermal method was used by 68.3 % and 82.7% of the people, respectively; other people used the Billings method. 'There is no doubt, therefore, that NFP has proved as efficient as modern contraceptive methods, in some instances more efficient, and can be used effectively by both uneducated and educated couples'[25].

MATERIALS FOR TEACHING, EVALUATION AND FOLLOW-UP

Abundant and diversified materials exist to teach natural family planning methods, such as video (for example 'Fertility' from Oxford University[26], available in Spanish), slides, posters, the material from WHO mentioned above, NFP teacher's book, charts, puzzles and so on.

For the follow-up, every teacher needs an archive containing the history of the user, a copy of her charts and a code to analyze the charts. When a woman explains her difficulties with the method in special circumstances (for example charts of breastfeeding, long cycle, post-pill and so on), it is easy for the teacher to show her a similar case to encourage her, in this first and difficult phase of learning.

The initial interview discusses whether the purpose of the learner is to space or to limit her family. A teacher sometimes teaches NFP to achieve pregnancy. The user knows the most fertile days for every cycle, but this is not the aim of this talk.

ADVANTAGES AND DIFFICULTIES OF NATURAL CONTRACEPTION

Natural family planning is the cheapest birth-control method, and it helps users to understand the menstrual cycle and combined fertility of men and women. Charts indicating signs of fertility and infertility help to detect some abnormalities in ovarian activities (anovulatory cycles, deficient corpus luteum, repetitive atresias) or diseases of the cervix and vaginal tract. Basal body temperature is the cheapest method by which to diagnose pregnancy.

The present author remembers that the Institute for Reproductive Health[23] believes that modern natural contraception is a 'good option' and that physicians should propose modern NFP as an alternative form of contraception to enable women to have the chance of making an informed choice according to the Beijing Declaration and Platform for Action No.96:

> *'Reproductive health is a state of complete physical, mental and social well-being and not merely the absence of disease or infirmity, in all matters relating to the reproductive system and to its functions and processes. Reproductive health therefore implies that people are able to have a satisfying and safe sex life and that they have the capability to reproduce and the freedom to decide if, when and how often to do so. Implicit in this last condition are the right of men and women to be informed and to have access to safe, effective, affordable and acceptable methods of family planning of their choice, as well as other methods* [in Mexico[27], specified 'including natural family planning'] *of their choice for regulating of fertility which are not against the law, and the right of access to appropriate health-care services that will enable women to go safely through pregnancy and childbirth and provides couples with the best chance of having a healthy infant'.*

Knowledge brings with it responsibilities, and some people are afraid to choose, preferring ignorance and that others have the responsibility of choosing. Fromm wrote: 'Can freedom become such a heavy load for people that they do their best to avoid it? Why is it then that for many freedom is a desired goal, while for others it is nothing but a threat? Might it not be that together with an innate desire of freedom, there is an instinctive longing for submission[28].' Could we paraphrase Fromm by substituting 'fertility' for 'freedom'? Could this instinctive longing for submission explain difficulties in regularly using contraception methods, or in having intercourse only during the infertile phases of the cycle. Couples who have difficulties with periodic abstinence or women with casual sexual encounters may think that NFP alone is not adequate for them.

Stress and drugs can postpone normal follicle development and cause long cycles with repetitive symptoms of fertility but not followed by an infertile phase.

CONCLUSIONS

There is a need for research into a remedy for irregular cycles. The option of natural contraception is the right of women and couples. Natural contraception is an innocuous method that can be learnt by everybody (even the illiterate). Some methods are very effective and cheap. Autodiagnosis of fertility is also helpful for subfertile couples.

ACKNOWLEDGEMENTS

The author would like to thank Sean Murphy and Jesus de Andres for their help with the definitive version of the text.

REFERENCES

1. World Health Organization. *Natural Family Planning, A Guide to Provision of Services.* Geneva: WHO, 1988; 82
2. Ferin M, Jewelewicz R, Warren M. Hypothalamic–pituitary–ovarian communication. In *The Menstrual Cycle.* Oxford: Oxford University Press, 1993: 42–61
3. World Health Organization and BLAT. *Family Fertility Education, A Resource Package for Teachers of Natural Family Planning Methods.* Geneva: WHO and BLAT, 1982
4. Döring GK, Sollfrank R. Wann die Liebe am schösten ist. Gibt es ein eindeutiges Libido-Maximum im Zyklus der Frau? *Sexualmedizin* 1988; 17: 8–13
5. Guy F, Guy M. *Présentation des schémas d'anatomie et de physiologie.* Grenoble: B20 IREC, 1977: 26
6. Barranco E, Garcia E, Sánchez MJ, Soler F. Sugerencias pedagogicas para la introducción al autoconocimiento de la fertilidad. In Barranco E, Caño A, eds. *Hacia el Autoconocimiento del Cuerpo Femenino, Fertilidad y Métodos Naturales Feminae 11.* Granada: University of Granada, 1994: 27–67
7. Flynn AM, Brooks M. *A Manual of Natural Family Planning.* London: Unwin Paperbacks Women's Health, 1985: 27
8. Ryder B, Campbell H. Natural family planning in the 1990s. *Lancet* 1995; 346: 233–4
9. Wilcox AJ, Weinberg CR, Baird DD. Timing of sexual intercourse in relation to ovulation. *N Engl J Med* 1995; 333: 1517–21

10. Rötzer J. *Family Planning the Natural Way*. Old Tappan, NJ: Fleming H, Revell Co, 1981: 123
11. Parenteau-Carreau S. *Love and Life Ottawa 1989*. Montreal: Serena, 1992
12. Freundl G, Suberg D, Flynn AM, Diemer AM, Diemer HP. Natural family planning (sympto-thermal method) and objective ovulation parameters – a pilot study. *Geburstshilfe Frauenheilkd* 1984; 44: 368–74
13. Ghosh AK, Saha S, Chatterjee D. Symptothermia vis a vis fertility control. *J Obstet Gynecol* 1982; 3: 443–7 and *Natura Med* 1986; 13: 14–18
14. CLER. *La Fertilité de l'Homme et de la Femme et ses Points de Repère*. Paris: CLER: 36
15. Action Familiale. *La Conduite de la Fécondité*. Kinshasa: Archid. de Kinshasa, 1987: 40
16. Lepault P. *Approfondissement et enseignement de la méthode Billings*. Grenoble: Fac. de Méd., 1989: 118
17. Clubb E, Knight J. *Fertility a Comprehensive Guide to Natural Family Planning*. London: David and Charles Publishers, 1987: 34
18. Parenteau-Carreau S, Infante-Rivard C. Self palpation to assess cervical changes in relation to mucus and temperature. *Int J Fertil* 1988 (Suppl.): 10–16
19. Natürlich und sicher Natürliche Familienplanung – ein Leitfaden-Arbeitsgruppe NFP Ehrenwirth München 1987, p. 59
20. Torres P. Regulación de la fertilidad y educacion. Una aproximación práctica. In Barranco E, Caño A, eds. *Hacia el Autoconocimiento del Cuerpo Femenino, Fertilidad y Métodos Naturales Feminae*. II. Granada: University of Granada, 1994: 151–9
21. Jennings V. Difusione dei metodi naturali del mondo. In *La Regolazione Naturale della Fertilità: Scienza, Cultura, Esperienza Verso il 2000*. Milan: Camen, 1995
22. Ryder B, Campbell H. Author's reply. *Lancet* 1995, 346: 775–6
23. Institute for Reproductive Health, Georgetown University School of Medicine. *Natural Family Planning, A Good Option*. Washington: Institute for Reproductive Health, Georgetown University School of Medicine, 1989: 15
24. Klann N, Hahlweg K, Hank G. Psychological aspects of NFP practice. *Int J Fertil* 1988; 33 (Suppl.): 65–9
25. Flynn AM. Natural family planning in developing countries. *Lancet* 1992; 340: 309
26. Clubb E, Knight J. *Fertilidad, una guia para la planificación familiar natural*. Video Claret, ed. Barcelona: Roger de LLúria
27. Recommendation No. 26, International Conference on Population, Mexico City, August 1984
28. Fromm E. *The Fear of Freedom (El Miedo a la Libertad)*. Paidos, 1978: 352

12 Importance of intrauterine contraception

H.E. Van Kets

INTRODUCTION

Recently, the medical and lay worlds were shaken by papers in the *Lancet*[1] which claimed that oral contraceptives containing desogestrel and gestodene doubled the risk of venous thrombosis and embolism. As often happens, history tends to repeat itself and the message in these papers was not very different from what we have known since 1968[2,3].

Although the use of intrauterine devices (IUDs) is progressing both in developing and developed countries[4], oral contraceptives account for the greatest share of the highly efficient methods of family planning used in Western Europe, ranging from 40% in Germany to 12% in Spain[5].

Even if we accept that the risks of deep venous thrombosis have been grossly overestimated, nobody can deny that even a short spell of taking low-estrogen contraceptive pills doubles the always present risk for this complication[6].

Malcolm Potts[7] once developed a very original approach to the problem of health safety considering various events in a woman's life. He calculated how long a woman would live if she had to die from only one isolated cause. The risks of being hit by lightning or a falling airplane are so small that she could live several millions of years. Using oral contraceptives as sole risk gives her 63 000 years to live but, using an IUD, she would reach the blessed age of 200 000 years.

Apart from being amusing which unfortunately does not happen very often in medical papers – Malcolm Potts' calculations illustrate that IUD-use is three times safer than taking the pill which, in itself, is a relatively harmless threat for life-expectancy.

REASONS FOR LIMITED IUD USE

The limited IUD use, specifically in the developed world, can be ascribed to various causes: the first lies with the pharmaceutical industry. One should be aware that the pill market is of great economic importance. This is the single drug that is taken by the greatest number of healthy women in the world. Once initial research into steroids is completed, production costs of pills are low and earnings high. It would be frankly unfair to blame the industry for trying to achieve its main purpose: commercial viability.

A second reason can be found within the medical profession: prescribing oral contraceptives is much easier and less time- and energy-consumingthan inserting an IUD. Moreover, not all practitioners have acquired the skills to perform a correct insertion which guarantees the best possible results[8].

Women themselves are often very poorly informed, and fear that inserting a piece of plastic and metal into their uterus has to be painful and may bring an unknown risk of infection and even cancer.

The media have never been very kind to IUDs and have often neglected their many advantages, but are still repeating the old stories of the ill-fated Dalkon Shield.

It is probable, however, that the side-effects of IUDs themselves may be responsible for the fact that IUDs represent a minority in the group of contraceptives. These side-effects are: a generally slightly higher pregnancy rate than with the pill, increased spotting and menstrual bleeding sometimes accompanied by expulsion and pain.

IUD USE IN EUROPE

The percentage of IUD use differs from country to country. In Germany, 40% of women at risk of pregnancy use oral contraceptives, 9% have an IUD and 10% rely on barriers. In The Netherlands, 8% of suitable candidates have IUDs versus 34% pill users[5].

In the UK, contraceptive pills are used by 26% of women, but only 5% use an IUD whereas sterilization (18%) and barrier methods (14%) are popular[5].

France shows keen pill use by 34% of women, but also shows the second highest percentage (19%) of IUD use with relatively few (6%) sterilizations and a low percentage (3%) of barrier methods[5].

Norway and Scandinavia in general have highest use of the IUD with 30% of eligible women using IUDs versus 21% taking the pill[9]. Countries with a stronger Catholic influence suffer from the consistent claim that the IUD is an abortifacient and, in Italy, 21% of women use contraceptive pills, 6% have an IUD, 21% use barrier methods and 30% use coitus interruptus, but a minority of 4% relies on the only Rome-approved method of periodic abstinence[10].

Finally, Spain uses the pill in 12% of women, the IUD in 8% and appears to take great risks with 16% of women using no contraception at all[5]. These figures have been collected from a limited number of questionnaires carried out between 1988 and 1995 and are only intended as indicative figures[5,11].

THE IUD TODAY

The medical profession should realize that intrauterine contraception is important for the developed world, and even more for developing countries because of the limited involvement of the recipient and the low cost. It is a long lasting – 5–10 years – method[12,13] with a good contraceptive performance. It requires not more than a few minutes for insertion, which can be performed at interval or immediately after an abortion, a vaginal delivery[14] or a Cesarean section[15,16]. Follow-up visits are desirable to detect an expulsion, but are not an absolute requirement for demographic control[17]. The IUD requires no coitus-related action and does not jeopardize women's health, providing the well-established contraindications are observed[18].

The long-claimed relation between the use of IUDs and pelvic inflammatory disease (PID) has since been disclaimed[19,20]. Only exposure to sexually transmitted diseases increases the risk for both IUD-users and non-users.

A feeble risk of infection occurs at insertion, and shows within approximately 20 days after the procedure. An aseptic technique should be used, and the vagina and cervix must be cleansed and swabbed before attempting the insertion[21]. Prophylactic administration of antibiotics has not influenced the rare occurrence of a PID after insertion[22]. In long-term users of copper IUDs, reversibility of the contraceptive effect after removal of the device was proven to be complete[23]. These findings imply that nulliparity cannot any longer be quoted as a contraindication[20].

Recently, the side-effects have been successfully decreased[24]. The norgestrel IUD (Figure 1) is as reliable or better than the pill for contraception, and reduces the duration of the menses and the quantity of blood loss[25–27].

Smaller, atraumatic and more flexible IUDs, such as the Cu-Safe 300®, make the push-in insertion extremely simple and devoid of pain. Its user-friendly qualities make this device suitable for many nulligravidas[28].

The GyneFix®, finally, has completely done away with any form of skeleton, which avoids incompatibility and, hence, reaction between the cavum uteri and the device. The fixation mechanism, a tiny knot tied in the supporting thread, is easily implanted into the myometrium at insertion and accounts for the extremely low expulsion figure[29,30]. Knowing that many accidental pregnancies occur in IUD users after an unnoticed expulsion, the contraceptive efficacy of the GyneFix® is high, and the atraumatic frameless design reduces the requests for removal because of bleeding and pain. The design also allows a thin applicator to be used, which is an advantage in the presence of a nulliparous cervix.

CONCLUSION

It is due time for the medical profession to realize that contraception does not equal oral contraception. The correctly inserted IUD in correctly evaluated recipients has come of age, has eliminated a great deal of its previous disadvantages, has received a clean bill of health[20] and offers an economically and medically justified choice.

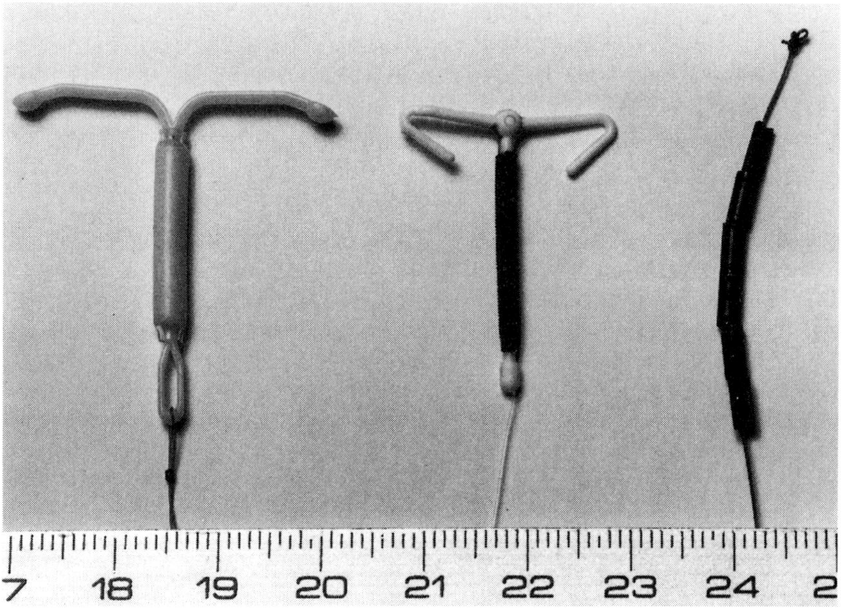

Figure 1 The levonorgestrel IUD (left) has a clearly visible silastic hormone reservoir on the vertical stem. The small, thin and flexible Cu-Safe 300 (center) has curved horizontal arms to minimize uterine trauma and the GyneFix (right) needs only a surgical monofilament thread as a support for the copper collars: the fixation knot can be seen at the upper end

REFERENCES

1. World Health Organization. Venous thromboembolic disease and combined oral contraceptives: results of international multicentre case–control study. *Lancet* 1995; 346: 1575–82
2. Vessey MP, Doll R. Investigation of relation between use of oral contraceptives and thromboembolic disease. *Br Med J* 1968; 2: 199–205
3. Inman WHW, Vessey MP. Investigation of deaths from pulmonary, coronary and cerebral thrombosis in women of childbearing age. *Br Med J* 1968; 2: 193–9
4. Shah IH. The advance of the contraceptive revolution. *World Health Stat Q* 1994; 47: 9–15
5. Oddens B. Contraceptive use in developed countries. In Senanayake P, ed. *The Reproductive Revolution.* New York and London: Parthenon Publishing, 1994: 39–55
6. Farmer RDT, Preston TD. The risk of venous thromboembolism associated with low oestrogen oral contraceptives. *J Obstet Gynaecol* 1995; 15: 195–200
7. Potts M. Benefits and risks of oral contraception. In Halbe HW, Rekers H, eds. *Oral Contraception into the 1990s.* Carnforth, UK: Parthenon Publishing, 1989: 11–20

8. Thiery M, Van Kets H, Van Der Pas H, *et al.* The Dimélys IUD. *Adv Contracept* 1987; 3: 43–7
9. Skjeldestad FE. Choice of contraceptive modality by women in Norway. *Acta Obstet Gynaecol Scand* 1994; 72: 48–52
10. Spinelli A, Grandolfo M, Donati S, *et al.* Family Planning in Italy. *Adv Contracept* 1993; 9: 153–60
11. Senanayake P, Potts M. *An Atlas of Contraception*. New York and London: Parthenon Publishing, 1994; 51
12. Sivin I. Should intrauterine devices be replaced before eight years? *Br J Fam Plann* 1992; 18: 9–11
13. Diaz J, Bahamondes L, Diaz M, *et al.* Evaluation of the performance of the Copper TCu380A IUD up to ten years. Is this IUD a reversible but potentially permanent method? *Adv Contracept* 1992; 8: 275–80
14. Xu JX, Reusche C, Burdan A. Immediate postplacental insertion of the intrauterine device: a review of Chinese and the World's experiences. *Adv Contracept* 1994; 10: 71–82
15. Van Kets H, Thiery M, Van Der Pas H. IUD insertion during cesarean section. *Adv Contracept* 1985; 1; 337—40
16. Chi IC, Farr G. Postpartum IUD contraception – a review of an international experience. *Adv Contracept* 1989; 5: 127–46
17. Janowitz B, Hubacher D, Petrick T, *et al.* Should the recommended number of IUD revisits be reduced? *Stud Fam Plann* 1994; 25: 362–7
18. Rivera R, Chi IC, Farr G. The intrauterine device in the present and future. *Curr Opin Obstet Gynecol* 1993; 5: 829–32
19. Ory HW. Ectopic pregnancy and intrauterine devices: new perspectives. *Obstet Gynecol* 1981; 57: 137–44
20. Chi IC. A bill of health for the IUD: where do we go from here? *Adv Contracept* 1994; 10: 121–31
21. Andolsek L. Round table discussion – intrauterine contraception. *Eur J Obstet Gynecol Reprod Biol* 1994; 55: 57–9
22. Sinei SKA, Schulz KF, Lamptey DA, *et al.* Preventing IUD-related pelvic infection: the efficacy of prophylactic doxycycline at IUD insertion. *Br J Obstet Gynaecol* 1990; 97: 412–19
23. Van Kets H, Thiery M, Van Der Pas H, *et al.* Long-term experience with Multiload intrauterine devices. *Adv Contracept* 1989; 5: 179–88
24. Bromham DR. New developments with IUDs: devices, patients and their management. *Br J Fam Plann* 1991; 15 (Suppl): 34–41
25. Chi IC, Farr G. The non-contraceptive effects of the levonorgestrel-releasing intrauterine device. *Adv Contracept* 1994; 10: 271–85
26. Luukkainen T. The levonorgestrel-releasing IUD. *Br J Fam Plann* 1993; 19: 221–4
27. Andersson K, Odlind V, Rybo G. Levonorgestrel-releasing and copper-releasing IUDs during five years of use. *Contraception* 1994; 49: 56–72
28. Van Kets H, Van Der Pas H, Delbarge W, *et al.* A randomized comparative study of the TCu380A and Cu Safe 300 IUD. *Adv Contracept* 1995; 11: 123–9
29. Van Kets H, Wildemeersch D, Van Der Pas, *et al.* IUD expulsion solved with implant technology. *Contraception* 1995; 51: 87–92
30. Van Kets H, Vrijens M, Van Trappen Y, *et al.* The frameless GyneFix intrauterine implant: a major improvement in efficacy, expulsion and tolerance. *Adv Contracept* 1995; 11: 131–42

3 Mechanism of action of intrauterine devices

B. Rojnik

INTRODUCTION

The majority of intrauterine device (IUD) research published in the last few decades deals primarily with the clinical performance of IUDs, while the mechanism of action of IUDs has received much less attention. Extensive data sets on the safety and efficacy of IUDs have enabled them to become the most widely used reversible method of contraception worldwide with approximately 100 million users at the dawn of the third millennium. However, understanding the mechanisms of action of the IUD remains a source of much controversy. This is mainly for two reasons: the difficulty of conducting definitive research in this area, and the sensitivity of this question to both users and the population at large.

MODE OF ACTION OF IUDs

The belief that IUDs are abortifacients is still a matter of major concern in Catholic countries and remains a barrier to their use in these settings. Recent research, however, no longer supports the idea that IUDs exert their primary action through impairing implantation or destroying embryos. In the 1980s, new aspects of IUD contraceptive action were identified[1–5] indicating their non-abortive nature.

A thorough literature review on the mode of action of IUDs reveals that, in animals, IUDs exert their contraceptive effect through different mechanisms which vary from one species to another[6]. Thus, a variety of synergistic mechanisms probably accounts for the contraceptive effect in a single species, including humans.

Current copper- and hormone-releasing IUDs exert a range of actions that prevent pregnancy in women far before implantation takes place[3]. It remains unclear, though, to what extent a single mode of action contributes to the anti-fertility effect, overall[6]. IUDs alter the reproductive process by affecting the endometrium, Fallopian tubes and cervical mucus. By interfering with sperm motility and survival[1], IUDs prevent fertilization. Also, many fewer ova were detected in IUD users compared to non-users, implying several possibilities about its effect on ovum transport[2,4].

All IUDs – be they inert, copper- or hormone-releasing – stimulate a foreign-body reaction in the endometrium. Cellular and humoral components of the local inflammatory reaction disturb the functioning of the endometrium and myometrium, changing the microenviroment of the uterine cavity and, eventually, that of the oviduct and cervix. Increased numbers of leukocytes affect sperm through phagocytosis. Degraded products spread by reflux from the uterine cavity to the tubes and the cervix[6], thus affecting different steps of the reproductive process. Medicated devices seem to exert the most profound effects.

In studies searching for spermatozoa in different segments of genital tract, authors reported decreased numbers or absence of spermatozoa in IUD users[2]. Because copper is spermicidal and cytotoxic, it adds to the inhibition of sperm migration[7]. Sperm tail-head separation has also been observed in copper IUD users[2], which affects the fertilizing capacity of sperm. Nevertheless, the fertilizing capacity of spermatozoa in IUD users has not fully been determined[3].

Steroid-releasing IUDs have several modes of action[8]. Levonorgestrel-releasing IUDs provoke specific morphological changes in the endometrium. Endometrial glands become atrophic, the epithelial cells grow inactive and the stroma is decidualized[9]. Levonorgestrel blocks estrogen and progesterone receptors; this effect is dose-dependent. The currently available levonorgestrel (LNg) 20 μg IUD affects ovarian function in a variety of ways[10]. However, systematic interference of ovarian function seems to be less common with long-term use of this device, as, after the first year of LNg 20 μg IUD use, most cycles are ovulatory[11]. Steroid-releasing IUDs also profoundly inhibit sperm transport by reducing the penetrability of mucus to sperm.

In 1987, a World Health Organization scientific group addressed whether or not the fertilized ovum in IUD users reaches the endometrial cavity at the same rate as in non-users[3]. If preventing implantation was the main mode of contraceptive action, then embryos would develop normally before they enter the uterine cavity and would enter the uterus at a frequency comparable to that observed in non-IUD users[4]. Studies were undertaken to search for ova in different parts of the genital tract. In a study of surgical sterilization patients, authors found no ova in the uterine cavities of IUD users, and significantly fewer eggs were recovered from the Fallopian tubes of IUD users compared to non-users. Thirty-nine per cent of 56 women with an IUD had eggs compared to 56% of 115 women using no contraception; the difference was most profound in copper IUD users[4]. As no ova were recovered from the uterus of any of the IUD users, contraceptive action was assumed to have occured before the ovum reached the uterus. In addition, no ova showed normal preimplantation development, and normally developed embryos (or eggs) reached the uterus at far lower rates. This finding supports the belief that the principal mode of action of IUDs is by a means other than the destruction of embryos[4]. The reduced probability of fertilization along the way to the uterine cavity indicates that IUDs interfere with steps of the reproductive process that normally take place outside the uterus. This probably can be attributed to the facts that: spermatozoa do not reach the site of fertilization; if they do arrive, they are not able to penetrate the oocyte, and/or oocytes are damaged by an adverse tubal environment[4].

Another piece of evidence demonstrating the extrauterine mode of action of the IUD is the lower levels of detection of β-human chorionic gonadotropin (hCG) in IUD users compared to non-users. Numerous studies have measured the levels of β-hCG among IUD users to determine whether implantation routinely occurs in the presence of an IUD[12]. Findings have been conflicting owing to sensitivity and specificity problems with the available kits. In a study using a more valid assay, a single episode of β-hCG elevation was detected among 107 cycles in 39 IUD users which is clearly less than would be expected if the IUD had no effect before implantation[12].

Apart from clinical and experimental studies mentioned above, further evidence to support the non-abortive nature of IUDs comes indirectly from epidemiological studies of ectopic pregnancies. Ectopic pregnancies implant before the blastocyst reaches the uterus, so if the IUD was an abortifacient, acting only through the prevention of implantation, the rate of ectopic pregnancies expected would be at least as high as in non-contraceptors[13]. This is not the case with modern IUDs (inert, copper and high dose progestin devices); much lower ectopic pregnancy rates are reported in IUD users compared to non-users[14–17]. The differences in ectopic pregnancy rates with medicated devices vary with the copper surface area or with the daily hormonal release[16]. Copper IUDs have much lower proportions of pregnancies that are ectopic compared to LNg 20 μg IUDs; the ectopic pregnancy ratios calculated from randomized IUD trials was 39 vs. 250 per 1000 pregnancies respectively[16]. The extremely low pregnancy rates associated with medicated devices correlate with their low rates of ectopic pregnancies. The ectopic pregnancy rate of the LNg 20 μg IUD is 0.2 per 1000 women years vs. 0.5 per 1000 with copper devices[16]. The above findings indicate that by preventing fertilization, IUDs protect women not only against ectopic pregnancies, but also against infertility associated with ectopic pregnancies. This is in contrast with the previous opinion that IUDs present a risk factor for ectopic pregnancies.

Because IUDs have a certain contraceptive failure rate, fertilization and implantation may occur with an IUD *in situ*. Implantation is rare, though, and prevention of implantation may be considered as a redundant back-up mechanism to support the major contraceptive modes of action of IUDs[18].

IUDs are not officially approved for postcoital contraception although they are effective as emergency contraception when inserted within 5 days of unprotected intercourse. The mode of action with postcoital insertion remains unclear, yet preventing implantation may in this case be more likely. The use of IUDs as emergency contraception should be reserved for couples who accept the possibility that, in such cases, an IUD may interrupt implantation. Still, it should be emphasized that this mechanism alone is not regarded to intervene as the main mode of action in long-term IUD users. This is of great importance, as postcoital IUD insertion is of greater benefit for women who consider continuing the use of an IUD for long-term contraception.

CONCLUSIONS

Getting closer to understanding the mechanism of action of IUDs goes beyond the purely scientific question. According to recent research, it is now believed that the high contraceptive efficacy in IUD users results from a combination of actions prior to fertilization. Therefore, IUDs are not deemed abortifacients. This notion will hopefully make IUDs an acceptable and viable solution for many women who previously believed otherwise. Identification of additional mechanisms of action of IUDs will continue. Clearly understanding the mode of action may lead to an improvement in IUD design that may help alleviate the most common side-effects with IUDs and further improve IUD continuation rates.

REFERENCES

1. Aref I, Kandil A, El Tagi A, *et al.* Effects of non-medicated and copper IUDs on sperm migration. *Contracept Deliv Syst* 1983; 4: 203–6
2. Ortiz ME, Croxatto MB. The mode of action of IUDs. *Contraception* 1987; 36 (1): 37–53
3. World Health Organization. 1987. *Mechanism of Action, Safety, and Efficacy of Intrauterine Devices.* Technical Report Series 753. Geneva: WHO, 1987
4. Alvarez F, Brache V, Fernandez E, *et al.* New insights on the mode of action of intrauterine contraceptive devices in women. *Fertil Steril* 1988; 49 (5): 768–73
5. Sivin I. IUDs are contraceptives, not abortifacients: a comment on research and belief. *Stud Fam Plann* 1989; 20 (6): 355–9
6. Croxatto MB, Ortiz ME, Valdez E. IUD mechanisms of action. In Bardin CW, Mishell DR, Newton MA, eds. *Proceedings from the Fourth International Conference on IUDs.* Boston: Butterworth-Heinemann, 1994; 44–59
7. Middleton JC, Kennedy M. The biological action of endouterine copper. *Contraception* 1975; 11: 209–25
8. Barbosa I, Bakos O, Olsson SE, *et al.* Ovarian function during use of a levonorgestrel-releasing IUD. *Contraception* 1990; 42: 51–66
9. Silverberg SG, Haukkamaa M, Arko H, *et al.* Endometrial morphology during long-term use of levonorgestrel-releasing intrauterine devices. *Int J Gynecol Pathol* 1986; 5: 235–41
10. Luukkainen T, Toivonen J. Levonorgestrel-releasing IUD as a method of contraception with therapeutic properties. *Contraception* 1995; 52: 269–76
11. Nilson CG, Luukkainen T, Arko H. Endometrial morphology of women using a d-norgestrel-releasing intrauterine device. *Fertil Steril* 1978; 29: 397–401
12. Wilcox AJ, Weinberg CR, Armstrong GE, *et al.* Urinary human chorionic gonadotropin among intrauterine device users: detection with a highly specific and sensitive assay. *Fertil Steril* 1987; 47: 265–9

13. Sivin I, Greenslade F, Schmidt F, *et al. The Copper T 380 Intrauterine Device. A Summary of Scientific Data.* New York: The Population Council, 1992
14. Ory, HW and The Woman's Health Study. Ectopic pregnancy and intrauterine devices. *Obstet Gynecol* 1981; 57:137–43
15. Gray RH. A case–control study of ectopic pregnancy in developed and developing countries. In Sciarra JJ, ed. *Intrauterine Contraception: Advances and Future Prospects.* Philadelphia: Harper & Row, 1985; 354–64
16. Sivin I. Dose- and age-dependent ectopic pregnancy risk with intrauterine contraception. *Obstet Gynecol* 1991; 78: 291– 8
17. Sivin I. Extrauterine pregnancies and intrauterine devices reassessed. In Bardin CW, Mishell DR, Newton MA, eds. *Proceedings from the Fourth International Conference on IUDs.* Boston: Butterworth-Heinemann, 1994; 195–209
18. Guillebaud J. *Contraception: Your Questions Answered.* London: Churchill Livingstone, 1993

14 Pelvic inflammatory disease in intrauterine device users

R.J.C.M. Beerthuizen

HISTORICAL REVIEW

Pelvic inflammatory disease (PID) has been associated with the use of intrauterine devices (IUDs) ever since they were introduced as a method for contraception in women. In the beginning of this century the transcervical intrauterine device – known as Sterilett – made from several metals such as gold and silver, was used as a contraceptive device. The stem of the device was situated in the cervical canal. On the cervical side there was a kind of button present. The device was kept in place by two divergent ends causing local pressure on the endometrium. The continuous pressure on the uterine wall caused local atrophy and ulcerations, leading to serious complications such as pelvic infections, sepsis and death[1–4]. To avoid the pressure of the diverging arms, Pust developed an intrauterine ring made from silk, and connected through a silk tail with an extracervical button made from Jena glass[5]. After the experience in one of their patients that the extracervical button had no function at all for contraceptive efficacy, intrauterine rings without a tail were developed by Gräfenberg in Germany[6] and Ota in Japan[7]. In experienced hands the side-effects were acceptable in carefully selected patients. However, after publications of serious side-effects with the use of rings[8], Gräfenberg was banished from his country and emigrated to New York.

During a period of nearly 30 years, hardly any attention was paid in the literature to intrauterine contraception. However, some clinicians continued using intrauterine rings in carefully selected patients. Favorable results with the Gräfenberg ring[9] as well as with the Ota ring[10] were published in 1959. In order to find out scientifically the value of intrauterine contraception, the Population Council initiated the first international conference on intrauterine devices in 1962 in New York[11]. The method turned out to be safe and effective with minor side-effects. During this conference devices made from polyethylene were introduced, and worldwide family planning programs were started afterwards. The continuous improvement of the devices as well as the favorable efficacy and acceptability led to a continuous increase in the use of the devices worldwide.

Serious problems associated with the use of the Dalkon Shield during the 1970s[12–14] caused worldwide concern about the safety of all devices. Following this concern the World Health Organization (WHO) convened a scientific group on the mechanisms of action, safety and efficacy of intrauterine devices in December 1986[15]. One of the most important conclusions in this report was that the risk of PID related to IUD use has been exaggerated due to persistent epidemiologic biases in published reports. Current IUDs provide safe, highly effective contraception at a low cost.

EPIDEMIOLOGY

Pelvic inflammatory disease (PID) is a broad diagnosis including endocervicitis, endometritis, pelvic peritonitis and pelvic abscess[16]. This broad diagnosis causes problems interpreting the different studies in relation to intrauterine device use.

Most of the studies concerning the relationship between PID and the use of IUDs are retrospective hospital-based case–control studies. In those studies the incidence of PID was suggested to be as high as three- to ninefold in IUD users compared to non-users[17,18]. Those studies might be susceptible to one or more of the following methodological flaws: (1) selectivity in obtaining IUD-use history in PID cases; (2) over-diagnosis of PID in IUD users; (3) over-referral of IUD users having PID to tertiary hospitals; (4) use of inadequate comparison (control) groups, consisting of users of the oral pill and barrier methods (both methods have some protective effects against PID); (5) failure to separate potentially confusing variables, especially the woman's sexual behavior, in their analyses[19].

Later epidemiological prospective studies showed a considerably lower risk of PID when comparing different types of contraception. Compared to non-contraceptive users, the relative risk ranged from 1.8 in patients with copper-containing IUDs to 3.3 in patients using the older inert IUDs like the Dalkon Shield[20]. Recently, comparison of the case–control and cohort studies used to indict the Dalkon Shield, with the findings of the Dalkon Shield clinical trials, offered convincing evidence that the case–control and cohort studies show methodological biases as mentioned above. The 71 clinical trials show that when the Dalkon Shield was inserted by an experienced clinician, it proved to be a safe and effective contraceptive method comparable with other IUDs used at the time. No evidence of an increased risk of PID was found in these clinical trials[21]. A re-analysis of the copper 7 intrauterine contraceptive device clinical trial and the incidence of PID showed annualized rates of PID between 1 and 2%, similar to the PID rates reported for fecund, sexually active women. Life-table PID rates were not different between nulliparous and parous women[22]. In a review of 35 clinical studies from 13 countries, including substantial numbers of nulliparous women using copper IUDs, PID rates in nulliparae did not indicate a risk of PID that was substantially different from that in parous women. A higher PID rate in younger women, regardless of parity, correlated with the age-related STD rates[23].

THE ROLE OF CURRENT IUD USE IN THE PATHOGENESIS OF PID

In over 50% of PID cases *Chlamydia trachomatis* and *Neisseria gonorrhoeae* are involved as causative pathogen. In one of the few prospective trials of laparoscopically proven PID, *C. trachomatis* was found to be the most important etiological agent in 43% of all cases, *N. gonorrhoeae* in 17% and *Mycoplasma hominis* in 13 % of cases[24]. A large prospective study including patients diagnosed with acute PID demonstrated the presence of sexually transmitted disease (STD) organisms in 65% and of non-STD organisms in 30% of cases. Current IUD use was negatively associated with STD pelvic inflammatory disease (odds ratio 0.26; 95% CI 0.09–0.77) and positively associated with non-STD pelvic inflammatory disease (odds ratio 3.87; 95% CI 1.30–11.53). The role of current IUD use in the pathogenesis of non-STD-related PID remains unclear, and continuing research on this topic is important[25]. The negative association of current IUD use and STD-related PID could possibly be the consequence of excluding subjects at risk for STD as candidates for intrauterine contraceptive devices.

FOREIGN-BODY REACTION

The introduction of an intrauterine device produces an effect on the endometrium. In the areas of the endometrium immediately underlying the device compression, edema, vascular distension and mononuclear leukocytic infiltration are consistent findings[26]. The response of the endometrial tissue to the device is similar to a foreign-body reaction in other tissues[27,28].

In the oviducts of IUD users inflammatory changes have been found, similar to those found in the endometrium in patients using inert IUDs and in patients fitted with a copper-containing IUD[29–31]. No changes have been found in the oviducts in Progestasert users, suggesting an influence of the progesterone on the foreign-body reaction[32]. In all but one of these studies microbiological investigations have been performed. No correlation was discovered between the micro-organisms found in some specimens and the morphological changes in the oviducts.

DEVICES WITH OR WITHOUT TAIL

After reports in the 1970s of septic abortions and maternal deaths associated with an intrauterine device *in situ* during pregnancy, especially with the Dalkon Shield[12], the possibility of a causal relationship between the structure of the tail of the IUD and pelvic sepsis was considered. The tails or appendages of the five IUDs used at that time – Lippes Loop, Saf-T-Coil, Dalkon Shield, Copper 7 and Copper T – were examined visually and with a scanning electron microscope. The tails in each of the devices except the Dalkon Shield consisted of either a single or a double segment of monofilament plastic thread. The tails of the

Dalkon Shield however consisted of a bundle of monofilaments enclosed freely within a thin plastic sheath. The structure of these tails suggested that they might function as wicks in ascending infections, especially in case of pregnancy. In *in vitro* studies it was shown that bacteria could indeed grow within the sheath and in the spaces between the filaments[33].

Clinical studies however show conflicting results in pelvic inflammatory disease rates between women wearing devices with or without tails. Most of the studies comparing IUDs with and without tails noted no differences in PID rates[34] even in laparoscopically verified diagnosis of PID[35]. In two recent randomized studies, however, again conflicting results were found. No difference in PID rates was found after a 12-month follow-up in 1265 women randomly allocated to either a TCu-200 IUD with or without marker strings[36]. Women inserted with either the Nova-T or TCu-200 Ag without tails had a lower ($p = 0.07$) 5-year gross cumulative termination rate for infection (1.3 per 100 users) than those inserted with tailed IUDs (3.7 per 100 users)[37]. As the overall PID rates in IUD users are very low, a greater number of patients is needed to reach statistically significantly data.

THE IMPORTANCE OF CAREFUL INSERTION

Recently the results of data collection from twelve randomized and one non-randomized study have been published to evaluate the risk of PID in IUD users. These studies were carried out under the auspices of the World Health Organization (WHO) and involved a total number of 22 908 insertions and 51 399 years of follow-up.

Pelvic inflammatory disease risk is substantially higher in the first 20 days after insertion, with an incidence rate of 9.66 per 1000 woman-years, than at all other times, when the incidence rate was 1.38 per 1000 woman-years. The rate of PID was lowest in recent insertions, most likely attributable to more appropriate selection of women for IUD insertion, with increasing awareness of STD risk as a contraindication to IUD use. The PID incidence rate after 20 days is similar to the incidence rate found in the general population[38]. The higher incidence during the first 20 days after insertion is the result of brief, transient microbiological contamination of the uterine cavity following IUD insertion[39].

As the insertion *per se* provides a risk for infection, efforts have been made to produce an antiseptic-releasing IUD. However, no differences in bacteriological contamination of the uterine cavity were found between the bacteriological results of two groups with medicated IUDs (coated with chlorhexidine acetate) and non-medicated devices[40].

The prophylactic use of antibiotics at the time of IUD insertion did not reduce the risk of PID significantly. In three randomized studies, 200 mg of either doxycycline or placebo was given 1 h prior to insertion. The difference in the 3-month PID rates between the doxycycline and the placebo group was not statistically significant in any of these studies[41–43]. For women with cervical gonorrheae benefit appeared evident, but given the small incidence of cervical gonorrheae in the study group, statistical significance could not be reached. No benefit at all was found in women with cervical *C. trachomatis* infection[41]. This difference could be the consequence of the different rates of growth of *N. gonorrhoeae* and *C. trachomatis*, as the gonococcus replicates in a matter of hours, compared with several days for *C. trachomatis*[44]. For that reason the prophylactic antibiotic in the study of Walsh and colleagues was changed to a 500 mg dose of azithromycin with a serum half-life of 68 h, nearly three times that of doxycycline with a serum half-life of 24 h[43]. Results of this latter study have not yet been published.

In a population or region at high risk for STD and with good access to public health services (as is the case in most developed countries) a screening for organisms like *C. trachomatis* and *N. gonorrhoeae* should be considered in women seeking IUDs and, if positive, treated adequately before insertion of the IUD[45].

To reduce the infection risk at the time of insertion it is of the utmost importance to insert the IUD after cleansing the cervix and the cervical canal with an appropriate antiseptic compound like povidone–iodine or chlorhexidine. The latter compound is active against yeasts (*Candida albicans*), a range of viruses and protozoal species (*Trichomonas vaginalis*)[46].

ACTINOMYCES AND IUD USE

Since the first case report of severe pelvic actinomycosis related to the use of an intrauterine device[2], over 300 cases have been reported in the world literature[47]. New case reports are still being published[48].

Pelvic actinomycosis remains a rare condition and is described mostly in relation to long-term use of inert IUDs. Actinomyces is a common saprophyte of the oropharynx and the intestinal tract and is under normal circumstances incapable of penetrating intact anatomical barriers. Trauma has been shown to be a predisposing factor in the development of infection caused by Actinomyces. Infection is dependent on synergistic facultative anaerobic bacteria. *In vitro* cultures of Actinomyces show an inhibiting zone around copper IUDs.

Actinomyces-like organisms (ALOs) diagnosed in Pap smears are a more frequent entity. No difference was found in the prevalence of ALO-positive cervical smears between copper and inert IUD users. Patients with ALO-positive smears are asymptomatic and after removal of the IUD all Pap smears return to normal within 3 months without additional treatment. The presence of ALO on smears was not a clinically significant finding in the asymptomatic patient, and as such was of limited importance[49].

THE LEVONORGESTREL-RELEASING DEVICE

The levonorgestrel-releasing intrauterine device has proven to be a highly effective contraceptive method that combines the advantages of both hormonal and intrauterine contraception[50]. In order to evaluate the risk of PID with use of levonorgestrel-releasing IUDs and copper-releasing IUDs, a multicenter randomized comparative trial was carried out in five European countries. Altogether, 1821 women had the levonorgestrel IUD and 937 women had the copper Nova T IUD inserted. During the first year of study there was the same low rate of infection with both devices[51]. After 3 years of use, the gross cumulative rate of PID in levonorgestrel IUD users was as low as 0.5 and significantly lower than that of 2.0 associated with the Nova T[52]. After 5 years of use the gross cumulative removal rates for PID were 2.2 in the Nova T and 0.8 in the levonorgestrel IUD group ($p < 0.05$). The lower infection rate was most marked in the age group of 17–25 years, where the gross cumulative PID rate was 5.6 for the users of copper IUDs and 0.3 for the users of levonorgestrel IUDs ($p < 0.01$)[53]. Thickening of cervical mucus and reduced bleeding may be the protective mechanisms against PID during the use of the latter device.

THE FRAMELESS INTRAUTERINE IMPLANT SYSTEM

Another remarkable new intrauterine copper-releasing contraceptive is the frameless GyneFix® implant system. An ongoing, multicenter randomized comparative WHO study, conducted in over 4000 women, compared the frameless device with the Standard TCu380A. The 3-year data reported only one woman with PID with the frameless device and nine with the TCu380A[54]. In another 3-year, international, multicenter study conducted by the International Study Group on Intrauterine Drug Delivery at the University of Ghent, Belgium, involving 1039 women (including a large proportion (26%) of nulligravid/nulliparous women at low risk for STDs), not one case of PID was registered[55]. The virtual absence of PID in both these studies confirms the importance of behavioral factors in the occurrence of PID. The optimal design characteristics and the fact that the device is completely contained in the inserter at the moment of insertion may contribute to the low risk of PID with the frameless device.

CONCLUSIONS

Pelvic inflammatory disease among IUD users is related to the insertion process and to the background risk of sexually transmitted disease.

Women most at risk of developing sexually transmitted diseases are those below the age of 25 years with multiple sexual partners regardless of parity. If other forms of contraception are contraindicated in this high-risk group the additional use of barrier methods should be strongly advised if the contraceptive method of choice is the IUD.

Careful screening before insertion is of utmost importance. The device can only be inserted after adequate desinfection of the cervix and the cervical canal.

Replacement of devices must be limited. If the IUD user is doing well with her device, prolonged use beyond the recommended replacement interval could be considered[56].

REFERENCES

1. Reist A. Die gefahren der zur Konzeptionsverhütung intrauterin eingeführten sogenannten Sterilette oder Obturatoren, sowie des Fructuletts von Nassauer. *Schweiz Med Wschr* 1925; 5: 650–7
2. Draper JW, Studdiford WE. Report of a case of actinomycosis of the tubes and ovaries. *Am J Obstet Gynecol* 1926; 11: 603–8
3. Tietze K. Sieben Fälle schwerster Schädigung durch Intrauterinpessare. (Ein Fall von isolierter Genitalaktinomykose). *Dtsch Med Wochenschr* 1930; 56 (II): 1307–9
4. Jones HO. The cervical pessary – a menace to health and life. *J Am Med Assoc* 1932; 98: 1738
5. Pust. Ein brauchbarer Frauenschutz. *Dtsch Med Wochenschr* 1923; 29: 952–3
6. Tatum HJ. Intrauterine contraception. *Am J Obstet Gynecol* 1972; 112: 1000–23
7. Ota T. A study on the birth control with an intrauterine instrument. *Jpn J Obstet Gynecol* 1934; 17: 210–14
8. Sommer K. Konzeptionsverhütung durch Graefenbergring. *Zbl Gynaek* 1931; 55: 2547–9
9. Oppenheimer W. Prevention of pregnancy by the Graefenberg ring method. *Am J Obstet Gynecol* 1959; 78: 446–54
10. Ishihama A. Clinical studies on intrauterine rings, especially the present state of contraception in Japan and the experiences in the use of intrauterine rings. *Yokohama Med Bull* 1959; 10: 89–105
11. Tietze C, Lewit S, eds. *Proceedings of the Conference of Intra-Uterine Contraceptive Devices*, New York, April/May, 1962. Amsterdam: Excerpta Medica, 1962; International Congress Series No 54
12. Christian CD. Maternal deaths associated with an intrauterine device. *Am J Obstet Gynecol* 1974; 119: 441–4
13. Cates W, Ory HW, Rochat RW, *et al.* The intrauterine device and deaths from spontaneous abortion. *N Engl J Med* 1976; 295: 1155–9
14. Kahn HS, Tyler CW. An association between the Dalkon Shield and complicated pregnancies among women hospitalized for intrauterine contraception device-related disorders. *Am J Obstet Gynecol* 1976; 125: 83–6
15. World Health Organization. *Mechanism of Action, Safety, and Efficacy of Intrauterine Devices*. Technical Report Series 753. Geneva: WHO, 1987
16. Moors A, Thomas EJ. Pelvic inflammatory disease. *Adv Obstet Gynaecol* 1994; 9: 11–16
17. Westrom L, Bengtsson LP, Mardh P. The risk of pelvic inflammatory disease in women using intrauterine contraceptive devices as compared to non-users. *Lancet* 1976; 2: 221–4
18. Targum SD, Wright NH. Association of the intrauterine device and pelvic inflammatory disease: a retrospective pilot study. *Am J Epidemiol* 1974; 100: 262–71
19. Rivera R, Chi I, Farr G. The intrauterine device in the present and future. *Curr Opin Obstet Gynecol* 1993; 5: 829–32

20. Buchan H, Villard-Mackintosh L, Vessey M, *et al.* Epidemiology of pelvic inflammatory disease in parous women with special reference to the intrauterine device. *Br J Obstet Gynaecol* 1990; 97: 780–8
21. Mumford SD, Kessel E. Was the Dalkon Shield a safe and effective intrauterine device? The conflict between case–control and clinical trial study findings. *Fertil Steril* 1992; 57: 1151–76
22. Roy S, Azen C. A reanalysis of the Cu-7 intrauterine contraceptive device clinical trial and the incidence of pelvic inflammatory disease: a paradigm for assessing intrauterine contraceptive device safety. *Am J Obstet Gynecol* 1994; 170: 1606–16
23. Struthers BJ. Comparison of PID rates in parous and nulliparous women using copper IUDs. Summary of clinical studies. *Adv Contracept* 1990; 6: 257
24. Stacey CM, Munday PE, Taylor-Robinson D, *et al.* A longitudinal study of pelvic inflammatory disease. *Br J Obstet Gynaecol* 1992; 99: 994–9
25. Jossens MOR, Schachter RNJ, Sweet RL. Risk factors associated with pelvic inflammatory disease of differing microbial etiologies. *Obstet Gynecol* 1994; 83: 989–97
26. Morese KN, Peterson WF, Allen ST. Endometrial effects of an intrauterine contraceptive device. *Obstet Gynecol* 1966; 28: 323–8
27. Moyer DL, Mishell DR, Bell J. Reactions of human endometrium to the intrauterine device. *Am J Obstet Gynecol* 1970; 106: 799–806
28. Moyer DL, Mishell DR. Reactions of human endometrium to the intrauterine foreign body. II: Long-term effects on the endometrial histology and cytology. *Am J Obstet Gynecol* 1971; 111: 66–80
29. Beerthuizen RJCM, Van Wijck JAM, Eskes TKAB, *et al.* IUD and salpingitis: a prospective study of pathomorphological changes in the oviducts in IUD-users. *Eur J Obstet Gynecol Reprod Biol* 1982; 13: 31–41
30. Vanlancker M, Dierick AM, Thiery M, *et al.* Histologic and microbiologic findings in the Fallopian tubes of IUD users. *Adv Contracept* 1987; 3: 147–57
31. Wollen A, Sandvei R, Mork S, *et al.* *In situ* characterization of leukocytes in the Fallopian tube in women with or without an intrauterine contraceptive device. *Acta Obstet Gynecol Scand* 1994; 73: 103–12
32. Smith MR, Soderstrom B. Salpingitis: a frequent response to intrauterine contraception. *J Reprod Med* 1976; 16: 159–62
33. Tatum HJ, Schmidt FH, Phillips D, *et al.* The Dalkon Shield controversy, structural and bacteriological studies of IUD tails. *J Am Med Assoc* 1975; 231: 711–17
34. Treimau K, Liksin L. IUDs – a new look. Population Report 1988; Series B No 5, B1–32
35. Buchman MI. A study of the IUDs with or without an extracervical appendage or tail. *Fertil Steril* 1979; 21: 348–55
36. Potts DM, Champion CB, Kozuh-Novak M, *et al.* IUDs and PID: a comparative trial of strings versus stringless devices. *Adv Contracept* 1991; 7: 231–40
37. Batar I, Lampe LG, Allonen H. Clinical experience with intrauterine devices inserted with and without tail. *Int J Gynecol Obstet* 1991; 36: 137–40
38. Farley TMM, Rosenberg MJ, Rowe PJ, *et al.* Intrauterine devices and pelvic inflammatory disease: an international perspective. *Lancet* 1992; 339: 785–8
39. Mishell DR. The intrauterine device: a bacteriologic study of the endometrial cavity. *Am J Obstet Gynecol* 1966; 96: 119–26
40. Jackson R, Newton JR, Emens MJ, *et al.* Effects of chlorhexidine-coated intrauterine device on the bacteriology of the uterine cavity. *Adv Contracept* 1991; 7: 55–65

41. Sinei SKA, Schulz KF, Lamptey PR, *et al.* Preventing IUCD-related pelvic infection: the efficacy of prophylactic doxycycline at insertion. *Br J Obstet Gynaecol* 1990; 97: 412–19
42. Lapido OA, Farr G, Otolorin E, *et al.* Prevention of IUD-related pelvic infection: the efficacy of prophylactic doxycycline at IUD insertion. *Adv Contracept* 1991; 7: 43–54
43. Walsh TL, Bernstein GS, Grimes DA, *et al.* Effect of prophylactic antibiotics on morbidity associated with IUD insertion: results of a pilot randomized controlled trial. *Contraception* 1994; 50: 319–27
44. Thompson SE, Washington AE. Epidemiology of sexually transmitted *Chlamydia trachomatis* infections. *Epidemiol Rev* 1983; 5: 96–123
45. Sprague D, Bullough C, Rashid S, Roberts S. Screening for and treating *Chlamydia trachomatis* and *Neisseria gonorrhoeae* before contraceptive use and subsequent pelvic inflammatory disease. *Br J Fam Plann* 1990; 16: 54–8
46. Denton GW. Chlorhexidine: a WHO essential drug. *Lancet* 1984; 1: 517
47. Keebler C, Chatwani A, Schwartz R. Actinomycosis infection associated with intrauterine contraceptive devices. *Am J Obstet Gynecol* 1983; 145: 596–9
48. Blohmer JU, Hufnagl HU, Kürten A, Bollmann R. Die Intra-uterinpessar-assoziierte genitale Aktinomykose. *Fortsch Med* 1994; 112; 305–7
49. Singh MM, Ingham HR, Wadehra V, *et al.* Endometrial culture in IUD users with actinomyces-like organisms (ALOs) on cervical smears. *Br J Fam Plann* 1989; 15: 3–6
50. Luukkainen T, Toivonen J. Levonorgestrel-releasing IUD as a method of contraception with therapeutic properties. *Contraception* 1995; 52: 269–76
51. Luukkainen T, Allonen H, Haukkamaa M, *et al.* Effective contraception with the levonorgestrel-releasing intrauterine device. 12-month report of a European multicenter study. *Contraception* 1984; 30: 443–56
52. Toivonen J, Lukkainen T, Allonen H. Protective effective of intrauterine release of levonorgestrel on pelvic infection. Three years comparative experience of levonorgestrel- and copper-releasing intrauterine devices. *Obstet Gynecol* 1991; 77: 261–4
53. Andersson K, Odlind V, Rybo G. Levonorgestrel-releasing and copper-releasing (nova-T) IUDs during five years of use: a randomized comparative trial. *Contraception* 1994; 49: 56–72
54. UNDP, UNFPA and WHO Special Programme of Research, Development and Research Training in Human Reproduction. World Bank: IUD Research Group. The TCu380A and the frameless IUD 'The Flexigard®': interim three-year data from an international multicenter trial. *Contraception* 1995; 52: 77–83
55. Van Kets H, Vrijens M, Van Trappen Y, *et al.* The frameless GyneFix intrauterine implant: a major improvement in efficacy, expulsion and tolerance. *Adv Contracept* 1995; 11: 131–42
56. Toivonen J. Intrauterine contraceptive device and pelvic inflammatory disease. *Ann Med* 1993; 25: 171–3

This paper has been reproduced from *Eur J Contracept Reprod Health Care* 1996; 1: 237–43

5 The new generation of copper intrauterine devices

F. Martinez and P. Barri

INTRODUCTION

Modern high-load copper intrauterine devices (IUDs), i.e. TCu380A/Ag and Multiload 375 (MLCu375) provide high contraceptive efficacy with annual pregnancy rates lower than 1.0 for the best performing among them. Conversely, the use of IUDs is adversely influenced by relatively high expulsion rates or high discontinuation rates due to pain and/or bleeding.

To minimize these events, many attempts have been made over the past few decades, by researchers worldwide, to design IUDs which are better tolerated, with the aim of improving their acceptability and continuation of use. Three of the devices will be analyzed in more detail on the basis of results of recently conducted clinical trials with the respective IUDs. The Institut Dexeus collaborated in several of these research activities.

GYNEFIX® FRAMELESS INTRAUTERINE IMPLANT

The GyneFix® IUD is a remarkable newcomer because of its revolutionary design characteristics. The device was developed to minimize problems which frequently occur with conventional IUDs: displacement, expulsion, abnormal bleeding and pain complaints[1]. The rationale behind the development of the GyneFix was simple: owing to the great variation in size and shape of uterine cavities, aggravated by functional changes which occur during the menstrual cycle, only a string-shaped, frameless and flexible device, on which copper elements (cylinders) are fixed, can guarantee a perfect harmony with the uterine cavity. In order to retain the device in position, an anchoring system was invented: a simple knot made in the upper extremity of the thread (Figure 1). This knot is implanted in the myometrium of the uterine fundus with a specially designed inserter, thereby permanently securing the implant in the uterine cavity (Figure 2). The total surface area of copper is 330 mm^2.

Since the initial clinical investigations, which started in the mid-1980s, more than 10 000 woman-years of experience and up to 10 years of follow-up in international multicenter, non-comparative and comparative clinical trials have been collected. Because it was expected that the implant system would be well tolerated by nulliparous women, it was decided to include those young nulliparous

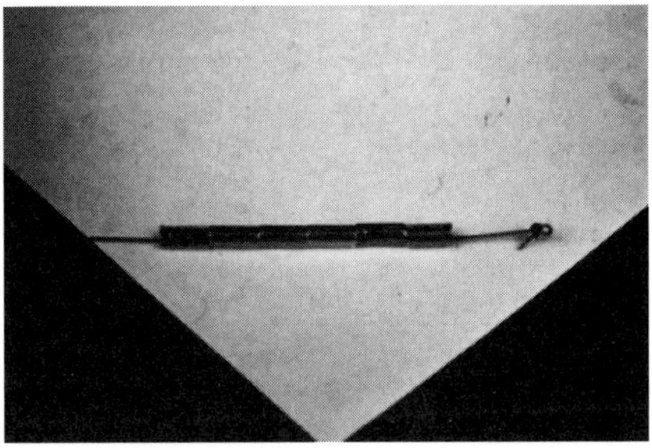

Figure 1 The GyneFix® intrauterine device

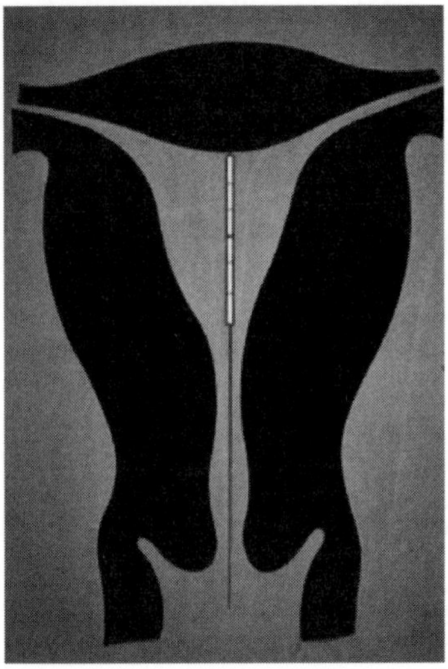

Figure 2 GyneFix® intrauterine device (IUD) in position with knot implanted in the myometrium of the uterine fundus

women who had a low risk for sexually transmitted diseases in some of the studies.

The main multicenter randomized comparative clinical trials were conducted by the World Health Organization (WHO) in over 4000 women, and compared the frameless IUD (Flexigard IUD) with the Standard TCu380A[2]. Although the trials were conducted with a highly inadequate Flexigard-insertion instrument, which resulted in a significant number of insertion failures and expulsions due to improper anchoring, and in interruption of the trials on several occasions, the results showed that the frameless device, if properly anchored, is at least twice as effective as the TCu380A. The comparative study also showed the high tolerance, high continuation rate and the virtual absence of infectious complications with the frameless device (only one case, vs. nine cases with TCu380)[2].

Parallel with the comparative studies, multicenter clinical trials were conducted in parous and nulliparous women (26% of the total number of insertions) with an optimized insertion system (GyneFix inserter) to minimize the insertion and expulsion problems and to evaluate the ease of use and reliability of the new inserter[3]. The new inserter was found to be easy to handle, allowing a reliable insertion of the anchor without the thread becoming snared during removal of the inserter, which occurred in the comparative studies. Apart from a few insertion failures due to unfamiliarity with the new concept, expulsion of the GyneFix implant was almost completely eliminated. The study also showed that insertion skill was easily acquired[3].

It was concluded from these studies that the GyneFix implant is highly effective (cumulative pregnancy rates less than 0.5 at 3 years) and that its design characteristics account for the absence of expulsion (cumulative expulsion rate less than 0.6 at 3 years), its optimal tolerance (cumulative removal rate for medical reasons 3.8 at 3 years) and consequent high continued use. The cardinal event rates were not significantly different between parous and nulliparous women.

The anchoring of the device results in a roughly 10-times lower expulsion rate compared to conventional IUDs. Indirectly, the optimal tolerance of the GyneFix explains why many women have complaints with conventional IUDs. The optimal IUD/endometrial cavity relationship, the absence of transverse arms, and the fact that the frameless device is completely retained in the inserter at the moment of insertion, are considered to be causally related to the almost total absence of infectious complications and the absence of ectopic pregnancies.

GyneFix has recently been approved for marketing in the European Union and is currently available in Belgium and France.

Cu-SAFE 300 IUD

The Cu-Safe 300 IUD was designed with the specific purpose of preventing damage to the endometrium and the design characteristics were derived from the results of cavimetric studies conducted in numerous parous and nulliparous women.

The average width of the fundal transverse dimension of the uterine cavity is less than the width of the transverse arms of the plastic T-platform. This dimensional incompatibility can lead to damage of the uterus. It has been shown that pointed IUD projections commonly become embedded in the uterine wall or the uterine ostia of the Fallopian tubes and can cause tissue proliferation and serious damage to the endometrial areas where the IUD projections have penetrated[4].

The plastic frame of the Cu-Safe IUD is made of very resilient material and is T-shaped with a copper wire wound around its vertical stem (Figure 3). The total copper surface area is 300 mm^2. The transverse arms of the device are 23 mm wide and the ends are bent to avoid endometrial trauma and with the intent to obtain a fundal seeking effect. The vertical stem is 2.5 cm long ending in a plastic tail which is moulded into the lower part of the stem. The applicator has an outer diameter of 3.1 mm and contains no plunger. Insertion is performed by the push-in technique which is facilitated by the resilience of the horizontal arms of the device.

In a randomized comparative study, the Cu-Safe was compared with the Standard TCu380A. The improved tolerance for the Cu-Safe device was demonstrated (cumulative removal rate for bleeding/pain 10.4 at 3 years vs. 15.6 at 3 years for TCu380A), however, at the expense of a significantly higher expulsion rate (6.8 for Cu-Safe vs. 2.7 TCu380A at 3 years). The pregnancy rate was slightly higher in the Cu-Safe patients compared to the TCu380A patients (cumulative rates at 3 years, 2.5 and 1.5 respectively). The apparent main advantage of Cu-Safe was its easy insertion and removal[5].

It was concluded from these studies that the Cu-Safe presents both advantages and disadvantages in comparison with the TCu380A. The device is less effective than the TCu380A which is probably the result of its tendency to be displaced downward due to the exertion of expulsive forces on its very flexible plastic frame. It is known that an IUD is maximally effective if the copper ions are delivered in the uppermost part of the uterine cavity. Once the stem is located in the cervical canal, the Cu-Safe IUD is more easily expelled due to the high flexibility of the plastic frame.

The main advantage of the Cu-Safe IUD over the TCu380A IUD is its enhanced tolerance which can be ascribed to its advantageous design characteristics.

TCu380 SLIMLINE IUD

The TCu380 Slimline (GyneT®380 Slimline) was developed to facilitate the insertion of the Standard TCu380A. The plastic frame is identical to the Standard TCu380A but the 'slimmer' copper tubes are placed at the end of the cross-arms of the T, instead of in the middle, making insertion in the insertion tube easier (Figure 4). The passage through the cervical canal is thereby also easier.

Because of the slight differences between the GyneT Slimline and the Standard GyneT, the devices were compared in a multicenter comparative study conducted by the Population Council[6]. The performance of the Slimline and Standard models of the GyneT380 were measured over 4 years in a comparative study involving 996 women, 70% of whom were randomized to the Slimline device. The 4-year pregnancy rate of the Slimline was exceptionally low (0.3 for the Slimline vs. 3.9 for the Standard GyneT). This low rate was attributed to a statistical anomaly, although the optimal placement of the copper collars near

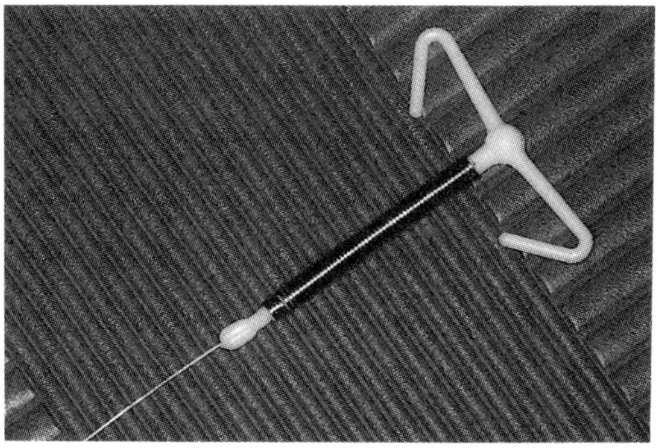

Figure 3 The Cu-Safe 300 intrauterine device

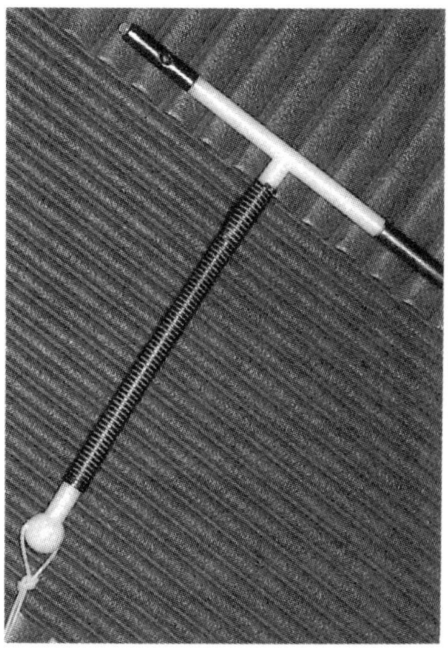

Figure 4 The TCu380 Slimline intrauterine device

the oviducts could also be the reason. The 4-year expulsion rate of the Slimline (cumulative expulsion rate of 8.6 at 4 years), however, was significantly higher than the 4-year comparable rate of the Standard GyneT (cumulative expulsion rate of 4.4 at 4 years) which is below the usual expulsion rate for the device.

The cumulative removal rates for medical reasons did not significantly differ between the two devices (36.0 for the Slimline vs. 32.6 for the Standard GyneT). However, as expected, there was a significant difference between 'prior IUD users' and 'no prior IUD users'. The removal rate was lower in the prior users, indicating satisfaction with the method. The cumulative pelvic inflammatory disease (PID) rates in this study were quite high (2.5 for the Slimline vs. 3.0 for the Standard GyneT); PID occurred mainly during the first 2 years. The two GyneT models did not show significant difference between continuation rates.

It was concluded that the Slimline variant, apart from its easier insertion, does not appear to alter the performance characteristics of the Standard Gyne T 380 IUD.

CONCLUSION

The new concept of the frameless GyneFix implant is particularly attractive when compared with other developments in the field of intrauterine contraception because of its advantageous features allowing universal intrauterine adaptation even when the cavity size is small as in nulliparous women. Because of its anchoring in the uterine fundus, the frameless device is well retained in the uterus, in contrast with the Cu-Safe IUD which floats freely in the uterine cavity. Skilful insertion, however, is a prerequisite. The anchoring technology offers new perspectives (i.e. for immediate post-abortal and post-placental insertion). It is our experience that this new method could result in improved acceptability and use of intrauterine contraception in general.

REFERENCES

1. Wildemeersch D, Van der Pas H, Thiery M, *et al.* The Copper-Fix (CuFix): a new concept in IUD technology. *Adv Contracept* 1988; 4: 197–205
2. UNDP, UNFPA, and WHO Special Programme of Research, Development and Research Training in Human Reproduction, World Bank: IUD Research Group. The TCu380A and the frameless IUD 'the FlexiGard': interim three-year data from an international multicenter trial. *Contraception* 1995; 52: 77–83
3. Van Kets H, Vrijens M, Van Trappen Y, *et al.* The frameless GyneFix® intrauterine implant: a major improvement in efficacy, expulsion and tolerance. *Adv Contracept* 1995; 11: 131–42
4. Kurz KH. Cavimeter uterine measurement and IUD clinical correlation. In Zatuchni GI, Goldsmith A, Sciarra JJ, eds. *Intrauterine contraception: Advances and Future Prospects*. Philadelphia: Harper & Row, 1984: 142–62
5. Van Kets H, Van der Pas H, Delbarge W, *et al.* A randomized comparative study of the TCu380A and Cu-Safe 300 IUDs. *Adv Contracept* 1995; 11: 123–9
6. Sivin I, Diaz J, Alvarez F, *et al.* Four-year experience in a randomized study of the GyneT® 380 Slimline and the standard GyneT® 380 intrauterine copper devices. *Contraception* 1993; 47: 37–42

16 Post-abortal IUD insertion: the challenge to minimize expulsion

I. Batár, D. Wildemeersch, W. Delbarge. M. Vrijens, M. Vekemans and H. Van Kets

INTRODUCTION

Even in the early years of the renaissance of intrauterine contraception, attempts were made to insert intrauterine contraceptive devices immediately after induced abortion[1]. The rationale of this is based on different factors:

(1) After evacuating the uterine cavity, pregnancy is excluded as one of the main contraindications for intrauterine device (IUD) insertion;

(2) The cervical canal, having been dilated, is sufficiently open enough to fit the device easily;

(3) The insertion of an IUD is almost always associated with some spotting/ bleeding and, because pregnancy termination also results in similar signs, these inconveniences caused by the insertion will be masked;

(4) An IUD fitted at the time of abortion provides effective protection even if the first sexual intercourse follows soon after the procedure;

(5) The hospital environment, especially when an unwanted pregnancy has just been terminated, provides a strong positive motivation towards contraception, and the insertion of an IUD suggests an optimal solution to the problem.

The method, however, did not become a routinely accomplished, widely accepted form of contraception. Conservative counter-arguments opposed the approach of immediate post-abortal IUD insertion, claiming that.

(1) The presence of an IUD prevents the proper involution of the evacuated uterus;

(2) Due to the insertion, bleeding problems will increase;

(3) The foreign body put into the uterine cavity could be a source of ascending infection resulting in endometritis, salpingitis, adnexitis or severe pelvic inflammatory disease (PID);

(4) Because of this, prolonged hospitalization is expected after a post-abortal insertion; and consequently

(5) The need for medication is increased.

These concerns did not prove to be well-established[2–4] and, in the 1970s, post-abortal IUD insertion became an accepted method of intrauterine contraception.

Studies conducted in both developed and developing countries confirmed the earlier findings, that expulsion rates after first-trimester abortion IUD insertion are usually not increased when compared with interval insertion[5]. However, the expulsion rate of conventional IUDs amounts to 5–10% or greater during their use[6]. The highest IUD expulsion rates are registered following second-trimester abortion[7] and when an IUD is inserted after delivery[8].

Since a significant proportion of these expulsions result in accidental pregnancies, often followed by induced abortions, the number of avoidable pregnancies and abortions, on a worldwide scale, would be huge if it were possible to reduce the expulsion rate of IUDs to almost zero. Of a total of 100 million IUD users in the world today, this would represent roughly 1.5 to 3.0 million fewer accidental pregnancies and 500 000 to 1.0 million fewer induced abortions, surmising that one-third of the IUD expulsions would result in accidental pregnancies and one-third of the accidental pregnancies were terminated (which is the case in China[9]). From this calculation, it is clear that every effort to reduce the number of expulsions would be highly rewarding (Table 1).

HISTORICAL ATTEMPTS AND USE OF CONVENTIONAL IUDs IN POST-ABORTAL PERIOD

At the Family Planning Center of the Department of Obstetrics and Gynecology of the University Medical School of Debrecen (UMSD), more than 40 000 IUDs have been inserted since 1972, the year of introduction of the intrauterine device in Hungary. In the 1970s, insertions of two non-medicated devices, the Szontágh-IUD[4] and the Spring Coil[10] were tested in the post-abortal period (see Figure 1).

Table 1 The cost of intrauterine device (IUD) failure

Number of IUD users in the world	100 million
Number of IUD failures due to expulsion	5–10 million
Estimated number of accidental pregnancies due to IUD expulsion	1.5–3.0 million
Estimated number of induced abortions due to these accidental pregnancies	0.5–1.0 million

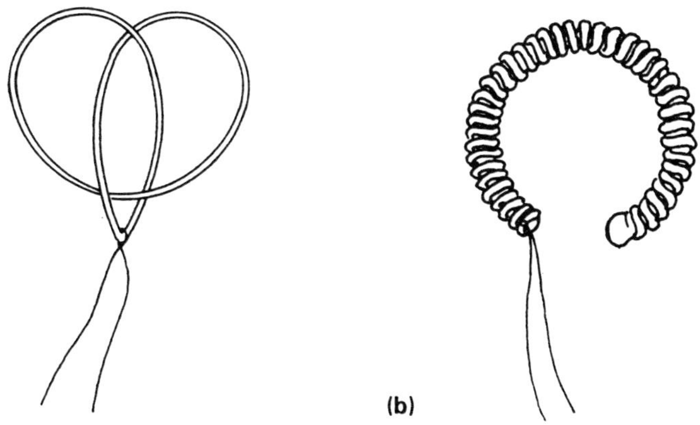

(a) (b)

Figure 1 Two non-medicated intrauterine devices (IUDs), **(a)** the Szontágh-IUD and **(b)** the Spring Coil, were tested for post-abortal insertion in the 1970s

The Szontágh-IUD study

This device, which is no longer in use, was a Hungarian IUD made of a simple nylon fishing-line[11]. The 160 mm long thread of 1 mm diameter was joined together at the two ends into a loop-like shape giving the device a suitable flexibility in two dimensions. In this way it could be accommodated to the given intrauterine space. Because of this feature, it seemed to be good for post-abortal insertion. Owing to the slimness of the nylon thread, the surface area was relatively small: 500–520 mm^2.

Between 1973 and 1974, in a 15-month period, 940 devices were inserted immediately after completing a first-trimester induced abortion. From these, data relating to 545 cases were legible for life-table analysis (Table 2). In a 1 year follow-up period, 22 IUDs were expelled, representing 26.5% of the terminations. This corresponds with a net cumulative life-table rate of 5.1 per 100 women[4]. The same rate with interval insertion was, however, only 3.1%[12]. The difference is statistically significant. No other relevant termination rates showed statistically significant differences[13]. Although the overall performance of the Szontágh-IUD in post-abortal insertion was almost the same as was experienced with fitting in the interval period, the device did not fulfill expectations as far as expulsion was concerned.

The Spring Coil

This device is a moulded linear alathon-20 polyethylene-barium coil, 80 mm in length with 50 turnings. The surface area is 1755 mm^2. The head of the IUD is closed and rounded to facilitate its passage into the uterine cavity and to avoid endometrial injury[14]. Without detailing the rather difficult insertion procedures, it should only be mentioned that, in a post-abortal situation, the results of the

Table 2 Results of a 1-year trial of two non-medicated intrauterine devices (IUDs) in post-abortal insertions (Family Planning Center, UMSD, Debrecen, Hungary, 1973–75)

	Szontágh-IUD		*Spring coil*	
	n	*Rate*	*n*	*Rate*
Number of insertions	545	NA	811	NA
Woman-months of use	3920	NA	4298	NA
Terminations				
Pregnancy	16	5.7	5	1.1
Expulsion	22	5.1	134	24.4
Removal for				
bleeding/pain	31	7.8	86	18.5
other	14	4.4	32	25.6
Total terminations	83	23.0	257	51.1

NA, not applicable

device proved to be poor and the Spring Coil remained in a clinical trial phase never to be introduced into routine use.

In 1973, during a 6-month period, 1086 devices were inserted *post menstruationem* and *post abortum*. The first-year results with 811 post-abortal cases showed an excellent protection rate (1.1), but the expulsion as well as the removal rates for bleeding/pain were unacceptably high (Table 2)[10]. Out of the 257 terminations, there were 134 expulsions (52.1%) and 86 bleeding/pain removals (33.5%). These figures did not at all encourage continuation of the post-abortal insertions.

World Health Organization study

In an international multicenter randomized study conducted by the World Health Organization (WHO)[15] in which three devices were tested (TCu 220C, Lippes Loop D and Copper 7), the 390 days cumulative net probability of expulsion (which refers to the 1-year gross rate used by Potter[16] and Tietze and Lewit[17]) was 4.4, 9.6 and 13.1, respectively. The differences were statistically significant. The findings indicated that expulsion of the device had remained a problem to be solved, especially in second-trimester abortions.

Lippes Loop D

One of the latest publications, which is probably the very first randomized 10-year comparison in the literature, Randic and co-workers[8] investigated the non-medicated Lippes Loop D and the same device with the addition of 200 mm^2 of copper in the form of copper sleeves. This 10-year evaluation showed a 1-year expulsion/displacement life table rate of 4.49 and 12.61, respectively, for the medicated and for the non-medicated version.

THE FRAMELESS 'ANCHORED' INTRAUTERINE IMPLANT SYSTEM

One of the recent developments, which has just been introduced in several European countries, is the frameless GyneFix®. This implant system has no frame. Instead, the proximal end of the non-absorbable surgical filament with six copper tubes threaded on it (Figure 2), is provided with an anchoring knot which is inserted in the myometrium of the uterine fundus with a specially designed inserter.

Since clinical studies conducted over the past decade with the GyneFix device for interval insertion demonstrated a very low expulsion, high efficacy and high tolerance rates[19], an international study was initiated in 1994 to evaluate the expulsion rate when the device is inserted in a postabortal situation. Additionally, the launch of the study was encouraged by the very favorable results of a similar international trial[8] in which the post-placental version of the device had been tested (Table 3). The device for post-abortal insertion is identical to the regular

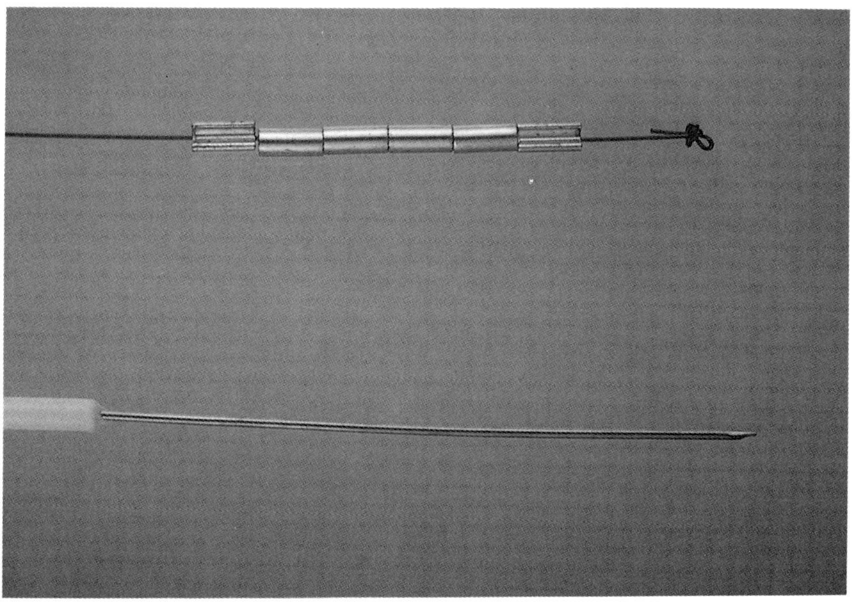

Figure 2 The frameless GyneFix® (top) has an anchoring knot which is inserted in the myometrium of the uterine fundus with a specially designed inserter (bottom)

Table 3 Results of an 18-month trial of post-placental GyneFix

	n	*Rate*
Number of insertions	73	NA
Woman-months of use	1101	NA
Terminations		
Pregnancy	1	1.5
Expulsion	2	3.1
Removal for		
bleeding/pain	7	10.8
other	0	0.0
Total terminations	10	15.4

NA, not applicable

device, except that the size of the knot is slightly larger to enhance the retention of the device while the uterus regains its normal size (see Figure 3).

To date, GyneFix devices have been inserted at three centers (Ghent, Brussels and Debrecen). The first insertion was done in October 1994 and the last one in Debrecen in August 1996. Sixteen devices were inserted in nulliparous women. Due to the relatively small number of cases and the short follow-up period, the data are not sufficient for life-table analysis (Table 4). There have been no pregnancies and no removals for medical reasons to date. Only one expulsion occurred at the beginning of the study, within the first month following insertion, in one of the centers that joined the study at a later stage. Our experience has shown that this case is in all probability a failed insertion, since retention of the anchor of the frameless device appears to be as good as when inserted post-menstrually. It is also noteworthy that no complications were found among those who had returned for follow-up. These data indicate that the post-abortal version of the GyneFix device appears to be as well retained in the post-abortal situation as when inserted post-menstrually.

CONCLUSION

Although the number of insertions is limited, the preliminary results indicate that similar low rates of expulsion can be obtained with use of the post-abortal device as is the case with the interval version of the implant system. This could be strategically important in reducing the number of accidental pregnancies and the high number of induced and repeat abortions. The fact that the frameless implant system is also well retained in the nulliparous uterus, and well tolerated, is of great importance, as many induced abortions occur in this group of women. In addition, insertion of the implant system is easy and appears to be safe.

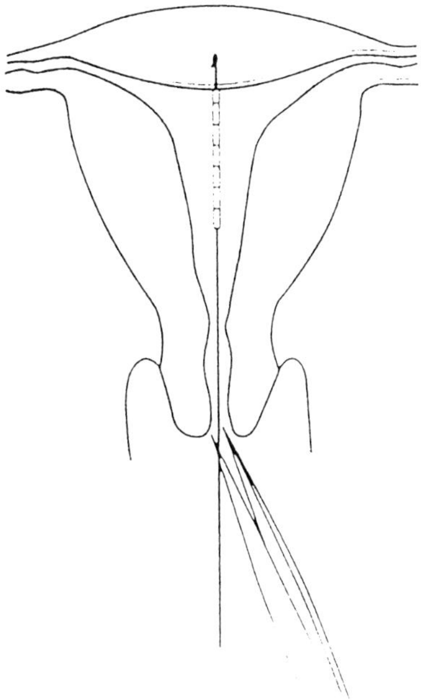

Figure 3 The GyneFix for post-abortal insertion has a larger knot than the regular device, to enhance retention while the uterus regains its normal size

Table 4 Preliminary results of trials of GyneFix post-abortion between October 1994 and August 1996

		Follow-up (n)		
Center	*Insertion (n)*	*> 3 months*	*> 6 months*	*> 12 months*
Belgium	39	12	10	4
Hungary	48	23	—	—

REFERENCES

1. Ishihama A. Clinical studies on intrauterine rings, especially the present state of contraception in Japan and the experiences in the use of the intrauterine rings. *Yokohama Med Bull* 1959; 10(2): 89–105
2. Andolsek L. Experience with immediate post-abortion insertion of the IUD. In Lewit S, ed. *Abortion Techniques and Services. Proceedings of a Symposium.* Amsterdam: Excerpta Medica, 1972; 63–7

3. Goldsmith A, Goldberg R, Eyzaguirre H, *et al.* IUD insertion in the immediate post-abortion period. In Goldsmith A and Snowden R, ed. *Proceedings of the Family Planning Research Conference. A Multidisciplinary Approach.* Amsterdam: Excerpta Medica, 1972; 56–67
4. Batár I. One-year clinical experiences with Szontágh-IUD. II Post-abortal insertions. *Magy Nöorv L* 1976; 39: 32–5 (in Hungarian)
5. Liskin L. *IUDs: an appropriate contraceptive for many women.* Population Reports, Series B, Number 4. Population Information program. Baltimore: The Johns Hopkins University, July 1982
6. Van Kets H. Clinical performance of intrauterine devices (dissertation). Faculty of Medicine, State University of Gent, Belgium, 1990
7. Treiman K, Liskin L. *IUDs – a new look.* Population Reports, Series B, Number 5. Population Information program. Baltimore:The Johns Hopkins University, March 1988
8. Van Kets H, Parewijck W, Van der Pas H, *et al.* Immediate postplacental insertion and fixation of the CuFix postpartum implant system. *Contraception* 1993; 48: 349–57
9. Kaufman J. The Cost of IUD failure in China. *Stud Fam Plann* 1993; 24: 194–6
10. Batár I, Thomas M, Lampé L. One-year experiences with Spring Coil in post-abortal insertions. *Magy Nöorv L* 1976; 39: 81–6 (in Hungarian)
11. Szontágh F, Zelenka L, Szereday Z. Contraception with a simple new intrauterine device. *Preventive Medicine. Family Planning.* Hartford: Austin and Sons 1967; 127
12. Batár I. One-year clinical experiences with Szontágh-IUD. I Interval insertions. *Magy Nöorv L* 1975; 38: 495–9 (in Hungarian)
13. Batár I. One-year clinical experiences with Szontágh-IUD. Comparison of the different types of insertions. *Magy Nöorv L* 1976; 39: 133–8 (in Hungarian)
14. Ragab MI. Intrauterine devices (IUDs) on trial. In Hasegava T, *et al.* ed. *Proceedings of the VII World Congress on Fertility and Sterility.* New York: Excerpta Medica, 1973; 958
15. WHO Task Force on Intrauterine Devices for Fertility Regulation, Special Programme of Research, Development and Research Training in Human Reproduction. IUD insertion following termination of pregnancy: a clinical trial of the TCu 220C, Lippes Loop D, and Copper 7. *Stud Fam Plann* 1983; 14(4): 99–108
16. Potter RG. Application of life table techniques to measurement of contraceptive effectiveness. *Demography* 1966; 3: 297
17. Tietze C, Lewit S. Recommended procedures for the statistical evaluation of intrauterine contraception. *Stud Fam Plann* 1973; 4: 35
18. Randic L, Haller H, Perovic M, *et al.* The effect of adding copper onto Lippes Loop IUDs: results from a ten-year study in Yugoslavia. *Contraception* 1997; 43(3): 229–39
19. Van Kets H, Vrijens M, Van Trappen Y, *et al.* The frameless GyneFix® intrauterine implant: a major improvement in efficacy, expulsion and tolerance. *Adv Contracept* 1995; 11: 131–42

17 Misconceptions about intrauterine devices

D. Wildemeersch, W. Parewijck, H. Van Kets, W. Delbarge, M. Vrijens and M. Thiery

INTRODUCTION

Although intrauterine devices (IUDs) are the most widely used modern reversible contraceptives worldwide, with about 100 million users, they are underused because they are misunderstood. It may surprise many people that the IUD is as safe or safer than other forms of contraception. Despite this fact, however, the IUD struggles to shake off its legacy of the past. Since the Dalkon Shield was removed from the US market in 1975, because of its links with pelvic inflammatory disease (PID), and later the Copper 7, Copper T and Lippes Loop, removed for purely economic reasons, the public perception and that of the media and many physicians around the world, is still that the IUD is bad for women's health. It was not understood that decisions to stop marketing IUDs in the USA were not made because of medical problems. Precisely because of this misunderstanding, the World Health Organization (WHO) gathered together a scientific group in 1986 to address the safety, efficacy and mechanism of action of IUDs. This panel of experts concluded that today's IUDs are among the safest and most effective contraceptives available[1].

The efficacy of the newer high-load copper IUDs has indeed improved manyfold over the previous generation of plain plastic IUDs[2], and the recently introduced frameless intrauterine implant system has shown an even greater efficacy (annual pregnancy rates down to 0.2 per year), a very good retention (expulsion rate of almost zero) and optimal tolerance (annual removal rate for medical reasons: ± 2%)[3].

As a consequence of the enhanced performance of modern IUDs, and the improved acceptability and retention of the frameless implant system, the number of IUD users worldwide should drastically increase in the coming decade. However, apart from improving patient acceptance, due attention should also be given to keeping the medical, scientific, and programmatic communities informed about the characteristics of the IUD and about new developments in this field, in comparison to other methods[4].

The purpose of this paper is to provide current scientific information about a number of misconceptions related to intrauterine contraception: mechanism of action, use in young nulliparous women, insertion-related aspects, safety aspects (PID, ectopic pregnancy), IUD effectiveness, etc. with the aim to reduce concerns many women have with regard to selecting an IUD for contraception.

MECHANISM OF ACTION: COPPER IUDs BLOCK FERTILIZATION

The primary contraceptive effect of copper IUDs is the prevention of fertilization and implantation by interfering with sperm motility and survival, and with egg development. The IUD reaction with the endometrium activates the release of leukocytes and prostaglandins which act not only in the uterine cavity but also in the oviduct and cervix to impede sperm and egg development. The copper ions delivered by the copper IUD enhance this effect. Studies conducted in women wearing a copper IUD have shown that copper is hostile to sperm. A reduced number of live sperm are found after intercourse compared with those found in non-users.

The following actions are attributed to the copper effect:

(1) Effect on sperm migration: the interruption of sperm migration starts at the level the cervix and continues in the uterus and oviducts. Researchers found no sperm·15–30 min after insemination in the oviducts of copper IUD wearers while sperm were detected in all women not using an IUD[5].

(2) Spermicidal effect: studies have also shown that copper acts as a spermicide and found that the sperm heads were detached from the tails in a majority of sperm cells[6].

(3) Effect on fertilization: fertilization is affected due to action on the unfertilized eggs. When searching for ova by flushing the uterus on the fifth day after ovulation, researchers found eggs in one-third of 36 women using no contraceptives, while only one egg was recovered among 22 users of inert IUDs that contain no copper and none in 43 users of copper IUDs[7]. A comparison of copper IUD users and women using no contraception showed that none of the eggs from the copper IUD users were fully developed or fertilized, in contrast to more than one-half of the eggs recovered from the non-contraceptive users[8].

(4) Effect on egg development and transportation: copper IUDs reduce the development and transportation of eggs. When tested for the appearance of the pregnancy hormone hCG prior to implantation of a fertilized egg, few IUD users tested positive for the hormone[9].

PELVIC INFLAMMATORY DISEASE: IUDs DO NOT CAUSE INFECTION

One of the important lessons drawn from the Dalkon Shield tragedy is the importance of selection and screening of patients for IUD insertion. In the

1970s, IUDs were prescribed to women with a high risk for sexually transmitted diseases (STDs). Since the Dalkon Shield had a multifilament tail which acted as a wick for bacteria, PID cases ensued. Modern IUDs have a monofilament tail which minimizes the ascent of bacteria. Recently, a better understanding of PID etiology has prompted questions about sexual behavior and other lifestyle factors in studies of IUD users. The findings indicate that PID risk is minimal in women who are at low risk for STDs, in other words among couples in monogamous sexual relationships. Age alone is not a contraindication for the use of an IUD and family planning providers should help clients understand how they can protect themselves in case of risk behavior. Certain women, who are at higher STD risk, have a higher risk of developing PID and should be discouraged from using an IUD or use a backup method (condom) for added protection.

Data from a long-term WHO study which started in 1975 indicate that the risk of PID is higher only during the first 3 weeks following insertion and that the risk does not increase with long-term use[10]. The reason for the increased risk of infection after IUD insertion is that bacteria in the vagina can be transported through the cervical canal into the uterine cavity. It is important to point out that the lactobaccilli that occur naturally in the vagina can result in infection if they are transferred to the uterine cavity. The WHO Scientific Group who reviewed the literature pointed out a number of methodological problems with earlier published reports, specifically the use of the wrong comparison group (e.g. pill users), overdiagnosis of PID in IUD users and failure to control for confounding variables. Re-analysis of the data in the USA found that IUD users at low risk for acquiring STDs were unlikely to develop PID[11].

It is also important to tell the IUD user that for the majority of IUD users, fertility is restored immediately after removal of the device, irrespective of whether the IUD was used for a few months or for many years[12].

There are certain basic principles which should be respected with regard to the use of IUDs in general. An IUD should not be inserted in a woman with certain lower genital tract infections, i.e acute mucopurulent cervicitis, gonorrhea and chlamydia. All potential users should be screened for at least the signs and symptoms of these infections and women should be given additional laboratory tests if necessary. Patient counselling about risks and symptoms, practicing aseptic insertion techniques and conducting a follow-up examination at 1 month are additional safeguards to prevent infectious complications in IUD users[13,14].

IUD USE IN NULLIPAROUS WOMEN: INTRAUTERINE CONTRACEPTION HAS DISTINCT ADVANTAGES

Another misconception is that women over 25 years or older are the best candidates for IUD use, and women over 35 years the ideal candidates. This misconception stems from studies conducted in the 1970s and early 1980s which showed that PID is more frequent in nulliparous users compared to women using other methods of contraception[15]. This recommendation, based on the fear of PID and the potential for resulting infertility, is no longer justified. There is no biological reason to conclude that a young woman is at higher risk than an older woman if they have the same sexual behavior.

Intrauterine contraception offers important advantages over other forms of contraception in nulliparous women because IUDs are non-hormonal, require minimal compliance, are long-lasting, are more effective than the pill, and because fertility return is immediate.

The main reason for the high accidental pregnancy rate in young women in industrialized countries is because they rely on methods that are dependent on daily administration. A high proportion of young women using oral contraceptives discontinue further use because of hormonal side-effects and menstrual problems. Others do not use the method correctly[16]. Methods which avoid non-compliance have been shown to be much more effective than the pill in preventing pregnancy in young women[17].

When considered for use by nulliparous women, conventional IUDs should be used with caution because of the higher risk of expulsion and PID (as discussed above in the previous section). Dimensional incompatibility is a major concern in IUD users in general because disharmony leads to reduced effectiveness owing to displacement of the IUD, and a higher removal rate for medical reasons. These potential problems are more likely to occur in nulliparous women. Traumatic lesions to the endometrium and myometrium owing to disharmony have been repeatedly demonstrated, and documented by hysteroscopy and histological examination[18,19]. Researchers have also suggested that these lesions may enhance the risk of infection.

When selecting an IUD for nulliparous women, the consequences of disharmony between the IUD and the uterine cavity should be taken into consideration. The low tolerance rate and significantly lower rate of performance of 'framed' IUDs in nulliparous women have contributed to the low acceptance of IUDs in general and the bad name attributed to IUDs in the media. The 'frameless' IUD (GyneFix® implant), developed by our group, possesses advantageous features (fixed to the uterine fundus, frameless and, therefore, totally flexible), resulting in improved performance and high tolerance, and should be recommended, therefore, as the first choice intrauterine contraceptive in nulliparous women[3] (see also Table 1).

CONCERNS ABOUT IUD EFFECTIVENESS AND SIDE-EFFECTS

Effectiveness

Copper IUDs protect against both intrauterine and ectopic pregnancy, in contrast to the general belief. Epidemiological analysis clearly shows that users of modern IUDs are at low risk of ectopic pregnancy[21].

Table 1 Intrauterine device (IUD) use in nulliparous women: 'framed' IUDs vs. the 'frameless' IUD. Data from reference 20

	Rate at 1 year per 100 users	
	Conventional IUDs	*Frameless IUDs*
Pregnancy	1–3 (or more)	< 1
Expulsion	high (up to 10–14)	low (< 1)
Total medical removal	high (up to 10–20)	low (< 5)

Similarly, physicians and the general public are often poorly informed about the effectiveness of IUDs and the effectiveness of contraceptive methods in general. The commonly held opinion is that oral contraceptives are more effective than IUDs. Yet, clinical studies show that IUDs are more effective than oral contraceptives in everyday practice[22]. Figure 1 shows the effectiveness of different contraceptive methods.

Displacement, partial expulsion and total expulsion

Displacement, partial expulsion and total expulsion of conventional IUDs are mainly caused by geometric factors and are important factors in the occurrence

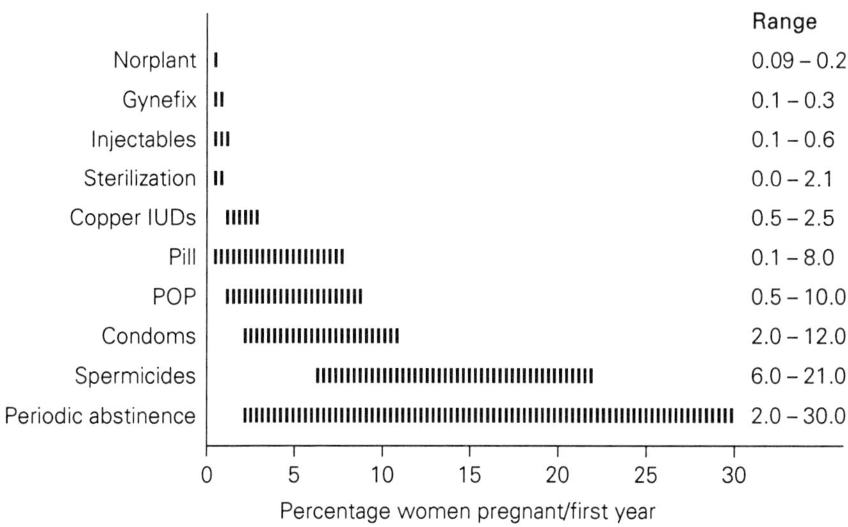

Figure 1 Protection against pregnancy: effectiveness of contraceptive methods at 1 year. Data from references 3, 23 and 24. POP, progestin only pill

of accidental pregnancy. Also, the insertion skill of the provider is important. However, an IUD which is too large or too small will, almost by definition, become expelled or displaced because the uterus will react to the 'non-fitting' foreign body. It is impossible to know the size and volume of the uterine cavity by performing a pelvic examination alone. A large or enlarged uterus can have a relatively small cavity, and a relatively small uterus on pelvic palpation can hide a big cavity[25,26]. Moreover, the uterus contracts differently from one woman to another during the menstrual cycle.

While it is clear that a totally expelled IUD exposes the woman to accidental pregnancy, a displaced or partially expelled IUD also reduces the protection from pregnancy[27,28]. Partial and total expulsion occur in 5–10% of women during the first 3–5 years of use, with an increased risk in nulliparous women. The majority of the expulsions occur during the first months after insertion, with 1–2% per year thereafter. The frameless GyneFix implant reduces the risk of displacement and expulsion approximately 10-fold[29]. If the distance between the upper part of the IUD and the surface of the uterus is > 2 cm, the IUD should be replaced because of the greater likelihood of accidental pregnancy. The proper location of the IUD in the uterine cavity can be checked by ultrasound. The woman can also feel if the device is still in place by checking for the IUD string(s) attached to the bottom of the device. If an IUD is partially expelled, the stem of the IUD is felt at the cervical os. A displaced IUD, however, cannot be felt and will often remain undetected if no ultrasound check is done.

Side effects and complications

Bleeding

The copper released from the IUD affects the bleeding pattern and causes the endometrium to shed more frequently than normal. Abnormal bleeding is not usually a sign of a health problem.

Over the age of 35–40 years abnormal bleeding is frequently caused by hormonal imbalance (irregular bleeding and menorrhagia) and is an important reason for IUD removal. The amount and type of blood loss, however, also depends on: the size of the IUD, the flexibility of the IUD and the relationship of the IUD to the uterine cavity. If the IUD causes abnormal bleeding and pain, the majority of women will request its removal. Bleeding without pain is more readily accepted. Many of these bleeding problems can be treated adequately without the necessity to remove the IUD, using: estrogens, estro-progestogens, progestogens, non-steroidal anti-inflammatory drugs, anti-fibrinolytic drugs or ergometrin.

Owing to the possiblity of anemia in women with heavy bleeding associated with IUD use, women should be checked and iron supplements should be given if necessary.

Pain

One of the reasons for the underuse of the IUD is the fear of insertion pain. The insertion of an IUD is not usually a painful procedure. However, many women, nulliparous women in particular, fear insertion and this may be an important reason not to select an IUD. Comfort at insertion and during the use of the IUD is extremely important and is strongly related to the acceptability of the method as a whole. Women tend to reject the method more easily if they experienced severe discomfort during insertion of the IUD[30].

Several measures have been used to reduce patient discomfort during the insertion and removal of an IUD: premedication, topical intracervical anesthesia, and loco-regional anesthesia. Vasovagal syncope appeared to be less frequent when paracervical block (PCB) anesthesia is used and the method was described as safe and highly effective in minimizing discomfort for IUD retrieval/insertion[31]. However, the use of PCB anesthesia is feared by many physicians because of the danger of inadvertent intravascular injection, and the risk of convulsions and central nervous system depression. To prevent these potential problems, the use of dental equipment for the injection of a small amount of a local anesthetic drug into the uterine cervix prior to the insertion of an IUD has shown to be very effective, extremely simple, convenient, and safe for IUD insertion in nulliparous women and in parous women who desire analgesia. The use of local anesthesia not only minimizes or eliminates the discomfort of IUD insertion totally, but also minimizes the hazards such as vasovagal syncope and convulsions[32]. Attention to the comfort of women during IUD placement will undoubtedly increase the demand for intrauterine contraception.

Pain in IUD users is most often caused by incompatibility between the IUD and the uterine cavity, the rigidity of the IUD (sometimes due to penetration in the myometrium), and by displacement or partial expulsion.

CONCLUSION

In addition to proper fitting of an IUD, good screening and counselling of clients, including the provision of current scientific information, a proper pelvic examination and insertion, ultrasound control and post-insertion counselling, proper follow-up and management of side-effects are important issues to improve the acceptability of intrauterine contraception. The IUD provider must understand the following relationships and be able to transmit the information to the woman: (1) the relationship between IUD–cavity compatibility and effectiveness, expulsion and occurrence of side-effects; (2) the relationship between IUD use and sexually transmitted disease transmission and pelvic inflammatory disease; and (3) the relationship between IUD use and changes in menses.

This, together with the elimination of myths, will result in increased use of intrauterine contraception and enhanced acceptability of the method.

REFERENCES

1. World Health Organization. Mechanism of Action, Safety and Efficacy of Intrauterine Devices. Technical Report Series 753. Geneva: WHO, 1987
2. Sivin I, Greensdale F, Schmidt F, *et al. The Copper T 380 Intrauterine Device: A Summary of Scientific Data.* New York: The Population Council, 1992
3. Van Kets H, Vrijens M, Van Trappen Y, *et al.* The frameless GyneFix® intrauterine implant: a major improvement in efficacy, expulsion and tolerance. *Adv Contracept* 1995; 11: 131–42
4. Maulding WP, Segal SJ. IUD use thoughout the world: past, present and future. In Bardin CW, Mishell DR, Newton MA, eds. *Proceedings from the Fourth International Conference on IUDs.* Boston: Butterworth-Heinemann, 1994: 1–10
5. Tredway DR, Umezaki CU, Mishell DR, *et al.* Effect of intrauterine devices on sperm transport in the human being: preliminary report. *Am J Obstet Gynecol* 1975; 123: 734–5
6. Ortiz ME, Croxatto HB. The mode of action of IUDs. *Contraception* 1987; 36: 44
7. Ortiz ME, Croxatto HB. The mode of action of IUDs. *Contraception* 1987; 36: 55
8. Alvarez F, Brache V, Fernandez E, *et al.* New insights on the mode of action of intrauterine devices in women. *Fertil Steril* 1988; 49: 768–73
9. Wilcox AJ, Weinberg CR, Armstrong EG, *et al.* Urinary human chorionic gonadotropin among intrauterine device users: detection with a highly specific and sensitive assay. *Fertil Steril* 1987; 47: 265–70
10. Farley TMM, Rosenberg MJ, Rowe PJ, *et al.* Intrauterine devices and pelvic inflammatory disease: an international perspective. *Lancet* 1992; 339: 785–8
11. Lee NC, Rubin GL, Borucki R. The intrauterine device and pelvic inflammatory disease revisited: new results from the Women's Health Study. *Obstet Gynecol* 1988; 72: 1–6
12. Wilson JC. A prospective New Zealand study of fertility after removal of copper intrauterine devices for contraception and because of complications: a four year study. *Am J Obstet Gynecol* 1989; 160: 391–6
13. Curtis KM, Bright PL, eds. *Recommendations for Updating Selected Practices in Contraceptive Use: Results of a Technical Meeting.* Chapel Hill: Technical Guidance Working Group, U.S. Agency for International Development, 1994; Vol. 1
14. World Health Organization. *Improving Access to Quality Care in Family Planning: Medical Criteria for Initiating and Continuing Use of Contraceptive Methods.* Geneva: WHO, 1995
15. Westrom L. Incidence, prevalence, and trends of acute PID and its consequence to industrialized countries. *Am J Obstet Gynecol* 1980; 138: 880–92
16. Guillebaud J. *Oral Contraceptive Compliance.* London: Churchill Livingstone, 1995
17. Wildemeersch D, Van Kets H, Vrijens M, *et al.* Intrauterine contraception in adolescent women. The GyneFix intrauterine implant. *Ann NY Acad Sci* 1997; 817: 440–50
18. Sheppard BL. Endometrial morphological changes in IUD users: a review. *Contraception* 1987; 36: 1–10
19. Pizarro E, Schöenstedt G, Mehech G, *et al.* Uterine cavity and the location of IUDs following the administration of meclofenamic acid to menorrhagic women. Contraception 1989; 40: 413–23
20. Van Kets H. Clinical performance of intrauterine devices. Dissertation, Faculty of Medicine, State University Ghent, Belgium, 1990

21. Schmidt F, Sivin I, Waldman S. The Copper T 380 IUD. In Bardin CW, Mishell DR, Newton MA, eds. *Proceedings from the Fourth International Conference on IUDs*. Boston: Butterworth-Heinemann, 1994: 303–12
22. Wyeth-Ayerst Contraceptive Survey in Europe (WYCON). London: ISIS Research Ltd, 1993
23. Contraceptive method failure rates. *IPPF Med Bull* 1994; 28 (4)
24. Peterson HB, Xia Z, Hughes JM, Wilcox LS, Tylor LR, Trussell J for the US Collaborative Review of Sterilization Working Group. The risk of pregnancy after tubal sterilization: findings from the US Collaborative Review of Sterilization. *Am J Obstet Gynecol* 1996; 174: 1161–70
25. Hasson HM. Clinical studies of the Wing Sound II metrology device. In Zatuchni GI, Goldsmith A, Sciarra JJ, eds. *Intrauterine Contraception: Advances and Future Prospects*. Philadelphia: Harper & Row, 1984; 126–41
26. Kurz KH. Cavimeter uterine measurements and IUD clinical correlation. In Zatuchni GI, Goldsmith A, Sciarra JJ, eds. *Intrauterine Contraception: Advances and Future Prospects*. Philadelphia: Harper & Row, 1984; 142–62
27. Kaivola S. Postremoval assessment of the intrauterine position of the IUDs: an analysis of 1012 removals with special reference to pregnancy risk and dislocation. Presented at the *Annual Meeting of the Society for the Advancement of Contraception*, Singapore, 1990
28. Anteby E, Revel A, Ben-Chetrit A, Rosen B, Tadmor O, Yagel S. Intrauterine device failure: relation to its location within the uterine cavity. *Obstet Gynecol* 1993; 81: 112–4
29. Van Kets H, Wildemeersch D, Van der Pas H, *et al.* IUD expulsion solved with implant technology. *Contraception* 1995; 51: 87–92
30. Smith P. Copper IUDs in nulliparous women. In Hafez ESE, van Os WAA, eds. *Medicated Intrauterine Devices*. Martinus Nijhoff 1980; 119–26
31. Thiery M. Pain relief at insertion and removal of an IUD: a simplified technique for paracervical block. *Adv Contracept* 1985; 1: 167–70
32. Delbarge W, Wildemeersch D, Van Kets H, *et al.* Intracervical anesthesia for IUD insertion in nulliparous women. 1997, in preparation

18 Contraceptive barrier methods: new developments

E.A. Hassan and G. Creatsas

INTRODUCTION

Barrier contraceptives (BCs), the oldest form of contraception, are still in use today despite the development of other methods such as oral contraceptives and intrauterine devices (IUDs), which are more effective in preventing pregnancy.

The various types of BC have their own characteristics and proponents. One of their main advantages is that they have no significant side-effects and they offer better protection against sexually transmitted diseases (STDs). They usually require the users to have a great deal of motivation to attain maximum effectiveness. Barrier contraceptives are currently one of the reliable methods for the protection against both pregnancy and STDs as vaccines are not yet available[1].

Safe and effective BCs are critically needed to reduce transmission of STDs, and their development is a global priority. There are increasing data that the use of BCs should reduce the risk of acquiring STDs. Evidence of the protective effect of BCs against the risk of STDs has been published, but there is a lack of quantitative assessment on the protection[2]. Another urgent priority is the development of new female-controlled BCs that combine bacteriostatic and spermicidal activity. The target is to develop safe antiviral, antibacterial and anti-protozoal substances[1,3].

TYPES OF BARRIER CONTRACEPTIVE

Condoms

Condoms, for the time being, are one of the most reliable methods for protection against pregnancy and STDs. The efficacy of condoms depends on the users' attitude. If they are consequently and properly used they offer highly effective protection. Male latex condoms are the most effective method in clinical practice and are used as the gold standard against which other BCs are tested. World Health Organization reports estimate the use of the male condom to be as high as 19% of all contraceptive methods employed in the developed countries, compared to 6% in less developed regions[1].

In spite of latex's disadvantages, latex condoms were the only form available until recently. A small percentage of users are allergic to latex. In addition, the safety of latex can be reduced with the use of lubricants and it can perish under conditions of excessive heat or light. Recently, new condoms have been developed from other materials such as polyurethane and other polymers. These products are expected to be more acceptable to users and it is anticipated that they will be more durable[1,4]. Several new male condoms are being developed in a way to increase acceptability and encourage more consistent use. Innovative designs of latex condom and formulations of non-latex condom are currently being researched. The new male condoms are designed to combine the ease of use and comfort, to be non-allergic, to offer a longer shelf-life and to be more efficient[5]. 'Avanti®', the first plastic male condom, is available in the USA and others will be appearing soon.

Female condoms

New female condoms have been developed in addition to the male variety. These offer women a measure of control over their risks of pregnancy and STD. The major concern at the present time is acceptability, which largely depends on convenience for women. No barrier is effective unless used consistently. Some find female condoms unappealing and a hindrance to foreplay if worn prior to intercourse. 'Reality®' is a very thin polyurethane female condom but it is still 40% stronger than a typical latex male condom. It is available in the USA and a similar product, 'Femshield®' is available in Europe[1]. Some reports on Femshield showed that the outer and inner rings caused discomfort during intercourse, plus the fact that the device could be expelled from the vagina during intercourse. Both partners stated that the outer ring and bag reduced sensitivity and sexual satisfaction[6]. Another female condom, which the developer expects to market soon in Canada and some parts of Europe, is the 'Bikini Condom' which is worn like a panty. 'Women's Choice' is another product requiring an applicator; this condom is currently undergoing tests for efficacy[1]. It appears that acceptability of the female condom is increased with persistent use and that this device has a role in broadening the choice of contraception open to women. However, it appears that many individuals still want simple methods of contraception and do not want to think about device availability or following instructions at a critical moment[7].

Diaphragms

The first diaphragm available was a rubber cup and no new varieties have appeared in the market for several decades. Currently, new forms of diaphragms are being tested. The disposable diaphragm, a product that released spermicide, has not been found to be practical. As some diaphragm users often have urinary tract infections, continuous use is not recommended for all women. *Escherichia coli* was detected twice as frequently in the vagina of diaphragm users[1,8] and women suffering frequent urinary tract infections should seriously consider using other types of contraception. Several types of silicone diaphragms and caps have been developed in order to eliminate the physician's involvement. A new product, 'Lea's shield®', combines the features of a diaphragm and cervical cap. Recent studies of its efficacy when used with spermicide were very promising[9]. The 'Femcap®' is another new product, a silicone cervical cap including spermicidal material. Femcap is made in three sizes small for women who have never been pregnant, medium for women who have been pregnant but did not deliver vaginally and large for women who have had at least one vaginal birth. In a preliminary clinical trial, the failure rate was as low as 4.8%. More extensive trials on the efficiency of the method are expected[1,10].

Spermicides

Spermicides offer additional protection when used in conjunction with other barrier methods. Originally, they were developed to prevent pregnancy; prevention of STDs was a subsequent consideration. The more the spermicide covers the vaginal epithelium, the more effective it is. A dual role and broader application for chemical barriers necessitates rapid tests to define their efficiency in preventing STDs as well as pregnancy. Duration of the effective level of spermicide remaining in the vagina, and, ability to spread over the entire vaginal and cervical surface constitute some properties of chemical barriers[1]. Acceptable chemical barriers should uniformly spread and distribute over the vaginal and cervical epithelium. They should maintain the normal microflora and pH of the vagina, inactivate various STD organisms, be effective, non-irritating and aesthetically acceptable. They should also be degradable and easily removed by natural and physiological actions after the desired time period.

The vaginal pH is acidic, varying from 3.5 to 4.5. This acidity immobilizes sperm, which have a slightly alkaline effect. Seminal plasma may raise the vaginal pH to a neutral level, and some sexually transmitted pathogens may reach target cells during this time. Chemical products that preserve the consistency of the vaginal pH may limit transmission of STDs.

Currently available spermicides include jellies, creams, foams, suppositories and films. The active ingredient of most commercially available spermicides is nonoxynol-9, a highly polar molecule that immobilizes sperm by disrupting the cell membrane. Laboratory investigations indicate that nonoxynol-9 inhibits a variety of sexually transmissible organisms, including those responsible for *Neisseria gonorrhea*, chlamydial infection, candidiasis, genital herpes, syphilis, trichomoniasis and the acquired immunodeficiency syndrome (AIDS)[11,12]. Nonnoxynol-9 at concentrations of ≥ 0–5% inactivated human T-cell lymphotrophic virus type III (HTLV-III) and human immunodeficiency virus type I (HIV-I) *in vitro*, while ≥ 1% reduced the live counts of the target lymphocytes[13,14]. Cholic acid (sodium cholate) was found to exhibit a strong spermicidal and antiviral (anti-HIV-I) activity, while benzalkonium chloride has a direct inhibitory effect on HIV-I *in vitro*[15,16].

Commercially available spermicides contain 1–5% nonoxynol-9 and are often included in contraceptive jellies and foams used by women, in combination with another barrier method. Certain pharmacological problems may be introduced by the local application of these compounds, such as local cytotoxic irritational effect on the vaginal mucosa, as well as systemic effects after absorption and transfer into the circulation. Such criticisms have been expressed, in particular, for nonoxynol-9 which is used in certain barrier contraceptives at high concentrations[17]. Chlorhexidine is a new, less irritating spermicide. Apart from its potential as a spermicide *in vivo*, it is also active *in vitro* against HIV in low concentrations[18]. The advantage of chlorhexidine is that it can diffuse into cervical mucus allowing more time in which to inactivate sperm and pathogens.

Far more research is now concentrated on producing contraceptive methods that give women more control, act probably at the vaginal or cervical level, and are safe and easily used. The goal today is the development of more effective and acceptable BCs. New chemical barriers which provide more options to women are under development. These are:

(1) C31G, (Biosyn, Philadelphia), a spermicidal, microbicidal and antiviral product, which, unlike nonoxynol-9, causes less irritation to the vaginal epithelium and diffuses into cervical mucus;

(2) 'Sulfated polysaccharide' (Population Council, New York City), a linear polysaccharide which prevents adherence of HIV and chlamydia to cells *in vitro*. The drug is not spermicidal;

(3) 'N-docosanol' (Lidak, La Jolla), a drug which has an extensive antiviral activity and may inhibit lipid-enveloped viruses. N-docosanol has also been shown to protect five out of six monkeys after vaginal exposure of simian immunodeficiency virus (SIV);

(4) 'Re Protect' (Johns Hopkins University, Baltimore), a buffering gel which preserves a low vaginal pH and does not irritate the vaginal flora; and

(5) 'Squalamine' (Magainin, Plymouth, Pennsylvania), a steroid-based compound which inhibits the sodium-hydrogen exchange on the cell surface and stops cell growth. Studies indicate that the compound is effective against *Neisseria gonorrhea*, Chlamydia, trachomatis, HIV and HSV. Squalamine appears to have a long-acting period and is well tolerated[1].

The following new chemical preparations are currently being tested: 'Triad' (University of Kentucky, Lexington) is an approach which combines a fast-releasing layer on the outer surface with intermediate-releasing granules and slow-releasing pellets, which allow rapid, but long-acting, spermicidal and anti-HIV effects. The 'Contraceptive gel' (Biotek, Woburn, Massachusetts) is a barrier, a harmless lipid substance which changes to a gel upon contact with the vaginal secretions. This gel physically and chemically blocks sperm within minutes of application[1].

Protection against sexually transmitted diseases

There are only a few procedures which women may follow to protect themselves from STDs and HIV. Most preventive strategies are designed around a limited number of partners and the use of latex condoms, but women cannot always reduce the number of partners, or male partners might not cooperate in the use of condoms. Barrier contraceptives provide protection against STDs and pelvic inflammatory disease and STD protection has a beneficial impact on the risk of tubal infertility and ectopic pregnancy. Toxic shock syndrome was found to be increased in women who use BCs, but the actual incidence is so rare that this risk is not clinically significant[19]. Barrier contraceptives may also protect against cervical diseases including cervical intraepithelial neoplasia[20].

Epidemiological studies and clinical trials should provide quantitative data from barrier method users and indicate which factors affect the level of protection. They should also indicate the method that combines the highest level of protection, ease of use and high acceptability, in order to promote their use in prevention campaigns. To evaluate the efficiency, protection, level of irritation and acceptability of two regimens of Protectaid®, a contraceptive vaginal sponge (Axcan Ltd, Mont St. Hilaire, Canada), we conducted a randomized clinical study. Both regimens were impregnated with an F-5 Gel, but with different doses of nonoxynol-9. F-5 Gel consists of benzalkonium chloride 1.0%, sodium cholate 0.5% and nonoxynol-9 0.5% in the first type, and nonoxynol 0.125% in the second. Dimethylpolysiloxane was used as dispersing agent and methylcellulose as a carrier. Sponges were prescribed to 35 women aged 20–35 years, who were randomly allocated into two groups. The first group consisted of 20 women and the first regimen (nonoxynol-9 0.5%) was given. The second group consisted of 15 women who were given the second regimen (nonoxynol-9 0.125%). All women showed normal ovulations and intact internal genitalia during the pretreatment examination.

During a 12-month period, the efficiency rate was 100% in both groups. At the 6-month interval, cervical cultures showed the presence of *Mycoplasma hominis* and *Candida albicans* in one and two cases, respectively, in the first group of women. In the second group, during the third month's tests, the cervical cultures showed *Gardnerella vaginalis* and β-*haemolytic streptococcus* in one and two cases, respectively. Patients were treated according to minor clinical symptoms. Colposcopical examination showed no cervical or vaginal lesion in either group. One case of irritation and one case of hyperemia of the vagina were found in the first group. No significant changes were found in the second group. The acceptability of the sponge was perfect with no complaints of inconvenience or discomfort. The Protectaid® contraceptive sponge with F-5 Gel is a modern contraceptive method, which allows easy insertion, fits the woman's vaginal shape and size, due to its supple construction, and maximizes comfort and discretion during sexual intercourse. Results do not indicate that the contraceptive sponge should be the only prophylaxis against STDs, since this substance does not protect all possible sites of infection. Although this regimen does offer a new and highly promising contraceptive method, the different concentrations of F-5 Gel indicate that a low content of nonoxynol-9 decreases the possibility of vaginal irritation but does not affect its contraceptive efficiency. The use of a sponge can be controlled by the sexually-active female who needs to profit by both spermicidal and anti-STD properties. In general, it allows a woman to be in control and enjoy discreet protection.

CONCLUSION

New, safe and efficient barrier contraceptive methods are needed to prevent pregnancy, as well as sexually transmitted diseases (STDs), and to improve compliance. The prevalence of STDs and human immunodeficiency virus (HIV) is still increasing. The HIV has become the most important sexually transmitted infection in the 1990s, and HIV prevention activities have become integrated into STD control programs. In addition to acquired immunodeficiency syndrome (AIDS), the long-term sequelae of STDs include infertility, ectopic pregnancy, pelvic inflammatory disease and cervical intraepithelial neoplasia. The impact of these diseases, in terms of financial cost and human suffering, has made STD control one of the nation's top public health priorities.

REFERENCES

1. Alexander N. Barriers to sexually transmitted diseases. *Sci Am Sci Med* 1996; 32–41
2. d'Oro LC, Parazzini F, Naldi L, Vecchia CL. Barrier methods of contraception, spermicides and sexually transmitted diseases: a review. *Genitourin Med* 1994; 70: 410–17
3. Richardson H. Recent developments in barrier methods of contraception. *Midwife, Health Visitor Comm Nurse* 1988; 24: 476–9
4. Stratton P, Alexander N. Prevention of sexually transmitted infections. Physical and chemical barrier methods. *Infect Dis Clin North Am* 1993; 7: 841–59
5. Hatcher R, Lee Warner D. New condoms for men and women, diaphragms, cervical caps and spermicides: overcoming barriers to barriers and spermicides. *Curr Opin Obstet Gynecol* 1992; 4: 513–21
6. Jivasak-Apimas S. Acceptability of the vaginal sheath 'Femshield' in Thai couples. *Contraception* 1991; 44: 183–90
7. Hickey M, Fraser IS. Contraception of the future. *Contemp Rev Obstet Gynecol* 1995; 7: 160–6
8. Hooton T, Hilier S, *et al. Escherichi coli* bacteriuria and contraceptive methols. *J Am Med Assoc* 1991; 265: 64–9
9. Hunt W, Gabbay L, Potts M. Lea's Shield, a new barrier contraceptive: preliminary clinical evaluations three-day tolerance study. *Contraception* 1994, 50: 551–61
10. Shihata A, Trussell J. New female intravaginal barrier contraceptive device: preliminary clinical trial. *Contraception* 1991, 44: 11–19
11. Allicotti GM, Jensen RH. Prophylactic properties of the Today contraceptive sponge. Presented at the *Annual Meeting of the Association of Planned Parenthood Professionals*, Seattle, USA, 1985

12. Jick H, Hannan MT. Vaginal spermicides and gonorrhea. *J Am Med Assoc* 1982; 248: 1619–21
13. Hicks DR, Martin LS. Inactivation of HTLV-111/LAV-infected cultures of normal human lymphocytes by nonoxynol-9 *in vitro*. *Lancet* 1985; 2: 1422–3
14. Polsky B, Baron P. *In vitro* inactivation of HIV-1 by contraceptive sponge containing nonoxynol-9. *Lancet* 1988; 2: 1456
15. Psychoyos A, Creatsas G, Hassan E, Georgoulias V, Gravanis A. Spermicidal and antiviral properties of cholic acid: contraceptive efficacy of a new vaginal sponge (Protectaid®) containing sodium cholate. *Hum Reprod* 1993, 8: 866–69
16. Wainberg MA, Spira B. Inactivation of human immunodeficiency virus Type 1 in tissue culture fluid and in genital secretions by the spermicide benzalkonium chloride. *J Clin Microbiol* 1990; 28: 156–8
17. Niruthisard S, Roddy R, Chutivongse S. The effects of frequent nonoxynol-9 use on the vaginal and cervical mucosa. *Sex Transm Dis* 1991; 176–9
18. Anonymous. Multipurpose spermicides. *Lancet* 1992, 340: 211–13
19. Schwartz B, Gaventa S, *et al.* Nonmenstrual toxic shock syndrome associated with barrier contraceptives: report of a case–control study. *Rev Infect Dis* 1989; 11: S43–5
20. Coker A, Hulka B, McCann M, *et al.* Barrier methods of contraception and cervical intraepithelial neoplasia. *Contraception* 1992; 45: 1–3

19 Female condoms

W. Bounds

Urgent need for a wider range of female-controlled barrier contraceptives that also protect against sexually transmitted diseases (STDs) has led to the development of female condom-like devices. However, the concept of a female condom is not new. Early versions, known as *Capote Blanco* and *Capote Anglaise*, were available in the 1920s[1] and in the 1960s[2], although not widely used. They consisted of a thick rubber tube to line the vagina and were held in position by a thick air-filled ring attached at the open end of the condom. It took the arrival of AIDS and a general rise in STDs to rekindle scientific interest in this type of barrier contraceptive. Several variants, often referred to as 'vaginal liners' or 'vaginal pouches', have been designed over recent years, although most are still in the very early stages of development and clinical testing. They include the Femidom (Reality), the Bikini Condom, Women's Choice and the Janesway condom. With the exception of Femidom, they are all made of latex rubber. The physical shapes of the Bikini Condom and the Janesway device have similarities in that both incorporate a pantie design, with the condom incorporated within the portion covering the vulva. The latter, however, differs from the Bikini Condom in that the latex condom section is detachable from the body of the pantie, which can be made of lace or other attractive fabric to enhance user-acceptability. No doubt, the aim of a Bikini-type design is to enable the woman to put on the garment well before initiation of intercourse, thus allowing more sexual spontaneity. To date, however, no published data on user-acceptability and efficacy in terms of contraception and STD prevention are available for Bikini-type condoms, nor for Women's Choice. The latter is similar in appearance to the *Capote Anglaise*, and is inserted by means of an introducer. Further development and clinical evaluation of the Bikini Condom and of Women's Choice is said to be 'on hold', and it remains to be seen whether these designs will become a realistic option for consumers.

Undoubtedly, the most advanced and widely tested female condom design is the Femidom, which is already in commercial use in the USA (where it is marketed under the trade name Reality) and in parts of Europe. Femidom was designed by a multidisciplinary team and is manufactured in the UK by Chartex International (now a subsidiary of Female Health Co., USA). Combining features of a male condom and a diaphragm, the condom consists of a soft, loose-fitting thermoplastic polyurethane sheath, 17 cm in length, the open end of which is attached to a 70 mm diameter flexible polyurethane ring. A separate removable polyurethane ring, 65 mm in diameter, lies inside the condom where it serves as an introducer and as a means of anchoring the device in the vagina. Once inserted, the outer ring lies against the vulva and protects it and the base of the penis during intercourse. A pilot study of user-acceptability by the Margaret Pyke Centre, UK in 1988[3], which involved testing a 15 cm long version with a separately applied inert lubricant in 24 self-selected married/cohabiting couples suggested that, with appropriate modifications in its structural design and method of use, Femidom could become a realistic contraceptive/STD prevention option. These preliminary findings led to the development of the 17 cm long, prelubricated condom, currently in use. In 1988, the same research group initiated a much larger prospective study, designed to assess contraceptive efficacy and user-acceptability during 12 months of observation, which involved a 17 cm long condom coated with a nonoxynol-9-containing lubricant. One hundred and six women, of whom 100 were eligible for efficacy evaluation, used Femidom for a total of 441 months[4]. Seven accidental pregnancies were documented, representing a typical-use (use-effectiveness) failure rate by life-table of 15% at 12 months (95% confidence interval 3.5–26). Of these, four conceptions are known to be associated with inconsistent use of Femidom in the relevant cycle, while the remaining three appear to be true method failures. To date, the only other published contraceptive efficacy study is a multicenter clinical trial conducted in the USA and Latin America, which involved observation of 328 women over 6 months of use[5]. Gross cumulative accidental pregnancy rates of 12.4% (USA) and 22.2% (Latin America) were documented for typical-use, while rates for perfect-use were 2.6% and 9.5% for the US and Latin American centers, respectively. These data indicate that Femidom provides contraceptive efficacy in the same range as other barrier methods, particularly if used consistently and correctly. Possible reasons for true method failures include the entire condom (including the outer ring) being accidentally pushed into the vagina during coitus, reported by 32% of women in the UK study to have happened on at least one occasion, and inadvertent insertion of the penis outside, rather than within, Femidom, reported by 25% of the study participants. Adding more lubricant, holding the condom in place and guiding the penis into Femidom may reduce these risks, although some patients in the UK study considered the need to be alert and guard against these events an unwelcome intrusion in their lovemaking. As is the case with other barrier contraceptives, there is a learning curve, and mishaps during Femidom insertion and use are likely to decline as users gain confidence and become familiar with the product.

How widely the female condom will be used as a contraceptive and/or for STD protection by the general public will also largely depend on its acceptability by the woman and her partner. Clinical trials to date have concentrated mainly on short-term acceptability, with volunteers being invited to express an opinion on the basis of having tried a small number of devices (e.g. 6–12) involving short periods of observation, while relying on another method of contraception[6–13]. Most of these studies reported 'acceptability' rates of approximately 60–100%. However, it remains to be seen whether such an initially favorable response can be shown during sustained longer-term use. The above-cited efficacy studies[4,5], which involved observations over periods of 12 and 6 months respectively, suggest more moderate levels of acceptability, as measured by continuation rates. For example, of the 106 women who started the use of Femidom in the UK study[4] (and who had selected themselves from approximately 1000 potential volunteers who had initially expressed interest in the study), only 10% were still using the condom 12 months later, the majority (56%) having abandoned the method because they had found aspects of its use unsatisfactory. Assuming that the 20 women (19% of the 106 recruited) who had to stop the use of Femidom prematurely on account of no further supplies being available from the manufacturer had continued its use, still only 29% would have completed the 12-month study. Somewhat higher continuation rates were observed in the US/Latin American study[5], where 66.5% and 44.9% of users completed the 6-month trial, respectively. Undoubtedly, there exists a subgroup of women and their partners who consider Femidom to be their most appropriate contraceptive and who will use it in the long term. Their comments that the loose-fitting polyurethane membrane causes less loss of sensitivity, compared with a male condom, should encourage further attempts to create loose-fitting condom variants, both for male and female use. Possible improvements in product design and increasing familiarity with the method as its availability increases may lead to more widespread use. This is particularly relevant for women considered at high risk of contracting STDs, especially AIDS. Although Femidom's clinical efficacy in STD prevention has not yet been widely investigated, preliminary evidence suggests a protective effect. An *in vitro* study, designed to test Femidom for permeability by the human immunodeficiency virus (HIV) and cytomegalovirus (CMV), showed no viral leakage in three trials for each virus[14], while another study, which investigated the incidence of semen leakage in the vagina through tears, leaks and spillage, documented a lower leakage rate for Femidom (3%) compared with a male condom (11.6%)[6]. To date, the only published clinical investigation into Femidom's efficacy in STD prevention is an American study, which looked at reinfection rates with trichomonas in women who had been treated for the infection immediately prior to study entry[15]. Of 54 women who were assigned to use Femi-dom, no reinfection occurred in the 20 women who had used the condom consistently, whereas 14.7% of non-compliant Femidom users and 14% of 50 controls were found to be reinfected within the predetermined 45-day period of observation. These findings are most encouraging and demonstrate the importance of consistent use in order to derive maximum protection. Similar studies, involving other STD-causing organisms, e.g. chlamydia, gonorrhea and HIV are urgently needed in order to provide clinical evidence of Femidom's prophylactic potential during actual use. In this respect, the results of several studies underway in the USA, Zimbabwe and Thailand are awaited with much interest.

In conclusion, the search for effective and acceptable female condoms is a welcome development, as it will increase the contraceptive and STD protection options open to women. Of the various models created to date, Femidom is the most advanced in terms of technical development and clinical testing and is the only product in commercial use. Femidom's contraceptive efficacy appears to be within the range reported for other barrier contraceptives, but more clinical studies are urgently needed to confirm its prophylactic potential against STDs. Its effectiveness will largely depend upon consistent and correct use and on the product's ability to maintain an effective physical barrier throughout penetrative intercourse. Potential users should familiarize themselves with the condom to determine whether it suits them before abandoning more effective non-intercourse related methods, e.g. the contraceptive pill or intrauterine device (IUD). As with most innovative contraceptives, curiosity and initial public acceptance, as documented in short-term acceptability studies, appear to be high, but longer-term acceptability, based on continuation rates, needs to be determined. If sustained and consistent use can be achieved, perhaps with the addition of possible further refinements of the current design, Femidom can play an important role in pregnancy and STD prevention.

REFERENCES

1. Stopes M. *Contraception: Theory, History and Practice.* London: Bale Sons and Danielson Ltd, 1923; 169–170
2. Consumers Association UK. Capote Anglaise. *Which?* June 9, 1966; 89
3. Bounds W, Guillebaud J, Stewart L, *et al.* A female condom (Femshield): a study of its user acceptability. *Br J Fam Plann* 1988; 14: 83–7
4. Bounds W, Guillebaud J, Newman GB. Female condom (Femidom). A clinical study of its use-effectiveness and patient acceptability. *Br J Fam Plann* 1992; 18: 36–41
5. Farr G, Gabelnick H, Sturgen K, *et al.* Contraceptive efficacy and acceptability of the female condom. *Am J Publ Health* 1994; 84: 1960–4
6. Leeper MA, Conrardy M. Preliminary evaluation of REALITY, a condom for women to wear. *Adv Contracept* 1989; 5: 229–35
7. Sakondhavat C, Potter L. Further testing of female condoms. *Br J Fam Plann* 1990; 15: 129–30
8. Jivasak-Apimas S. Acceptability of the vaginal sheath (Femshield) in Thai couples. *Contraception* 1991; 44: 183–90
9. Ray S, Bassett M, Maposhere C, *et al.* Acceptability of the female condom in Zimbabwe: positive but male centred responses. *Reprod Health Matt* 1995; 5: 68–79
10. Gollub EL, Stein Z, El-Sadr W. Short-term acceptability of the female condom among staff and patients at a New York City Hospital. *Fam Plann Perspect* 1995; 27: 155–8
11. Sapire KE. The female condom (Femidom) – a study of user acceptability. *South Afr Med J* 1995; 85: 1081–4

12. Masters L, Mostyn P, Bunting P, *et al.* How do attenders of a genitourinary medicine clinic feel about the female condom? *Br J Fam Plann* 1996; 21: 135–8
13. Ford N, Mathie E. The acceptability and experience of the female condom, Femidom among family planning clinic attenders. *Br J Fam Plann* 1993; 19: 187–92
14. Drew, WL, Blair M, Miner RC, *et al.* Evaluation of the virus permeability of a new condom for women. *Sex Transm Dis* 1990; 17: 110–12
15. Soper DE, Shoupe D, Shangold GA, *et al.* Prevention of vaginal trichomoniasis by compliant use of the female condom. *Sex Transm Dis* 1993; 20: 137–9

This paper has been reproduced from *Eur J Contracept Reprod Health Care* 1997; 2: 113–16

20 Lea® Contraceptivum: a new concept in female barrier contraception

H. Salzer, S. Jinniate and S. Tatschl

INTRODUCTION

The Lea® Contraceptivum is a new barrier contraceptive made of a soft, medical-grade rubber, and is intended to prevent pregnancy by its ability to cover the cervix.

Lea® Contraceptivum has a unique design comprising a cup-shaped voluminous bowl, designed to completely cover the cervix and, at the same time, by virtue of its thick posterior lip, to fully occupy the posterior fornix. The device is held in place by the vaginal walls and not by the cervix. The control loop, which is also an integral part of Lea® Contraceptivum, was designed to assist ease of placement and ease of removal. The device is manufactured in one piece. It is a 'one-size-fits-all' device and can be left in place for up to 48 h.

With good hygienic care, the new contraceptive can be used from 6 to 9 months before being replaced. It is recommended to use Lea® together with a spermicidal gel, to act as a lubricant and also to enhance the efficacy rate.

The new contraceptive was studied extensively in our clinic to evaluate its safety, tolerance and acceptability. Between May and November 1995, 89 women were enrolled in this study at the Wilhelminenspital/gynäkologisch-geburtshilfliche Department. Our clinic was chosen as one of the centers to perform a feasibility, safety and tolerance study to familiarize the physician community with this new device, as well as to confirm the clinical results obtained in the United States.

OBJECTIVE OF STUDY

The objective of the study was to evaluate the safety, tolerance and acceptability of the Lea® Contraceptivum, a new female barrier contraceptive device. In this study, the women were given no information or guidance by the physicians on how to insert the device. The Lea® Contraceptivum was given to them with the 'Instructions for Use' and they were told to use the device after reading the instructions. Although this study was not designed as an efficacy study, the

Table 1 Age and parity of women in study (%)

Age (years)	
< 20	0
20–25	9
26–30	26
31–35	44
36–40	10
> 40	11
Parity	
0	38
1	30
2	28
3	3
4	1

women were told to use the device as their only means of contraception. A secondary objective of this study was to familiarize Austrian physicians with this new means of contraception.

STUDY DESIGN

The women are regular patients in our clinic. In the interviews with them, the new device was described and they were told the study objectives. The women that consented to be included in this study were given Lea® Contraceptivum with the 'Instructions for Use'. No explanations were given to them with regard to the evaluation of the safety, tolerance and acceptability, or the general effectiveness of the device if used without the help of a health-care professional (as an over-the-counter product).

Although the women were at risk of pregnancy, this study was not designed fully to evaluate the failure rate of the device. The primary parameters for evaluation were the safety, tolerance and acceptability of the device.

MATERIALS AND METHODS

Study population

Between May and November 1995, 89 women were enrolled in the study at the Wilhelminenspital/gynäkologisch. The age of the women was between 20 and 44 years. Table 1 presents the different age groups of the study subjects. Most women were parous (62%) and 38% were nulliparous. The majority of the parous women had one or two children.

Table 2 Medical history of women in study (n = 89)

Uneventful	56
Prior surgery	15
Excessive bleeding	13
Herpes genitalis	6
Uterine prolapse	1
Ectopic pregnancy	4
Cesarean section	7
Ovarian cyst	5
Others	20

Table 3 Reasons for choosing new contraceptive (n)

Cannot tolerate contraceptive pill	20
Contraindication to contraceptive pill	5
Tiredness from contraceptive pill	20
Temporary pause from contraceptive pill	2
Worries about long-term hormonal effects	9
Post-partum/breast-feeding	19
Back-up method	11
Partner unwillingness to use condom	2
Desire to 'space' children	3
Dissatisfied with existing methods	2
Perimenopausal contraception	2
Recommended by physician	2
Price	1

Medical and surgical history at admission

Most women had no remarkable medical or surgical history (56 subjects). Fifteen had had prior surgery, 13 had a history of excessive menstrual bleeding, six had had herpes genitalis, one woman had had uterine prolapse, four had had ectopic pregnancy, seven had had Cesarean section, five had had an ovarian cyst and 20 had had miscellaneous unspecified problems (Table 2).

CONTRACEPTIVE REASONS FOR CHOOSING LEA® CONTRACEPTIVUM

Table 3 gives the different reasons for choosing a new contraceptive. Most of the women were former 'pill' users (56 subjects), 19 women were breast-feeding and 11 used the Lea® Contraceptivum as a back-up method (when they could not use the contraceptive pill.

USE OF LEA® CONTRACEPTIVUM

Of the 89 women who entered the study, 7% used the Lea® Contraceptivum more than twice a week, 48% used the device twice a week, 38% used the device approximately 4 times a month and 7% never used the device and were considered as discontinuations (six subjects).

RESULTS

Eighty-nine women entered the study and 83 women completed at least 3 months of use.

Women lost to follow-up

No subjects were lost to follow-up. The six women that did not use the Lea® Contraceptivum indicated their reasons for not using the device.

Discontinuations

Six women did not use the Lea® Contraceptivum for various reasons. One subject had difficulties understanding the 'Instructions for Use', one said the device was too bulky, one was afraid her partner might feel the device, two did not have sex for personal reasons and one woman said her partner objected to the use of the device.

SAFETY OF LEA® CONTRACEPTIVUM

Although the women were given the device without any special screening and used it frequently, no serious side-effects were reported after a few months of use. The only occurrence worth mentioning is that one woman had a urinary tract infection, but this was not necessarily caused by the device as 3% of women can have recurrent urinary tract infection even if they do not use any barrier method. One subject reported blood spotting on the bowl of the device which could have been a remnant of her menses. All other complaints were minor. No other side-effects were reported.

ACCEPTABILITY OF LEA® CONTRACEPTIVUM

The device was generally well accepted. Table 4 gives the general impressions of the 83 women who used the Lea® Contraceptivum and who commented about the device and its use.

Insertion

A total of 72% said they had no problems with insertion (very satisfied or satisfied); 28% said they had some difficulties or use of the device was unpleasant.

Table 4 Impression and comments after use by active users (n = 83)

	Very satisfied (%)	*Satisfied* (%)	*Dissatisfied* (%)
Insertion	47	25	28
Tolerance	52	32	16
Removal	26	41	33
Acceptability	39	30	31

Table 5 Natures of complaints by users (n)

Problems with insertion and removal	3
Removal unpleasant	1
Insertion might disturb spontaneity	1
Complicated manipulation	2
Suction too strong	1
Pressure on pubic bone	1
Abdominal pressure	3
Dullness in abdomen	1
Feeling of foreign body	3
Pain during sexual intercourse	3
Felt by partner during sexual intercourse	22
Subjective feeling about longer menstrual period	2
Blood spotting	1
Too big and too thick	5
Seemed unhygienic or malodorous	8
Difficult to clean	1
Urinary tract infection	1
Fear at time of bowel movements	1
Psychological barrier	2

Removal

Of the participants 67% had no problems with removal and 33% had some complaints, such as 'suction too strong'. All women were successful in removing the device in all instances. They soon learned how to break the suction.

Tolerance

Of the participants 84% tolerated the device very well; 16% did not like the device for one reason or another. Table 5 reports all the complaints or comments made by the users of Lea® Contraceptivum.

Acceptability

The study showed 69% of the participants to be satisfied with the Lea® Contraceptivum and 31% to be dissatisfied. A total of 51% said they would continue to use the device as a means of contraception; 45% said they would use it as the sole means, while 6% said they would use it as a back-up method. Another 7% said they might use the device and 42% said they would not.

DISCUSSION

This study was intended to test how well the Lea® Contraceptivum would be tolerated by and acceptable to women that had no training or explanation regarding the device from their physician. Clearly, this study has shown that the Lea® Contraceptivum is well tolerated and 51% of the couples questioned wished to continue to use this new means of contraception.

The women were chosen to enter the study with very liberal inclusion criteria, yet no apparent safety issues have been raised by their experience. Frankly, we did not expect to find such high acceptability. We were sceptical that one size of any device would fit all women, but this study has confirmed the 'one-size-fits-all' concept. It is also interesting to note that the age and parity of the subjects, as well as the position of the uterus or the shape of the cervix, had no influence on the insertion, removal or acceptability of the Lea® Contraceptivum.

When women were asked what they liked about the device, they responded that the Lea® Contraceptivum offered a better sense of safety than their current contraceptive and it allowed normal spontaneity as it can be used continuously for up to 48 h.

Disadvantages

Some women perceived the Lea® Contraceptivum as large and bulky. This concern seemed to be satisfied once the device had been used. There is a need to stress very clearly in the 'Instructions for Use' that experience shows that the volume of the device does not present a real problem and, furthermore, it is necessary for proper efficacy.

Another concern is the fact that some women did not understand the importance of breaking the suction before pulling out the device.

It will be interesting to compare such a group with a group of women that have received training by the physician. The acceptability can be considered as excellent in this study. It might even be higher if the users receive training by a health-care professional.

Indications for use and advantages of Lea® Contraceptivum

The following are the situations for which, in our opinion, the Lea® Contraceptivum can be used:

(1) For women who are dissatisfied with the available methods;

(2) For women who do not want to or cannot use hormones;

(3) For women who are post-partum and are breast feeding;

(4) For women who have infrequent sex (weekend partner) or do not have a steady partner;

(5) For women who want to be in control and their partners are unwilling to use the condom;

(6) As a back-up method (e.g. when women forget to take the 'pill' for a day or two);

(7) As a barrier method that covers the cervix; this method might have an advantage in reducing the transmission of sexually transmitted diseases (STDs) but probably not human immunodeficiency virus (HIV);

(8) For women who are on the 'pill' but, in certain stages of their reproductive life, should not take the 'pill' or are on 'holiday' from the 'pill'.

Efficacy

Although this study was not designed as an efficacy study, the women were at risk and it is significant that no women became pregnant while using the Lea® Contraceptivum. By the end of October 1995, the 83 women who used the device had accumulated 332 women months without any pregnancies. These results demonstrate that the effectiveness of the Lea® Contraceptivum is very high.

CONCLUSION

The Lea® Contraceptivum was well tolerated by the users. This study has reconfirmed the concept of 'one-size-fits-all' and that this new female contraceptive method can be successfully used by women after they have read the 'Instructions for Use'. The device seems to be very effective in preventing pregnancy. The device has an acceptability that is very high and it is a safe method.

The Lea® Contraceptivum should be a welcome alternative for women who are dissatisfied with existing contraceptive methods.

21 Methods of abortion in Europe during the first trimester of pregnancy

E. Aubeny

INTRODUCTION

Over the last 20 years in almost all of Europe, the legalization of abortion has eliminated clandestine abortions and their resulting serious complications. Today, abortions are performed by doctors on healthy women. Consequently, the techniques developed to treat those complicated procedures have been modified and improved in the last 20 years, thanks to new drugs and some medical teams interested in these problems.

At the present time, two abortion methods are used in Europe: the surgical method, which has been used for many years and has been greatly improved, and the medical method, a new method introduced in 1982.

THE SURGICAL METHOD

There are three steps in this method of abortion. All of them have been improved in the last few years.

Cervical dilatation

Cervical dilatation is the most critical step in the surgical method. Problems such as a uterine perforation or a torn cervix often occur at this time. At the present time, dilatation is sometimes peformed with laminaria placed in the cervix before the abortion, which is an efficient method but requires hospitalization for 24 h and causes severe pelvic pain. More often, the dilatation is performed at the time of the abortion using metallic dilators. This method of dilatation is effective and less painful, especially if local anesthesia has been given first, and requires no hospitalization.

In the future, dilatation of the cervix will be prepared and assisted by drugs ingested before the procedure. Two types of products are currently being investigated: the antiprogesterone mifepristone (RU 486) and prostaglandin analogs.

The antiprogesterone mifepristone (RU 486)

Many trials have been performed with RU 486 to investigate cervical dilatation by the drug. They all demonstrated its effectiveness. One of the most conclusive trials was performed by Lefevre and colleagues[1]. This trial shows that, from a dose of 100 mg, the mifepristone produces maximum dilatation of the cervix, after a 48-h delay. Mifepristone at a dose of 600 mg has been authorized for this purpose in the UK since 1993. In France, 200 mg mifepristone is often used for this procedure. At the Antoine Béclère and the Broussais hospitals (Paris), more than 5000 women have received 200 mg of mifepristone 48 h before undergoing a surgical abortion. In this way, mifepristone allows easy dilatation of the cervix and makes the abortion safer, as well as less painful. It also allows a fast aspiration, since the removed egg is drawn up without being broken, avoiding any retention.

This well-tolerated drug is very helpful, especially in abortion of primiparae and very early pregnancy.

The prostaglandin analogs

Different prostaglandin analogs have been tested for their effect on cervical dilatation. At the present time, two analogs are used predominantly: gemeprost and misoprostol. Research has been carried out to compare the efficacy of these two products. Platz-Clistenses and colleagues[2] have conducted a trial on this topic. Gemeprost was introduced into the vagina 3–5 h before the abortion procedure and misoprostol was taken orally either 17–19 h or 8–10 h before the abortion. The results showed that the effectiveness of the two products is comparable and that the secondary effects (digestive problems, pelvic pain) are identical. In addition, no difference in efficacy was shown between the misoprostol ingested 8–10 h prior to the abortion, and the misoprostol taken 17–19 h prior to the abortion. However, the misoprostol ingested earlier, before the procedure, induced spontaneous abortions and metrorrhagia. Consequently, the use of misoprostol taken later may be preferred as it has the advantage of being both less expensive and easier to administer.

Research has also been carried out to determine the optimal dose and the best way to administer misoprostol, vaginally or orally. Schaub[3] has compared misoprostol 200 μg taken orally with 400 μg of the drug administered vaginally and 400 μg taken orally, all given 12 h before the abortion. The greatest cervical dilatation was obtained with misoprostol 400 μg, administered vaginally. Secondary effects such as pain and digestive problems were equivalent in the three groups, and vaginal administration did not decrease them. Metrorrhagia and hemorrhage, however, were more prevalent when the product was vaginally administered.

In conclusion, misoprostol 400 μg, inserted vaginally 12 h prior to abortion, appears to be an appropriate dose.

Mantion (Amiens, France) has used misoprostol widely at a dose of 400 μg, ingested 12 h before the abortion (personal communication). A proportion of women had to undergo emergency curettage due to incomplete abortion during that lapse of time. Consequently, today, misoprostol is taken 4–5 h before the procedure and since the introduction of this regimen, no curetting has been required.

In summary, drug dilatation of the cervix prior to aspiration is an advantage, making abortion safer, quicker and painless. It should be used increasingly.

The evacuation of the uterine content

Before the legalization of abortion, women would often be admitted to hospital with infections caused by clandestine procedures. In these cases, curettage was deemed to be legitimate, permitting complete evacuation of the uterus and wide dilatation of the cervix to allow drainage. Today, this procedure is no longer justifiable since women are admitted to hospital before having received any intrauterine operation, and it has been replaced with a vacuum aspiration method developed in the 1970s. This method is as effective as curettage. It is less traumatizing for the uterus: disappearance of dilatation of the isthmus and decrease of the synechia of the uterine body. Furthermore, it is less painful and it allows the use of light anesthetic.

Anesthetics

At last, it is generally admitted that abortions should be painless. Pain should not be the price to pay for having an abortion; therefore, anesthetic may be considered as being part of the abortion. Two techniques of anesthetic are used primarily: local anesthetic and general anesthetic.

Local anesthetic

Use of local anesthetic has increased over the last few years, benefiting from the replacement of the curettage by aspiration, a less painful technique. Local anesthetic is performed either by use of xylocaine alone or by use of adrenalized xylocaine at 1/200 000. The dose varied between 10 and 15 ml. It is para- or intracervically injected, or both techniques are used together.

Local anesthetic (LA):

(1) Is effective: it enables women to have a good analgesia;

(2) Is much safer than general anesthetic. There are 0.15 deaths for every 100 000 patients (four times less than with general anesthetic). The immediate complications are also less frequent than under general anesthetic (GA) (uterine perforation: LA 0.13%, GA 0.29%; hemorrhage: LA 0.32%, GA 0.54%)[4];

(3) Is economic since the xylocaine is not expensive;

(4) Enables patients to spend less time at the hospital (from 30 min to 3 h if there has been premedication), which is also economic.

Local anesthetic appears to be the correct alternative for women who accept involvement in their abortion.

General anesthetic

Thanks to the progress in anesthetics, abortions can and must be performed in ambulatory patients, with 6 h of hospitalization being enough. A 24-h hospitalization is not justifiable, apart from exceptional cases. However, there is no risk-free anesthetic. Precautions must be taken as in any other anesthetic and a consultation performed by a physician must precede the procedure.

General anesthetic allows women less involvement in their abortion and to feel no pain. Consequently, some women prefer this kind of anesthetic and it is important that they can be offered the choice.

In summary, anesthetic is right for women, and is now performed in an ambulatory way. Local anesthetic is safer than general anesthetic. The distribution of these types of anesthetic varies widely in Europe from one country to another. Almost 100% of anesthetic techniques are general in the UK whereas nearly 100% are local in the Netherlands! Is it a question of physicians' habits or women's requests? This is a matter for debate; however, it seems important that women should be able to choose the method of anesthetic that they prefer.

Results of the surgical method

Results vary widely according to operator skills, but generally, international statistics show[5]:

(1) Effectiveness: ongoing pregnancies are between 1/1000 and 2/1000;

(2) Complications: it is important to underline that complications are less frequent between 8 and 10 weeks of amenorrhea. They are more frequent both before and after this period:

   (a) Perforations: between 1/1000 and 1/3000;

   (b) Serious perforations with lesion of adjoining organ: between 1/10 000 and 1/20 000;

   (c) Hemorrhages: transfusions necessary during a vacuum aspiration abortion under local anesthetic: 1/5000;

   (d) Local regional infections: 1%.

Prophylactic antibiotherapy is still subject to discussion.

In summary, thanks to technical progress made in the dilatation of the cervix, evacuation of the uterus and anesthetic, surgical abortion (if performed by trained physicians) is an effective, safe and painless procedure. Its safety is increased further if it is performed between the 8th and the 10th weeks of amenorrhea, and under local anesthetic.

MEDICAL ABORTION IN EUROPE

Women have always asked for a medical method of abortion. Mifepristone (RU 486) converted this wish into a reality. Its use is authorized in France (1989), in the UK (1992) and in Sweden (1993). It is also used in China.

Mifepristone is a potent antiprogestin synthesized by Roussel Uclaf in 1980. It prevents progesterone action by taking its place, at the receptor level, in the target cells. It has been used to prevent early pregnancy since 1983, at the instigation of Professor E.E. Baulieu.

The drug was administered alone, in clinical trials for pregnancies up to 42 days of amenorrhea, at a dose of 600 mg in one oral intake. The efficiency of this method was found to be 80%; however, this percentage was considered insufficient and the method was discontinued[6]. Thus, since 1987, at the suggestion of Professor Bigdeman, a very low dose of prostaglandin analog has been administered 48 h after mifepristone, in order to increase the rate of success.

The present regimen in the three countries where this method is authorized (France, Sweden and the UK) is as follows:

(1) Day 1: mifepristone (600 mg) taken at an authorized center.

(2) Day 3: 48 h later, administration of a prostaglandin analog in the center, followed by medical supervision in the center.

(3) Between days 10 and 14: check-up visit.

Prostaglandin analogs used are different, however, and consequently the maximum length of pregnancy at which each procedure is undertaken stands as follows: in France, misoprostol (Cytotec) up to 49 days of amenorrhea; in the UK and Sweden, gemeprost (Cervagem) up to 63 days of amenorrhea.

The procedure used in France

The prostaglandin analog used in France is misoprostol. Misoprostol (Cytotec), an oral prostaglandin E_1 analog, has been used since 1987 to prevent stomach ulcers in many other countries, at triple the dosage used in early abortion, and was used for 6 weeks at the lower dose without any major complication coming to light. The drug is easy to use because it is taken orally, it is easy to store since it does not need to be kept cool and its price is reasonable. Therefore, there are numerous reasons for using this product.

The first trial of this regimen, using mifepristone + misprostol was performed in 1991, in the Orthogenie Center, Broussais Hospital, Paris, followed by a successful multicenter study carried out by Roussel Uclaf. These trials were successful; consequently, in 1992, the agreement of the French Ministry of Health was given for this regimen which is now widely used in France.

The schedule of administration of mifepristone 600 mg + misoprostol 400 μg is as follows:

(1) Day 1: mifepristone 600 mg taken at an authorized center. Patients afterwards return home.

(2) Day 3: 48 h later, two tablets of misoprostol are taken at the center, with 4 h of monitoring at the center. After this time, the patients return home, whether expulsion has taken place or not.

(3) Day 8–12: the follow-up visit. Ultrasound scan or human chorionic gonadotropin measurement are performed if the expulsion has not taken place at the center.

The results of this trial are shown in Table 1.

Variation of the regimen

An alternative regimen is mifepristone 600 mg + misoprostol 400 μg + 400 μg misoprostol. Many teams give a second dose of 400 μg of misoprostol to the patients if they have not expelled 3 h after the initial dose of 400 μg of misoprostol. In the Orthogenie Center at Broussais Hospital, from 1994 to 1995, 903 patients were included in this protocol.

This variation of the regimen increases the rate of success (Table 2). This practice increased the number of patients who expelled at the hospital: expulsion within 3 h, 48.8%; expulsion in the 4th hour, 25.8%. In total, 74.64% of patients expelled at the hospital. It is important to underline that the women who expel at the hospital do not need an ultrasound examination to ensure that the procedure was successful. This regimen is used more and more often in France.

It is important to note that the agreement of the French Ministry of Health for administering mifepristone + misoprostol was given for pregnancy up to 49 days of amenorrhea; however, a trial conducted in 1992 by Roussel to evaluate the efficiency and tolerance of this combination up to 63 days of amenorrhea showed that, as pregnancy advanced, the efficiency of this combination decreased slightly between 49 and 56 days of amenorrhea, from 95.4% to 93.4%; significantly between 56 and 63 days of amenorrhea, from 93.4% to 86.8%; and the frequency of hemorrhage increased: 1% between 49 and 56 days of amenorrhea and 2.5% between 56 and 63 days of amenorrhea.

Therefore, in France, in order to ensure safety and efficiency for ambulatory women, this method is used only up to 49 days of amenorrhea.

Table 1 Results from the multicenter study of 1286 cases using 600 mg mifepristone + 400 μg misoprostol, managed by Roussel France at the request of the French Government in 1992[7]

Success rate (%)	95.4
Failure rate (%)	
total	4.6
ongoing pregnancies terminated by a surgical method	1.5
incomplete expulsion	2.8
needed for hemostatic procedure	0.3

Table 2 Results from the trial at the Orthogenie Center, Broussais Hospital, Paris. Mifepristone (600 mg) + misoprostol (400 μg) followed by a second dose of misoprostol (400 μg) were given to 903 patients

Success rate (%)	98.6
Failure rate (%)	
total	1.4
ongoing pregnancy	0.1
pregnancy stopped but not expelled	0.5
metrorrgahia treated with aspiration	0.7
hemorrhage treated with aspiration	0.1

The procedure in England and Sweden

The prostaglandin analog used is gemeprost (Cervagem), a vaginal prostaglandin E_1 analog which is very effective; no major problem has been reported with its use. It is efficient until 63 days of amenorrhea, but it is very painful with 30% of patients asking for painkillers and 4% of them needing opiate. It is also expensive and difficult to use (it must be kept in a freezer).

The schedule of administration is:

(1) Day 1: mifepristone 600 mg taken at an authorized center followed by 4 h of monitoring in the center.

(2) Day 3: 36–48 h later, one vaginal suppository of gemeprost is administered at the center followed by 6 h of monitoring.

(3) Day 12: control visit.

The rate of efficiency is 95.5%[9].

Table 3 Comparison of methods of medical abortion used in France, the UK and Sweden

		Dose regimen		
	Gestation limit (days of amenorrhea)	*Mifepristone (RU 486)*	*Prostaglandin analog*	*Hours spent in hospital*
France	49	600 mg	misoprostol 400 µg or 800 µg orally	RU 486 0 h misoprostol 4 h
UK, Sweden	63	600 mg	gemeprost 1 mg vaginally	RU 486 4 h gemeprost 6 h

Table 4 Comparison of abortion success rates and side-effects between the methods of medical abortion used in France, the UK and Sweden

	Abortion success rates	*Blood transfusion*	*Pelvic pain*
France	RU 486 + misoprostol 400 µg = 95.4%	0.1%	20% need painkillers, no opiate required
UK, Sweden	RU 486 + gestodene = 95.5%	0.9%	31% need painkillers, 21% need opiate

In summary, both techniques are:

(1) Efficient: 95.5% rate of success, more with 800 μg misoprostol (98.5%);

(2) Safe: no major problem has been reported since sulprostone has been stopped.

The techniques have an equivalent success rate to the surgical method. The French technique emphasizes the ambulatory aspect and the tolerance (painless, shorter time in the hospital) whereas the UK and Swedish technique gives more importance to the use of the procedure at a later stage of pregnancy.

Acceptability of medical abortion

Women choose the medical method of abortion because there is no surgery, no anesthetic, it is more natural and more confidential. This method is used increasingly and in 1995 accounted for 27% of abortions in France, 18% of abortions in Sweden and 8% of abortions in the UK (this low rate is due to extended waiting times for an abortion). In France, more than 200 000 women have used this procedure.

CONCLUSION

Since the 1970s, women have been offered methods of abortion which have greatly improved and diversified, which have become safe, effective and painless and which may be used in an ambulatory way. The challenge for the year 2000 is that women should have the right to choose freely the method which suits them best. However, these improvements cannot solve the painful moral problem of abortion.

REFERENCES

1. Lefevre Y, Proulx L, Elie R, Poulin O, Lanza E. The effects of RU 486 on cervical ripening. Clinical studies. *Am J Obstet Gynecol* 1990; 162: 61–5
2. Platz-Christensen JJ, Nielsen S, Hamberger L. Is misoprostol the drug of choice for induced cervical ripening in early pregnancy termination. *Acta Obstet Gynecol Scand* 1995; 74: 809–12
3. Schaub B, Fuhrer P, Sainte Rose D. Le misoprostol par voie vaginale avant interruption volontaire de grossesse chez la nullipare. *Cont Fert Sex* 1996; 24: 67–71
4. Grimes D. Local versus general anesthesia: which is safer for performing suction curettage abortion? *Am J Obstet Gynecol* 1979; 135: 1030–6
5. Cesbron P. 20 ans d'expérience d'interruption volontaire de grossesse en France. Bilan et perspectives. ANCIC Moulin March 1996
6. Couzinet B, Le Strat N, Ulmann A. Termination of early pregnancy by the progesterone antagonist RU 486. *N Engl J Med* 1986; 315: 1565–70

7. Peyron R. Early termination of pregnancy with mifepristone (RU 486) and the orally active prostaglandin misoprostol. *N Engl J Med* 1993; 21: 1509–13
8. Aubeny E, Peyron R. Termination of early pregnancy up to 63 D.A. with mifepristone and increasing dose of misoprostol. *Int J Fertil*, Supplement 2, 1995
9. UK multicentre trial. The efficiency and tolerance of mifepristone and prostaglandin in first trimester termination of pregnancy. *J Obstet Gynecol* 1990; 97: 480–6

This paper has been reproduced from *Eur J Contracept Reprod Health Care* 1997; 2: 75–80

22 Post-abortion contraceptive counselling: a matter of attitudes

R.H.W. van Lunsen

INTRODUCTION

In The Netherlands, only 25% of all women asking for an abortion are pregnant because they did not use any contraceptive method and only 12.2% because they used an unreliable method (rhythm or withdrawal). Almost 60% became pregnant while they were using oral contraceptives, condoms or an intrauterine device (IUD)[1]. The majority of abortions, thus, is performed on women who used a contraceptive method that failed, either because of method failures or because something else went wrong (ruptured condom, missed pills, unnoticed expulsion of the IUD etc.). Of the women not using any contraceptive method prior to the unplanned pregnancy, the majority became pregnant after unexpected or even involuntary sexual contact. Some women who request termination of pregnancy become pregnant because they are ambivalent about having children. Others initially plan a pregnancy but change their minds because of unexpected changes in their socioeconomic status, such as being abandoned by their partner.

ATTITUDE TO ABORTION

The general attitude of the Dutch population and of Dutch health authorities is that abortion is a necessity which should be limited, therefore abortion is not viewed as a form of contraception, but as an emergency solution, as an ultimate last resort in case of contraceptive failure[2]. On one hand, this attitude towards abortion is the main explanation for the low abortion rates in The Netherlands. On the other hand, it might result in what Janet Hadly recently called the 'awfulization' of abortion[3]. Women who become pregnant unintentionally often regard themselves as being guilty and/or stupid. These women may also be confronted with health-care professionals who implicitly, or even explicitly, aggravate these feelings of guilt. The 'awfulization' of abortion, contrary to viewing abortion as a calculated risk, may easily lead to post-abortion contraceptive counselling consisting of advice to prevent 'accidents', or to switch to an alternative method of contraception, regardless of whether or not such advice is really what the women need. In many cases, the counselling can be limited to an empathic talk stressing the fact that the woman is the victim of a case of bad luck. What should be kept in mind is that every contraceptive method has its failure rates, even when there is a strong motivation of the user. Moreover, reliability of the method is not the only consideration in choosing a method. There may be very good medical, relational, psychological, religious, sexological or economic reasons for choosing a less reliable method.

ATTITUDE TO CONTRACEPTION

Owing to effective formal and informal information sources, the majority of Dutch women, nevertheless, choose very reliable methods, with remarkably few user-failures. The use of oral contraceptives, for instance, is far more effective in The Netherlands than in most other countries. Estimated failure rates of oral contraceptive use are about 0.4, while these rates in, for instance, the UK and the USA are at least 5–10 times higher[4]. In this respect, it seems even more patronizing to talk about 'compliance' as if the effective use of a contraceptive method is simply a question of doing what the doctor tells you to do. Effective contraceptive behaviour is mainly the result of a cultural climate in which women are empowered to make their own decisions on the basis of a high level of information. This situation can only be reached in societies where there is a general openness regarding matters concerning sexuality, contraception and reproductive health, as is shown, for instance, in studies of the Alan Guttmacher Institute[5].

If anyone is to blame for contraceptive failure, therefore, it is, those who are opinion leaders and publicity-makers in the field of reproductive health. Nevertheless, the Dutch example teaches us the lesson that even when contraceptive behaviour in a population can hardly be improved, unintended pregnancies will always occur simply because mistakes are human and accidents can happen.

In contraceptive counselling after termination of pregnancy, the main question to the woman, therefore, is not 'What did you do wrong?' or 'How do you want to prevent this happening again?' but, 'Do you think you should reconsider your choice of contraception?'

CONCLUSION

The choice of a contraceptive method is not simply a question of 'prescribing' the most reliable method, but letting the woman or couple choose the method that meets, as far as possible, the wishes and expectations of these individuals depending on their individual bio-psychosocial status. This might result in choosing a method in which the woman recognizes that she takes a calculated risk, knowing that if something goes wrong she can always try emergency contraception and/or rely on safe abortion services, provided by professionals who refrain from moralizing and patronizing attitudes that contribute to the stigmatization of women asking for termination of pregnancy.

REFERENCES

1. Rademakers J. *Abortus in Nederland* (Abortion in The Netherlands). Utrecht: Stimezo 1992; 27
2. Ketting E, Visser AP. Contraception in The Netherlands; the low abortion rate explained. *Patient Educ Couns* 1994; 23: 161–71
3. Hadley J. The 'awfulisation' of abortion. Presented at *Abortion Matters*, First International Congress on Abortion, Stimeso, Amsterdam, March 1996
4. van Lunsen RHW, Arnolds HT, van Maris MGM. Choices and changes in contraceptive behaviour, the role of information sources. *Patient Educ Couns* 1994; 23: 197–202
5. Jones EF, Forrest JL, Hemshaw SK, *et al. Teenage Pregnancy in Industrialized Countries.* New Haven and London: Yale University Press, 1986

23 Trying to prevent abortion

D.R. Bromham and E.J. Oloto

INTRODUCTION

Since antiquity it has been apparent that a proportion of women confronted with the dilemma of an unwanted pregnancy will, in most societies, choose the option of abortion as a means of resolving their problem. Ancient Greek sources including the Hippocratic texts regarded abortion as a eugenic instrument suitable for certain classes of women only[1,2]. In Western societies we have evolved an antipathy to abortion that is attributable to considerations of respect for fetal life in the Judaeo-Christian tradition. However, selective editing[3] and mistranslation[4] of ancient Greek and Arabic texts were instrumental in defining that attitude.

In spite of opposition from major religions, the use of abortion probably made a significant contribution to limitation of family size seen among the middle classes of developing Western societies in the 19th century[5,6]. Where contemporary objections to the use of abortion for such purposes were voiced, these were often in terms of potential risks and inconveniences to the women concerned[6]. In Eastern societies, where the major religions such as Hinduism and Shinto have been more neutral on the subject of fetal rights, the major objection to abortion has to be couched in terms of its impact on the woman concerned. However, political factors may in many cases override or modify other considerations[7].

For some time it has been acknowledged that mortality from safe, medically supervised abortion is comparable to that found with some of the more effective contraceptive methods. In spite of the safety of the procedure it is likely that most of us would welcome a reduction in numbers and rates of abortions as this would represent both fewer women confronting an unpleasant decision and less loss of fetal life. We will therefore examine some of the approaches that have been suggested for reducing the use of abortion and consider their value.

RESTRICTION OF ACCESS

Currently, the majority of the world's women live in societies where abortion is, to some extent, legal and where access to medically supervised and safer procedures is theoretically possible[7].

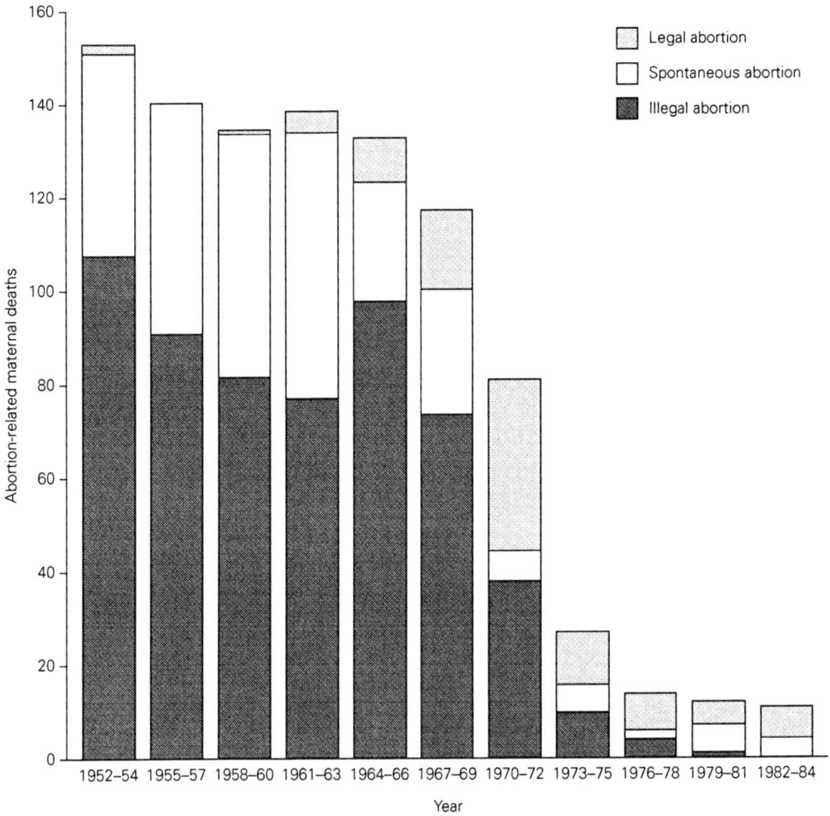

Figure 1 Numbers of abortion-related maternal deaths in England and Wales for each triennium 1952–54 to 1982–84[8,9]. Note that after the Abortion Act 1967 came into effect in 1968, deaths associated with both illegal and allegedly spontaneous abortions fell

In England, Wales and Scotland, but not the fourth part of Great Britain, Northern Ireland, the passage of a law (Abortion Act 1967), clarifying the circumstances under which induced abortion could be regarded as legal, led to a reduction in mortality from criminal abortion and a reduction in mortality from so-called spontaneous abortions (Figure 1). This preservation of maternal life is the main reason for the Act being referred to as 'one of the most outstandingly successful measures in preventive health care'[10,11]. The other phenomenon apparent from national statistics collected since the Act came into effect has been the increase in abortion numbers and rates (Figures 2 and 3). The initial rapid increase reflects the transfer of abortion from informal or criminal sectors to legal, and therefore monitored, services, but gives some idea of the size of abortion activity prior to the Act. Since then there have been periods of lesser, but still worrying increases in abortions. Some have argued that this

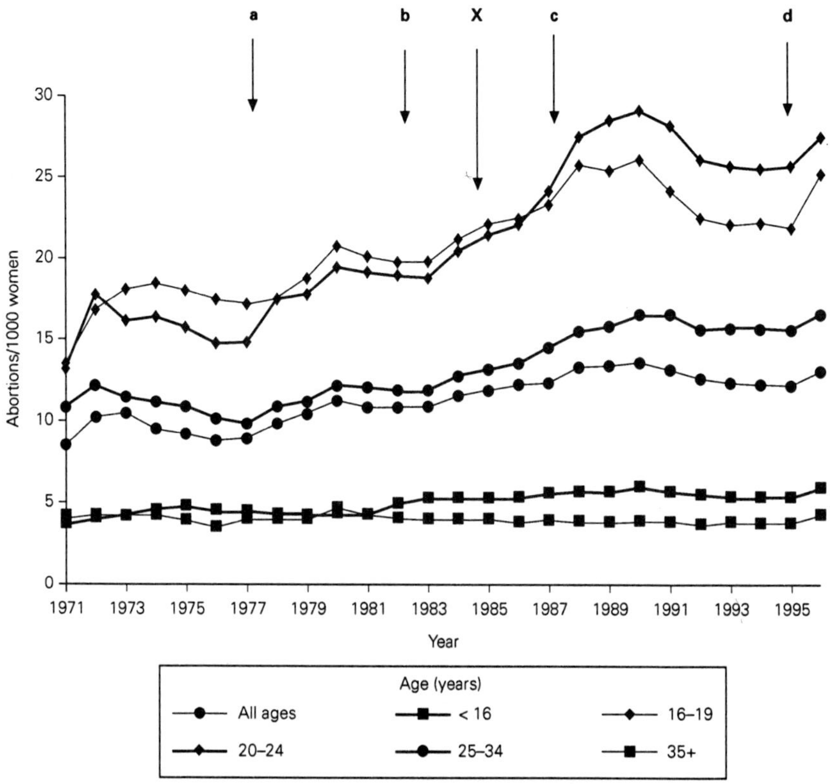

Figure 2 Age-related abortion rates for England and Wales 1971–96[12]. Note that there is an increase in abortion rates after each of the four major pill scares (a, b, c and d). The effect of the scare persists for several years in the case of a, b and c. In addition to scare 'c', the 20–24-age group, with high frequency of pill usage[13], would have been vulnerable to both scare 'c' and to the national campaign 'X' encouraging greater condom use (this did not emphasize the need for combined condom–pill use or for postcoital contraception). The 16–19-age group, initially more likely to be non-contraceptors[13], responded to the condom campaign[14] which in their case had a more beneficial effect. The different contraceptive use of these age groups and their consequent different vulnerabilities to factors 'c' and 'X' explain the change of positions of their graphs

represents excess recourse to abortion that is unwarranted and would justify recriminalization by repeal of the Abortion Act. However, the experiment has been conducted elsewhere and it would be a tragedy if we overlooked the results. At about the same time that Great Britain legalized abortion, the Ceausescu regime in Romania issued, because of pro-natalist concerns over rising abortion numbers and a declining birth rate, a decree forbidding both abortion and contraception[15]. The impact was immediate, with hospital

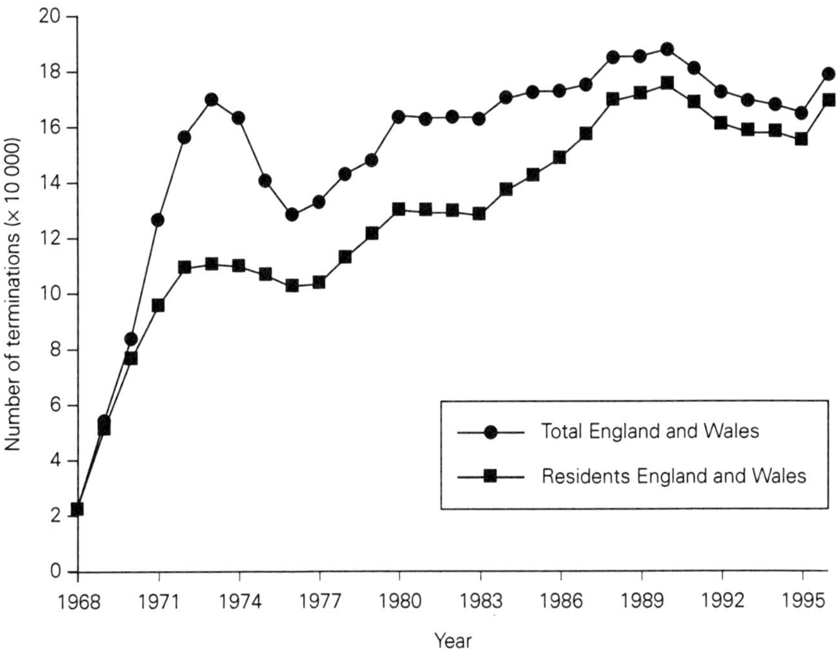

Figure 3 Number of terminations, 1968–96, England and Wales (total and residents)

admissions associated with abortion (induced and spontaneous) declining, and the birth rate rising. However, the effect was only transient, with the birth rate again declining and abortion admissions, supposedly due to 'spontaneous' events, increasing. The real tragedy was the impact on maternal mortality. The desire to avoid unwanted pregnancy had overcome the power of law, and abortions still took place. Arguably, as many fetal lives were ended, but through abortion in clandestine, criminal and entirely unsafe circumstances, an epidemic of maternal death arose. Fortunately the fall of the Ceausescu regime has led to just as dramatic a reduction in abortion-related maternal deaths[16].

It is to be regretted that access to safe procedures may not be as generally available for a population as might be expected by local law[17]. The procedure might be legal but it may be inaccessible for many who need to use it, often for financial reasons. Examples can be seen even within Great Britain. The proportion of procedures carried out under the National Health Service (NHS), free of charge to the woman, varies (4–90%) from district to district. When attempts are made to increase NHS provision they are often challenged as potentially encouraging abortion and increasing abortion rates. However, recent statistics for districts in Yorkshire, one of the English regions[12], show that there is no significant correlation between improved access to free, NHS-provided abortion and change in abortion rates (Figure 4). Indeed, the district with the greatest increase in NHS provision, Leeds, had one of the greater decreases in abortion.

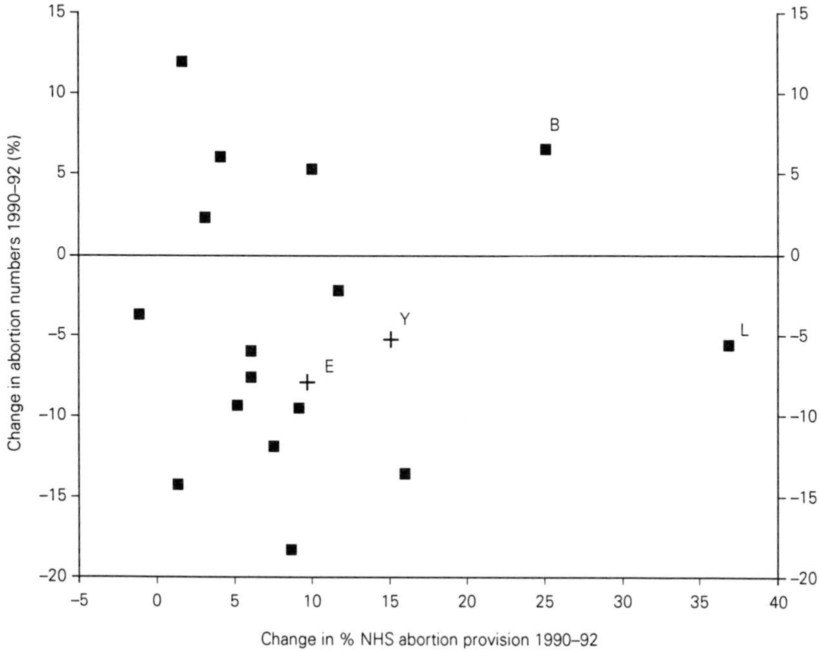

Figure 4 Effects of NHS abortion provision on number of abortions performed. Increasing the proportion of abortions performed free under the NHS does not increase numbers of abortions. Data for health districts in Yorkshire Region[12]. Between 1990 and 1992 most districts increased NHS abortion, provision particularly Leeds (L) and Bradford (B), but many, including Leeds, showed a marked reduction in abortions. Equivalent data for the Yorkshire Region (+Y) and for England and Wales (+E) are also shown

Consequently, if criminalization and restriction of access do not prevent abortion, but increase risks of maternal death, what other means are available to prevent or reduce abortion?

MORE EFFECTIVE MEASURES

International comparisons help to identify, in broad terms, some of the major factors. Examining teenage conception specifically, the Alan Guttmacher Institute[18] identified an index for 'open attitudes to sex' for selected societies. Based on such factors as frankness of discussions in the home, school and the media, availability of sex education and accessibility of contraception, this index correlated very well with teenage fertility rates: the more open the attitude of society the lower the number of conceptions (Figure 5).

We should not be surprised to find an inverse correlation between contraceptive use and abortion. This is observable when contraceptive use and

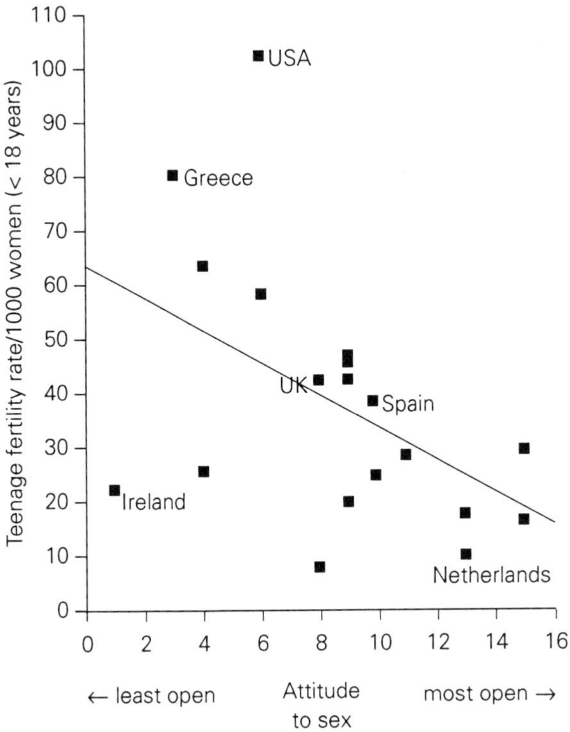

Figure 5 Fertility rates in women under 18 years of age and a score for open attitudes to sex in a range of industrialized countries[18]. With the exceptions of the USA and Ireland there is a close inverse correlation suggesting that teenage conceptions are commoner in those societies with the least openness in dealing with sexual matters. Among the other countries represented are Greece, the Netherlands, Spain and the United Kingdom (UK). Figure adapted from Ketting[19]

abortion rates are compared between countries, but the correlation is most marked when the considerable variation in the use of methods of varying efficacy is taken into account.

The dramatic changes that have been occurring in the countries of Eastern Europe also emphasize this point when changes within one country are considered. Thomas[16], for example, cites data from Russia and the Czech Republic where dramatic changes in abortion rates can be correlated with equivalent increase in the use of more effective contraceptive methods. Even in Western Europe, national abortion statistics may be sensitive to shifts in contraceptive usage. Figure 2 shows the apparent impact on abortion rates of four major 'pill scares' that occurred in the UK. We can see here how long an increase or acceleration in abortion rates takes to settle after such a scare. This phenomenon is not uniquely British and is observable in any society that has a high utilization of the combined pill, for example, in the Netherlands. Of course, it is not just pill-scares that can cause contraceptive revolution. Greater need for protection against sexually transmitted disease has encouraged increased usage of the male latex condom in most parts of Europe. In populations and sub-groups where contraceptive usage had previously been low this change had a reducing effect on abortions. British studies showed a considerable increase, from the mid-1980s, in condom use at the time of sexual debut amongst young people[14]. This group, teenagers predominantly aged 16–19 years, were, until then, the age group with the highest abortion rate, being largely non-contraceptors. However, as a greater proportion adopted the use of the condom they exchanged their 'league' position with 20–24-year-olds who had had a relatively high pill-usage and in whom this particular contraceptive revolution therefore had a negative effect (Figure 2). It is interesting that condom usage at first intercourse is highest, and non-contraception lowest, in those who mostly gained their sex education at school or from a relative[14], consistent with the findings on 'openness' discussed above.

Where changes in contraceptive practice for any group is likely to lead to reduced contraceptive cover, it is important to anticipate the need for alternative precautions. A number of British studies have demonstrated that a considerable proportion of women seeking abortion of unwanted pregnancies were aware of an increased risk of conception either through non-contraception or because of a condom accident, but that knowledge necessary to make the best use of post-coital, emergency or secondary contraception is inadequate in many who might have benefited from such preparations[13,20].

CONCLUSIONS

Nobody is 'happy' with the concept of abortion. That usually includes the woman confronted with an unintended and unwanted pregnancy for whom abortion may be the only option she can choose. However, much as we would prefer the situation if the numbers of abortions could be reduced, we have to be realistic about how this might be achieved.

My conclusions are simply this: reduction of abortion numbers and rates will not be achieved by criminalization, legal limitation of access or financial limitation of access. Reduction of abortion numbers and rates requires more openness regarding sex and sexuality, including good education programs, and greater access to the more effective methods of contraception including emergency or postcoital contraception.

REFERENCES

1. Filshie GM. Abortion. In Filshie GM, Guillebaud J, eds. *Contraception: Science and Practice*. London and Boston: Butterworth & Co., 1989; 250–74
2. King H. Making a man: becoming human in early Greek medicine. In Dunstan GR, ed. *The Human Embryo: Aristotle and the Arabic and European Traditions*. Exeter, UK: University of Exeter Press, 1990; 10–19

3. Green MH. Constantinus Africanus and the conflict between religion and science. In Dunstan GR, ed. *The Human Embryo:Aristotle and the Arabic and European Traditions.* Exeter, UK: University of Exeter Press, 1990; 47–69
4. Dunstan GR. The moral status of the human embryo. In Bromham DR, Dalton ME, Jackson JC, eds. *Philosophical Ethics in Reproductive Medicine.* Manchester, UK: Manchester University Press, 1990; 3–9
5. Hagenfeldt K. European and North American perspectives. In Bankowski Z, Barzelatto J, Capron AM, eds. *Ethics and Human Values in Family Planning.* Geneva: CIOMS, 1989; 184–207
6. McLaren A. *Reproductive Rituals.* London and New York: Methuen & Co., 1984; 89–112
7. Macklin R. Perspectives of different cultural and religious settings. In Bankowski Z, Barzelatto J, Capron AM, eds. *Ethics and Human Values in Family Planning.* Geneva: CIOMS, 1989; 68–85
8. Department of Health. *Report on Confidential Enquiries into Maternal Deaths in England and Wales 1970–1972.* London: HMSO, 1975
9. Department of Health. *Report on Confidential Enquiries into Maternal Deaths in England and Wales 1982–1984.* London: HMSO, 1989
10. McEwan J. Contemporary issues in family planning. In Byrne P, ed. *Health, Rights and Resources: King's College Studies 1987–8.* Oxford, UK: Oxford University Press, 1988; 128–65
11. Cochrane AL. *Effectiveness and Efficiency.* Rock Carling Fellowship. London: The Nuffield Provincial Hospitals Trust, 1971
12. OPCS. *Abortion Statistics England and Wales 1995.* Series AB no. 22. London: HMSO, 1997
13. Bromham DR, Cartmill RSV. Are current sources of contraceptive advice adequate to meet changes in contraceptive practice? – A study of patients requesting termination of pregnancy. *Br J Fam Plann* 1993; 19: 179–83
14. Wellings K, Bradshaw S. First intercourse between men and women. In Johnson AM, Wadsworth J, Field J, Bradshaw S, eds. *Sexual Attitudes and Lifestyles.* Oxford: Blackwell Scientific Publications, 1994; 68–109
15. Barron SL. Epidemiology of induced abortion. In Bromham DR, Dalton ME, Jackson JC, Millican PJR, eds. *Ethics in Reproductive Medicine.* Berlin and New York: Springer-Verlag, 1992; 145–60
16. Thomas L. The need for effective contraception: a global and European perspective. In Hannaford PC, Webb AMC, eds. *Evidence-guide Prescribing of the Pill.* Carnforth: Parthenon Publishing, 1996; 9–13
17. McLaurin KE, Hord CE, Noyes MW. Health systems' role in preventing maternal deaths related to abortion: the need for a pro-active response to abortion care. In Newman K, ed. *Progress Postponed: Abortion in Europe in the 1990s.* London: International Planned Parenthood Federation, 1993; 109–25
18. Jones EF. *Teenage Pregnancy in Industrialized Countries.* New Haven, Connecticut: Yale University Press, 1986
19. Ketting E. The contraceptive situation in Europe. In Newman K, ed. *Progress Postponed:Abortion in Europe in the 1990s.* London: International Planned Parenthood Federation, 1993; 7–30
20. Bromham DR, Cartmill RSV. Knowledge and use of secondary contraception among patients requesting termination of pregnancy. *Br Med J* 1993; 306: 556–7

This paper has been reproduced from *Eur J Contracept Reprod Health Care* 1997; 2: 81–7

24 How to handle repeat aborters?

B. Rojnik and I. Kirar-Fazarinc

Induced abortion is a tough, but inevitable, human reality, surrounded by much controversy, misunderstanding, guilt, stigma and disgrace. In spite of many efforts, unintended pregnancies remain a serious public-health problem for women worldwide. High numbers of abortions go hand-in-hand with increased numbers of repeat abortions. Repeat aborters complicate the already sensitive and controversial problem of abortion. They bring into focus the question of whether women use abortion to regulate their fertility, as a back-up procedure for contraceptive failure or for lack of a better alternative.

In many Eastern and Central European countries, the incidence of induced abortion is well above the world's average. Abortion rates have been high since the middle of the 20th century when abortion legislation was liberalized[1]. They range from 27.2 per 1000 women aged 15–44 years in the former German Democratic Republic to 112 per 1000 women aged 15–44 years in the former Soviet Union[2]. A thorough review of the abortion situation in Europe, that also summarizes the issues discussed at the 1990 Tbilisi conference *From Abortion to Contraception*, reveals that, in most European countries, about two-thirds of women have at least one unintended pregnancy by the time they reach the menopause[3]. Of pregnancies in the former Soviet Union, 55% were terminated by abortion[2], which suggests high repeat abortion rates in Eastern Europe. The proportion of repeat aborters in different countries of the world ranges from 17% in New Zealand to 49% in Hungary[2]. Women in the former Soviet Union were reported to undergo six or more abortions, on average, in their reproductive life[3], yet a high proportion of abortions are unregistered and performed illegally[4].

Numbers of repeat abortions, where available at all, need to be looked upon with caution, especially in countries with restrictive abortion laws. Women are very likely to under-report their previous experience or deny it altogether when having illegal abortions. Many abortions performed by private abortion providers or paramedical practitioners remain unrecorded. Repeat aborters are usually reported as the proportion of women with previous abortions[5]. Bias selection may be present in studies evaluating repeaters on the basis of retrospective data. As diverse situational characteristics are in play when deciding whether or not to abort, many unintended pregnancies are carried to term, making repeaters a non-representative sample of women experiencing an unwanted pregnancy. Once the threshold for first abortion is passed, women are more likely to have another abortion than women with no previous abortion history[5].

Several studies have examined women who have repeatedly undergone abortions; these have attempted to identify women who are at greater risk for subsequent abortions in regard to their psychological, demographic or social characteristics. These studies showed little in terms of psychological characteristics to differentiate repeat aborters from first-time aborters. Low incidence of adverse psychological sequels associated with abortion is reported[6].

Parity, age and marital status have strong correlation with use of abortion[7]. Abortions in Eastern Europe are more common among older women with two or more children[2], indicating that in these countries women use abortion to terminate their fertility or for spacing, rather than for delaying births. In the former German Democratic Republic, for example, women with two or more children accounted for 75% of all abortion procedures[4]. Fewer than one-fifth of women having abortions in Bulgaria, Czechoslovakia and Hungary had no children[2], yet the proportion of childless women having abortions increased for more than a decade.

Repeaters tend to be older than first-time aborters[8,9]. Young unmarried women frequently resort to abortion to delay the birth of the first child. As early child-bearing is acceptable in Eastern Europe, adolescents comprise a smaller proportion among first-time or repeat aborters[2]. A woman's satisfaction in her relationship also differentiates repeaters from first-time aborters[10], with dissatisfaction more often found among repeat aborters.

Data suggest that many more repeaters are using more effective contraception at the time of conception[9,11] than first-time aborters, implying that women learn from their own experience and are motivated to avoid further pregnancies. Studies also show that, on the whole, repeat aborters use methods of contraception with higher rates of efficacy – such as the pill and the intrauterine device (IUD) – than first-time aborters, but often discontinue owing to side-effects, lack of supplies or medical contraindications[11]. Poor contraceptive compliance and switching to less reliable contraception, therefore, are important characteristics of abortion seekers. Lack of contraceptive supplies, a condition that is especially severe in many Eastern European countries, adds to the problem of repeat abortions. Contraceptive failure alone is another common experience among women using current contraceptive technologies leading to repeat abortions.

Also, repeat aborters were found to be more sexually active[9,11] than women with no abortion experience. So, apart from contraception, there are several other factors in play, individually and/or in combination, that predispose women to use abortion.

To answer the question of how to handle repeat aborters, we need to realize that this is, in large measure, a social issue: how can we in the medical profession more effectively persuade policy makers and family-planning providers to adopt successful policies and practices in order to reduce the number of abortions to the lowest possible level? What can we do to better serve women who have poor compliance rates, discontinue methods due to side-effects or cannot reliably access effective methods?

This is a special challenge in the case of Eastern Europe, because of its high number of abortions. The tremendous political and economical changes that have recently taken place have also posed a challenge to health services. The fall of communism and the switch to a market economy have had a great impact on heath care and also have profoundly influenced family-planning programs. Many governments remain indifferent to the reproductive and sexual health of their people. In addition, family-planning providers often fail to recognize their pivotal role in changing women's and men's perceptions about their own reproductive health needs. This reluctance of family-planning providers, combined with the increasing power and influence of the church in the regulation of fertility, may further hinder access to effective reproductive health care unless an integrated societal approach is developed. Family-planning services should no longer be an erratic and non-integrated part of health care but should be organized to be available to any woman and couple in need, regardless of their socioeconomic status. This is a difficult task, especially with the transition to a market economy. In such circumstances, poor women are more likely to be denied access to family-planning services and, therefore, are left at increased risk of unwanted pregnancy and abortion.

In many Eastern European countries, where abortion was the only means to regulate fertility, the introduction and provision of modern contraceptives poses new demands for obstetricians and gynecologists. Some obstetricians and gynecologists will lose a profitable source of revenue, especially where abortions were illegal or hard to access. Such is the case, for example, in Romania[2].

Yet, on the other hand, apart from women, family-planning providers can be considered victims of abortions as well. Data from the former Soviet Union indicate that more than 3000 obstetricians and gynecologists performed abortions full-time[3]. Working in abortion clinics is stressful and is exacerbated by exposure to repeat abortions[10]. It is very likely that where clinic staff perform very high numbers of abortions per day, higher rates of abortion complications occur.

One of the important steps in reducing repeated abortions is to improve professional and public knowledge of the benefits and risks of contraceptive methods. Availability of modern contraceptives alone will not do much good unless effective and enthusiastic educational programs are implemented to shift health-care professionals' and clients' attitudes towards the use of effective and safe contraceptive methods. For society in general, however, contraceptive use saves health-care resources by preventing pregnancies. Cost–benefit analysis shows that preventing unwanted pregnancies is more cost–effective than paying for physical and physiological consequences of repeated abortions. Fear of side-effects associated with contraceptives significantly affects the underutilization of contraceptive methods and user compliance, although risks associated with pregnancy and abortion outweigh the risks associated with currently available contraceptives.

Health professionals must bear in mind that abortion is a physical and psychological trauma *per se*. Women are in dire need of sharing their burden of unwanted pregnancy with their health-care providers; for repeat aborters this is probably even more true. Many women undergoing their first abortion have never had any contraceptive counselling prior to the procedure. Proper counselling can decrease their risk of subsequent unwanted pregnancy and abortion. This is important because a majority of women who have had an abortion are sexually active and resume their usual sexual activity after pregnancy termination. Women are accepting of and motivated to use family planning at the time of abortion. Therefore, sympathetic and non-judgmental counselling needs to be a part of abortion providers' obligation. A scheduled follow-up must be arranged to discuss any possible problems with newly adopted contraceptive measures.

Immediate postabortion contraceptive delivery modalities are appealing from the programmatic and economic point of view. Sterilization at the time of abortion may be helpful, although it may not significantly reduce the overall rate of repeat abortions as women undergoing sterilization at the time of pregnancy termination are usually older and multiparous and do not substantially contribute to the numbers of repeat aborters. In Eastern Europe, concurrent sterilization at the time of abortion is known to be rare or non-existent[2].

Since the 1994 International Conference on Population and Development in Cairo, a shift has occurred from family planning to a more holistic approach to reproductive health. This places greater emphasis on male involvement and male responsibility for contraception. In so far as abortion indirectly affects males as well, men should be actively engaged in the problem of abortion, through other means than by decrying liberal abortion laws.

In addition, emphasis should be placed on evoking personal responsibility to adopt effective contraception and to prevent unwanted pregnancies. Education in family planning and sexuality can help decrease the numbers of induced abortions. Open discussion of sexual issues at a young age as well as special training of teachers in The Netherlands have decreased abortion to the lowest rates in the world[12].

In conclusion, as Christoper Tietze says, 'one should not expect perfection from human beings'. This does not mean that we do not need to strive for perfection. All sexually active people of reproductive age deserve to be able to have a child that is planned. They also deserve help to ensure that their sexuality becomes and remains an enriching experience, adding quality to their life. Every single abortion prevented will help people live a safer and happier life. An estimated 200 000 women die each year from complications related to clandestine abortions performed in unsafe conditions[13], which means that at least 550 women die needlessly every day. This is a tragic legacy for mankind, yet many people still argue that abortion legislation leads to the relaxation or abandonment of contraceptive use. Legislation of abortion does not mean the switch from contraception to abortion, but is an important step away from abortion to contraception. To achieve the goal embodied in the slogan from the Tbilisi conference in 1990[14], we must continue to act at all levels to move away from abortion.

REFERENCES

1. Frejka T. Induced abortion and fertility. *Int Fam Plann Perspect* 1985; 11: 125–9
2. Henshaw SK. Induced abortion: a world review, 1990. *Fam Plann Perspect* 1990; 22: 76–89
3. David HP. Abortion in Europe, 1920–91: a public health perspective. *Stud Fam Plann* 1992; 23: 1–22
4. Popov AA. Family planning and induced abortion in USSR: basic health and demographic chracteristics. *Stud Fam Plann* 1991; 22: 368–77
5. Skjeldestad FE. The incidence of repeat induced abortion – a prospective cohort study. *Obstet Gynecol Scand* 1994; 73: 706–10
6. World Health Organization. *Induced Abortion*, Technical report, No. 632. Geneva: World Health Organization, 1978
7. Steinhoff PG, Roy SG, Palmore JA, *et al.* Women who obtain repeat abortions: a study based on record linkage. *Fam Plann Perspect* 1979; 11: 30–8
8. Westfall JM, Kallail KJ. Repeat abortion and use of primary care health services. *Fam Plann Perspect* 1995; 27: 162–5
9. Berger C, Gold D, Andres D, *et al.* Repeat abortion: is it a problem? *Fam Plann Perspect* 1984; 16: 70–7
10. Berger C, Gold D, Andres D, *et al.* Repeaters: different or unlucky? In Sachev P, ed. *Abortion: Readings and Research.* Toronto: Butterworth, 1981: 159–70
11. Howe B, Kaplan RH, English C. Repeat abortions: blaming the victims. *Am J Publ Health* 1979; 69: 1242–6
12. Nyman V. Going Dutch – a pipe dream? *Br J Fam Plann* 1993; 19: 200–3
13. Maine D, Karkazis K, Bolan N. The bad old days are still here: abortion mortality in developing countries. *J Am Med Women's Assoc* 1994; 49: 137–42
14. World Health Organization, Regional Office for Europe Copenhagen. *From Abortion to Contraception.* Presented at the Tbilisi Conference, October 1990

25 Contraceptive options for adolescents

G. Creatsas

Adolescent contraception is related to adolescent sexuality, which recently has increased worldwide owing to the increased rate of premature sexual intercourse[1]. In the USA, by the age of 15, almost 25% of adolescents are engaged in harmful or dangerous behavior[2]. Many of them have already been exposed to danger as a result of their demographic background and in portrayal by the mass media. Boys start sexual intercourse earlier than girls; however, their knowledge of the complications of premature sexuality is very limited[3]. It is characteristic that most studies concern young women and no effort has been directed towards improvement of the sexual behavior of young men.

Adolescent contraception presents several differences compared with that of adults (Table 1). Many adolescents do not seek medical advice for contraception until they have been sexually active or have had at least one pregnancy. The major problem, however is that when adolescents start using a contraceptive method, the compliance is poor. Compliance depends on the sexual history, the previous history of contraceptive methods and socioeconomic and environmental factors as well as the sex education of the teenager. Compliance is also related to parental and physician's advice. Compliance is more problematic among immature teenagers and those having multiple partners[4]. It is expected to be higher when the suggested contraceptive method is also indicated for medical reasons, i.e. when oral contraceptives (OCs) are used to regulate the

Table 1 Characteristics of contraception during adolescence

No regular sexual intercourse
Menstrual irregularities
Incomplete education
Low compliance rate
Fear of parents and doctor
Friend's advice
Risk of sexually transmitted diseases
Condom versus oral contraception
Use of ineffective methods

Table 2 Contraceptive methods (%) used during adolescence in European countries, age 12–18 years. From reference 8

Country	PA/CI	OCs	IUD	Barrier	Other/no prophylaxis
Belgium	4.0	61.0	0	12.0	23.0
Denmark	NA	64.0	2.0	19.0	15.0
Finland	NA	32.0	0	50.0	18.0
France	NA	17.3	0.1	NA	NA
Germany	50.0	40.0	0	10.0	NA
Greece	30.5	40.5	3.8	20.7	4.5
Hungary	60.0	35.0	0	5.0	NA
Italy	39.2	7.9	0	31.2	NA
The Netherlands	7.0	56.0	0	29.0	8.0
UK	3.0	43.0	1.0	5.0	48.0

PA/CI, periodic abstinence/coitus interruptus; OCs, oral contraceptives; IUD, intrauterine device; NA, information not available

menstrual period. Consultation with a peer counsellor may also be more successful.

Contraceptive behavior is related to changing age structure and change in upper age limits for OC use. However, there are unpredictable factors affecting contraceptive use such as the publicity regarding OCs and breast cancer, and concern about sexually transmitted diseases (STDs) including human immunodeficiency virus (HIV) infection as well as abortion legislation[5]. In the USA, the number of women aged 15–19 years will change from 8.5 million in 1990 to 9.2 million in 2010. It is also estimated that OC use will not change significantly during these years. In 1990, 10.6 million women used OCs, while in 2010 these figures are expected to decrease to 10.2 million[5,6]. Choquet and Manfredi[7] carried out an epidemiological study among 4255 adolescents aged 11–19 years. A total of 31% had had sexual relations (43% of the boys and 20% of the girls). A large majority (79%) of the sexually active teenagers used some form of contraception (71% boys and 76% girls).

Hormonal and non-hormonal methods may be used for contraception during adolescence. Oral contraceptives seem to be a favorite method for use during adolescence. In a European multicentric study conducted by the International Federation of Infantile and Juvenile Gynecology (FIGIJ), it was found that in six out of 11 European countries contributing to the study, OCs were the most common contraceptive method used[8]. Among the barrier methods used, the condom was common (Table 2).

Creatsas and colleagues[9] evaluated the clinical and metabolic effects of the low-dose monophasic 'gestodene/ethinylestradiol' pill used for contraception

Table 3 Benefits of oral contraceptives when used during adolescence

Decrease risk of functional ovarian cysts
Regulate menstrual period
Improve dysmenorrhea
Prevent pelvic inflammatory disease

during adolescence. Among 50 adolescents who received the pill for contraceptive purposes for a 6-month period, no pregnancy occurred and no significant changes were seen in serum lipids and carbohydrate metabolism. The rate of intermenstrual bleeding was 0.7%. The authors concluded that the gestodene/ethinylestradiol OC results in good efficacy and minimum side-effects when used as an OC during adolescence.

A significant number of adolescents during the first 2 or 3 gynaecological years present menstrual irregularities. Oral contraceptives and especially those containing the new generation progestogens 'gestodene', '6-keto-desogestrel' or 'norgestimate' also have a favorable effect on regulation of the menstrual period[9,10]. The benefits associated with OCs when used during adolescence are summarized in Table 3.

Other hormonal contraceptive methods include the medroxyprogesterone acetate (Depo-Provera®, DMPA) and the Norplant subdermal implants. The DMPA is given in a standard dose of 150 mg intramuscularly every 3 months and yields a rate of 0–5.2 pregnancies per 100 women years; DMPA suppresses the preovulatory surge of luteinizing hormone and follicle-stimulating hormone and thereby inhibits ovulation[11,12]. The 'Norplant' subdermal implant system is an alternative hormonal injectable contraceptive method. The system contains six slow-releasing capsules or rods, which release levonorgestrel over 6–7 years. The World Health Organization (WHO) reported a pregnancy rate of 2.6 per 100 women years with this method[11,13].

Among the non-hormonal contraceptive methods, the condom is very popular. In many countries, it is offered by the family planning or other services. The correct use of the condom has to be introduced by the clinical staff of the center. Adolescents are advised to use lubricated latex condoms and possibly those equipped with spermicidal material.

Sexually transmitted disease has changed the sexual behavior of young teenagers and is also one of the reasons that the condom is popular among adolescents. In addition, the condom is easily available, has a low cost and presents no side-effects. In a study conducted by Weisberg and colleagues[14] it was found that, among 253 students from two high schools, girls appear to have more difficulty in asking how condoms are to be used. Elfenbein and co-workers[15] reported 69% condom usage among sexually active delinquent male adolescents admitted to a detection facility over a 6-month period. Review of the medical records of a similar group of detainees revealed a 44% condom usage, suggesting a marked increase in utilization. Brown and associates[16] reported that consistent condom use was more frequent in males, especially those with little history of risk behavior and stronger intentions to use this method in the future. Finally, it has to be mentioned that condoms protect from the transmission of both aerobic and anaerobic bacteria as well as *Chlamydia trachomatis* and mycoplasma.

Contraceptive sponges and other barrier methods are less commonly used during adolescence. Diaz and colleagues[17] reported the use of the sponge in 1.9% of 208 adolescents who completed a 54-item questionnaire. The authors concluded that the sponge may be a valuable contraceptive method. Psychoyos and co-workers[18] proposed the new vaginal sponge (Protectaid® containing sodium cholade with both spermicidal and antiviral properties. The authors reported a 100% efficacy with only two positive cervical cultures among 20 young women using the sponge for a 12-month period.

Intrauterine devices are not recommended during adolescence. In a study of 120 adolescents who received the Cu-7 intrauterine device satisfaction with the method was reported by 72% of the users and the pregnancy rate was 2.0 per 100 women years[19]. Finally, it should be mentioned that many adolescents use ineffective methods such as periodic abstinence, coitus interruptus and withdrawal prior to ejaculation.

It is suggested that adolescents, both boys and girls, should be properly informed on the methods of prevention of undesired pregnancies and STDs.

REFERENCES

1. Creatsas G. Sequelae of premature sexual life. *J R Soc Med* 1995; 88: 369–71
2. Hechinger FM. Fateful Choices: *Healthy Youth for the 21st Century*. New York: Carnegie Corporation 1992
3. Creatsas G. Adolescent sexuality in Europe: a multicentric study. *Adolesc Pediatr Gynecol* 1995; 8: 59–63
4. Brown RT, Cromer BA, Fischer R. Adolescent sexuality and issues in contraception. *Adolesc Pediatr Gynecol* 1992; 19: 177–91
5. Trussel J, Vaughan B. Contraceptive use projections: 1990 to 2010. *Am J Obstet Gynecol* 1992; 167: 1160–4
6. Spencer G. *Projections of the population of the United States by age, sex and race: 1988–2080*, Current population reports, Series p-25, No.1018. Washington, DC. Goverment Printing Office, 1989
7. Choquet M, Manfredi R. Sexual intercourse, contraception and risk-taking behavior among unselected French adolescents aged 11–20 years. *J Adolesc Health Care* 1992; 13; 623–30
8. Creatsas G, Vekemans M, Horejsi J, *et al*. Adolescent Sexuality in Europe. Multicentric study, International Federation of Infantile and Juvenile Gynecology, *Adolesc Pediatr Gynecol* 1995; 8: 59–63
9. Creatsas G, Adamopoulos P, Eleftheriou N, *et al*. Clinical and metabolic effects of the monophasic gestodene/ethinylestradiol pill for contraception during adolescence. *Adolesc Pediatr Gynecol* 1991; 4: 76–9

10. Creatsas G. Progestagens in reproductive endocrinology. *Eur J Obstet Gynecol Reprod* 1991; 41: 28
11. Shearin RB, Boehlke JR. Hormonal contraception. *Pediatr Clin North Am* 1989; 36: 697–715
12. Cromer BA. Depo-Provera: Wherefore art thou? *Adolesc Pediatr Gynecol* 1992; 5: 155–62
13. Miller M. Depot levonorgestrel (Norplant) use in teenagers. West J Med 1993; 158: 183
14. Weisberg E, North P, Buxton M. Sexual activity and condom use in high school students. Med J Aust 1992; 156: 612–13
15. Elfenbein DS, Weber T, Grob G. Condom usage by a population of delinquent Southern male adolescents. *J Adolesc Health Care* 1991; 12: 35–7
16. Brown LK, Diclemente RJ, Park T. Predictors of condom use in sexually active adolescents. *J Adolesc Health Care* 1992; 13: 651–7
17. Diaz A, Jaffe LR, Leadbeater BJ, *et al.* Frequency of use, knowledge, and attitudes toward the contraceptive sponge among inner city black and hispanic adolescent females. *J Adolesc Health Care* 1990; 11: 125–7
18. Psychoyos A, Creatsas G, Hassan E, *et al.* Spermicidal and antiviral properties of cholic acid. Contraceptive efficacy of a new vaginal sponge (Protectaid), containing sodium cholate. *Hum Reprod* 1993, 8: 866–9
19. Kulig JW. Adolescent contraception: nonhormonal methods. *Pediatr Clin North Am* 1989; 36: 717–30

26 Risks and benefits of adolescent contraception

S. Dexeus and F. Martinez

INTRODUCTION

Considering the tremendous socioeconomic and educational long-term consequences of unintended adolescent pregnancies, it is clear that the main benefit of adolescent contraception will be prevention of pregnancies. The decision process for choosing a contraceptive method must take into consideration two separate, but related, potential hazards of adolescent sexuality: pregnancy and sexually transmitted disease (STD). STD rates, particularly in the teenage population, seem to be escalating, and unintended pregnancy remains a very significant challenge both for individuals and for society.

While pregnancy rates among the young population are decreasing, as in the general population, mainly due to socioeconomic reasons, sexual activity rates among adolescents remain unchanged or are even increasing, without a parallel increase in protection against STD.

SCOPE OF THE PROBLEM

In 1990, a total population of 325 878 900 was estimated for the European Economic Community (EEC) of the 12 state members (data from Eurostat). Around 23 million would be female adolescents (15–20 years old) by 1995. In a multicentric European study undertaken by the International Federation of Pediatric and Adolescent Gynecology, it was found that the pregnancy rate among this age group ranged between 0.02% (Finland) and 21% (Germany) from 1985 to 1989[1]. Although the challenge of unintended adolescent pregnancy has been recognized for some time, the increasing prevalence of sexually transmitted diseases within the adolescent population is a major concern, as Genuis and Genuis have stated in a recent paper[2].

Rosenfeld[3] found that 38% of sexually active women, 13–21 years of age, were already infected with human papillomavirus (HPV), an incurable viral infection which has been linked to certain cancers of the genital tract. Although the full ramifications of HPV are not yet understood, this virus seems to facilitate the transmission of human immunodeficiency virus (HIV)[4].

The increasing number of individuals infected worldwide with *Chlamydia* has caused this pathogen to be considered the most common STD bacterial agent in many countries and has resulted in an increase in pelvic inflammatory disease, ectopic pregnancies and infertility in young women. As with many other STDs, *Chlamydia* infection is a significant factor affecting the adolescent population[2].

The infection that is causing most concern today, and which can be transmitted sexually, is HIV. It has been noted that half of all cases of HIV infection have occurred in young people under the age of 25 years. In addition to this primary epidemic, recent sequelae have been the alarming resurgence of active tuberculosis and the emergence of multi-drug-resistant tuberculosis. Women in their reproductive years are the fastest growing HIV-infected population in the United States[5].

Teenagers have the highest rates of hospitalization for pelvic inflammatory disease. The following statistics are cited with regard to adolescent young women in a study by Werner and Biro[6]:

(1) Of sexually active adolescent females, 8–25% are infected with *Chlamydia*;

(2) Infection with *Neisseria* accounts for 0.4–12%;

(3) Infection with human papillomavirus accounts for 15–38%;

(4) Abnormal Pap smears account for 16% of adolescents.

For these reasons, combined with the acquired immunodeficiency syndrome (AIDS) scare, an increase in the use of condoms has been reported among adolescents from the United States[7,8] and Europe.

In a study carried out in Barcelona[9], among 3139 adolescents aged 14–19 years (54% females and 46% males) found:

(1) Of all the adolescents, 12.9% had had intercourse and 31.1% were sexually active without intercourse;

(2) The mean age for first intercourse was 15.3 years for girls and 16.1 years for boys;

(3) The mean number of sexual partners was 1.8 for boys and 1.3 for girls; and

(4) Use of condoms was reported by 84.4% of boys and 68.8% of girls.

On the other hand, Poppen[10] reported an increase in self-reported condom use for very first intercourse, as well as first intercourse with current partner, between 1979 and 1989, indicating a trend towards 'safe sex' practices.

RISKS AND BENEFITS OF CONTRACEPTIVE METHODS FOR ADOLESCENTS

Oral contraceptives

The combined oral contraceptive is by far the most popular and most requested method of contraception by adolescents from the United States[7] and Europe[1].

This is appropriate because oral contraceptives are almost never medically contraindicated in healthy adolescents. The risk of death from oral contraceptive use by adolescents is virtually nil.

Benefits of oral contraceptives

The following benefits of oral contraceptives for adolescent females are of particular interest:

(1) High contraceptive effectiveness;

(2) Increased menstrual cycle regularity; a significant number of adolescents complained of menstrual irregularities during the first 2 or 3 gynecological years[1];

(3) Decreased incidence of menorrhagia, anemia, dysfunctional uterine bleeding, fibrocystic breast disease, ectopic pregnancy, pelvic inflammatory disease and its sequelae and functional ovarian cysts;

(4) Decreased incidence of dysmenorrhea and premenstrual syndrome;

(5) Decreased incidence of acne.

Adolescents are especially receptive to hearing about the beneficial impact of oral contraceptives on menstrual problems. Relief of dysmenorrhea in teenagers has been documented to be associated with better and more consistent use of oral contraceptives in a study by Robinson and colleagues[11].

Risks of oral contraceptives

Risks associated with oral contraception include:

(1) Poor compliance;

(2) Poor/no protection against STDs;

(3) Controversial future risk of breast cancer;

(4) Recent controversy about increased risk of deep venous thrombosis with oral contraceptive formulations containing gestodene or desogestrel.

A multinational survey of 10 000 European women, aged 16–30 years, revealed a direct correlation between poor patient compliance and unplanned pregnancies among oral contraceptive users, as Dr Mary Short reported during her presentation of the WYCON Survey, at the last European Society for Contraception Congress, in Dublin. Better compliance will be the end result of a properly informed adolescent, and this includes not only detailed instructions on beginning the therapy, but also open discussion of side-effects such as breakthrough bleeding, nausea and breast tenderness. It is important to discuss teenagers' fears and face concerns regarding oral contraception.

Impact on growth or reproductive tract

Before initiating oral contraceptive therapy in the adolescent, evidence of appropriate maturation of the hypothalamic–pituitary–ovarian axis is required (a minimum of three menstrual periods).

There have been reports suggesting that long-term treatment with oral contraceptives does not modify the bone mineral density but prevents the occurrence of the physiological peak of bone mass in young women[12]. A clinician can tell adolescents, with great confidence, that there is no impact on future fertility[13].

The cancer issue

According to Speroff and Darney[13], it seems appropriate to state that there is no definitive evidence demonstrating a link between breast cancer and oral contraception. On the other hand, patients deserve to know of our concern and about findings regarding long duration of use and the possible increased risk of early, premenopausal breast cancer.

Cervical cancer also continues to be a concern, although confounding factors have been difficult to control, and Pap smear surveillance must be emphasized[14].

Weight gain

It is worth emphasizing that studies with low-dose oral contraception in adolescents do not indicate a problem of weight gain, and that acne is usually improved[15].

Risk of cardiovascular events

The relative risk of cardiovascular events is increased for women of all ages who smoke and use oral contraceptives. Teenage smoking is still an important problem, however, because the incidence of cardiovascular disease (CVD) at this age is so low, there are no epidemiological data showing any significant increase of CVD risk. It is necessary to encourage teenagers to give up smoking. At the time of oral contraceptive prescribing to young smoking girls, it would be interesting to consider prescription of low-estrogen dose formulations.

Sexually transmitted diseases

Oral contraceptives do not protect against most STDs, although pelvic inflammatory disease rates have been shown to be decreased by up to 50%[16]. Because it is relatively common for young women to have changing relationships, through serial monogamy, a dual approach is recommended, combining the contraceptive efficacy and protection against pelvic inflammatory disease offered by oral contraception with the use of a barrier method for prevention of viral STDs.

Condoms

The main benefit of condom use among adolescents is obviously protection against STDs. One of the major disadvantages is the male partner's unwillingness to utilize this method. Even an increase in AIDS awareness has not substantially changed condom usage, possibly because the emphasis of HIV transmission via homosexual behavior has created a false sense of security in heterosexual teenagers[17].

The advantage of using condoms with a spermicide is that neither a prescription nor a consultation with a clinician is required. The problem is that of achieving sufficient education and motivation without the intervention of clinicians. Condom failures, unfortunately, are about ten times higher among teenagers than among older, married couples. Because of the risk of breakage or displacement, it is very important to give appropriate instructions about proper condom use and availability of emergency contraception. It should not be assumed that teenagers know how to use a condom.

Another complex issue of the dual approach with which reproductive health providers have to deal is that they must weigh factors such as cost and user compliance, as well as their relation to effective STD protection, among particular client populations, and changing priorities over time and among various relationships. It has been shown that HIV-infected women using the more effective methods of contraception were less likely to use condoms consistently than those using less effective contraceptive methods[18].

Diaphragm

The diaphragm is a relatively inexpensive form of birth control that still affords some STD protection. However, adolescents are not comfortable with body interventions, and diaphragm insertion interferes with the idealized 'natural' intercourse. This method requires privacy for insertion. Adolescents are discouraged by complicated methods. One reason the average teenager waits months to 1 year after initiating sexual activity before seeking contraceptive advice is fear about the pelvic examination. Furthermore, anxiety about the pelvic examination is a barrier to comprehending contraceptive instructions. Thus, letting teenagers know that the pelvic examination can be delayed until the 3rd or 6th month will encourage them to seek contraceptive advice. This approach is possible for oral contraceptives and condoms, but not for the diaphragm. There have been rare reports of toxic shock syndrome.

Intrauterine devices

Intrauterine devices (IUDs) are not considered a first-choice contraceptive method for the adolescent, mainly due to the risk of STDs. The IUD is associated with an increased risk of developing upper genital tract infection, primarily in the first month after insertion[19] and probably due to introduction of vaginal/cervical organisms into the uterus during insertion. On the other hand, low levels of pelvic inflammatory disease among women who have been enrolled in the studies suggest that concerns about the long-term effect of IUDs on upper genital tract infection may have been overstated, and proper user selection is the determining factor[18].

Exceptionally, an IUD might be the best choice in a mutually monogamous relationship, when hormonal contraceptives are contraindicated or are not tolerated, and always after exhaustive explanation of possible risks.

Norplant implants

Specific benefits of Norplant® (levonorgestrel) implants in the adolescent patient are:

(1) High contraceptive efficacy, with less than 1% failure rate;

(2) They require little compliance;

(3) They provide long-lasting contraception;

(4) They can be prescribed when estrogens are contraindicated by diabetes, hypercholesterolemia, hypertension and sickle cell disease, because no significant changes have been found in cholesterol, liver function tests or blood sugar in Norplant users[20];

(5) They are particularly well-suited for adolescents at postpartum or during breastfeeding; and

(6) Decrease in menstrual blood loss may be of particular interest.

Negative health risks include the potential for decreased condom use and increased incidence of STDs[21].

Norplant is less effective in heavier women because of the increased volume of distribution of levonorgestrel, producing a lower blood level; very overweight teenagers desiring Norplant should be counselled accordingly[22].

The higher continuation rate and lower failure rate for Norplant users have been reported in properly prepared adolescent mothers[23].

Depo-Provera

Although a long-acting method such as Norplant or Depo-Provera (medroxyprogesterone acetate) is an excellent alternative for contraceptive compliance problems, the numerous minor side-effects may contribute to a high rate of discontinuation among teenagers. Acne, weight change and irregular bleeding are more common among Norplant and Depo-Provera users, compared to those using oral contraception. Nevertheless, both long-acting gestagens have proved to be relatively popular and successful, especially among teenagers who have experienced previous pregnancies or have used oral contraceptives in the past. Effective counselling and education are critical for the successful use of these long-acting methods[24].

There is some concern that the blood levels of estrogen with the use of Depo-Provera are relatively lower over a period of time compared to a normal menstrual cycle, and therefore patients can lose bone mass to some degree[25]. Although the peak bone mass is influenced by heredity and endocrine factors, it is now recognized that there exists only a relatively narrow window of opportunity for acquiring bone mass. Almost all of the bone mass in the hip and the vertebral bodies will be accumulated by late adolescence. After adolescence, there is only slight gain in total skeletal mass that ceases around age 30 years, and in many individuals a decline in bone mass begins after age 18 years. Blair and colleagues[26] found a decrease in bone density among adolescents using Depo-Provera compared to an increase observed with Norplant or oral contraceptives. However, it has been reported that, after discontinuing Depo-Provera, bone mass density is regained, even after long-term use[27].

CONCLUSIONS

Because contraception affects not only the risk of unplanned pregnancy, but also that of sexually transmitted infection, the choice of a particular method is important to future fertility. Contraceptives with the best record of preventing pregnancy (oral contraceptives, Norplant, Depo-Provera and intrauterine devices) provide little protection against STDs, pelvic inflammatory disease or HIV, which are major threats to the fertility and well-being of adolescents who are sexually active and who have long reproductive and sexual lives ahead of them. Condom use needs to be strongly encouraged when counselling adolescents.

Adolescent contraception is a good opportunity to educate about 'responsible sexuality'. It has been claimed that, because of the established association between early initiation of sexual intercourse, unintended pregnancy and STDs, programs which result in the postponement of sexual involvement and a decrease in unintended adolescent pregnancies will also directly and significantly reduce the risk of STDs in the adolescent population.

Physicians must approach adolescent sexuality from the perspective of promoting optimal health-oriented decision making.

REFERENCES

1. Creatsas GK, Vekemans M, Horejsi J, Uzel R, Lauritzen C, Osler M, Athea N, Toublanc JE, Molnar A, Orley J, Bruni V, Rademakers J, Siegberg R, Widholm O, Stedman Y. Adolescent sexuality in Europe: a multicentric study. *Adolesc Pediatr Gynecol* 1995; 8: 59–63

2. Genuis S, Genuis SK. The challenge of sexually transmitted diseases in adolescents. *Adolesc Pediatr Gynecol* 1995; 8: 82–8
3. Rosenfeld W, Vermund SH, Wentz SJ, Burke RD. High prevalence rate of human papillomavirus infection and association with abnormal papanicolau smears in sexually active adolescents. *Am J Dis Child* 1989; 143: 1443–7
4. Lazzarin A, Saracco A, Musicco M, Nicolosi A. Man to woman sexual transmission of the human immunodeficiency virus: risk factors related to sexual behavior, man's infectiousness, and woman's susceptibility. *Arch Intern Med* 1991; 151: 2411–15
5. Boyer PJJ. HIV infection in pregnancy. *Pediatr Ann* 1993; 22: 406–10
6. Werner MJ, Biro FM. Contraception and sexually transmitted diseases in adolescent females. *Adolesc Pediatr Gynecol* 1990; 3: 127–30
7. Forrest JD, Singh S. The sexual and reproductive behavior of American women, 1982–1988. *Fam Plann Perspect* 1990; 22: 206
8. The Alan Guttmacher Institute. *Sex and America's Teenagers.* The Alan Guttmacher Institute, New York: The Contraception Report, 1994
9. Suris JC, Parera N, Puig C. *Encuesta de Salud a los Adolescentes de la Ciudad de Barcelona 1993.* Unitat d'Adolescents, Institut Universitari Dexeus
10. Poppen PJ. Adolescent contraceptive use and communication: changes over a decade. *Adolescence* 1994; 29: 503–14
11. Robinson JC, Plichter S, Weisman CS, Nathanson CA, Ensminger M. Dysmenorrhea and use of oral contraceptives in adolescent women attending a family planning clinic. *Am J Obstet Gynecol* 1992; 166: 578
12. Polatti F, Perotti F, Filippa N, Gallina D, Nappi RE. Bone mass and long-term monophasic oral contraceptive treatment in young women. *Contraception* 1995; 51: 221–4
13. Speroff L, Darney PH. *A Clinical Guide for Contraception.* Baltimore, USA: Williams & Wilkins, 1996
14. Buiattri E. Cervical smears: when to start and how often to do. In Hannaford PC, Webb AMC, eds. *Evidence-guided Prescribing of the Pill.* Carnforth, UK: Parthenon Publishing, 1996; 157–66
15. Carpenter S, Neinstein LS. Weight gain in adolescent and young adult oral contraceptive users. *J Adolesc Health Care* 1986; 7: 342
16. Sulak PJ, Haney AF. Unwanted pregnancies: understanding contraceptive use and benefits in adolescents and older women. *Am J Obstet Gynecol* 1993; 168: 2042–8
17. Grace E, Emans SJ, Woods ER. The impact of AIDS awareness on the adolescent female. *Adolesc Pediatr Gynecol* 1989; 2: 40–3
18. Cates W. Contraceptive choice, sexually transmitted diseases, HIV infection, and future fecundity. *J Br Fertil Soc* 1996; 1: 18–22
19. Farley MM, Rosenberg MJ, Rowe PJ, Chen J-H, Meirik O. Intrauterine devices and pelvic inflammatory disease: an international perpective. *Lancet* 1990; 339: 785–7
20. Fried-Oginski W, Hershlag A. The use of Norplant during teenage years. Literature reviews. *Adolesc Pediatr Gynecol* 1995; 8: 102–5
21. Rosenthal SL, Biro FM, Kollar LM, Hillard PJA, Ralph JL. Experience with side effects and health risks associated with Norplant implant use in adolescents. *Contraception* 1995; 52: 283–5
22. Sivin I. International experience with Norplant and Norplant-2 contraceptives. *Stud Fam Plann* 1988; 19: 81

23. Blumenthal PD, Wilson LE, Remsburg RE, Cullins VE, Huggins GR. Contraceptive outcomes among postpartum and post-abortal adolescents. *Contraception* 1994; 50: 451–60
24. Cromer BA, Smith RD, Blair JM, Dwyer J, Brown RT. A prospective study of adolescents who choose among levonorgestrel implant (Norplant), medroxyprogesterone acetate (Depo-Provera), or the combined oral contraceptive pill as contraception. *Pediatrics* 1994; 94: 687–91
25. Cundy T, Evans M, Roberts H, Wattie D, Ames R, Reid IR. Bone density in women receiving depot medroxyprogesterone acetate for contraception. *Br Med J* 1991; 303: 13
26. Blair JM, Cromer B, Mahan J, *et al.* Bone density in adolescent girls on Depo-Provera and Norplant. *J Adolesc Health* 1995; 16: 164–7
27. Cundy T, Cornish J, Evans MC, Roberts H, Reid IR. Recovery of bone density in women who stop using medroxyprogesterone acetate. *Br Med J* 1994; 308: 247

This paper has been reproduced from *Eur J Contracept Reprod Health Care* 1997; 2: 89–94

27 Hazards in perimenopausal contraception

H.P.G. Schneider

INTRODUCTION

Recently, Brambilla and colleagues[1] presented a method for defining the inception of perimenopause based on self-reported data. A large study sample (n = 15 050) was obtained from a 5-year longitudinal study of women aged 45–55 years. Responses to questions concerning timing of the last menstrual period, menstrual regularity and presence of menopausal symptoms allowed a definition of how to predict a menopause 3 years later. The two items that best defined the inception of perimenopause were:

(1) Self-report of 3–11 months of amenorrhea; and

(2) For those without amenorrhea, self-report of increased menstrual irregularity.

Thus, this proposed definition is consistent with a commonly accepted definition of natural menopause, which is 12 consecutive months of amenorrhea.

Early publications in 1975 highlighted an increased risk of myocardial infarction in combined pill users, especially in women over 40 years of age. However, in those studies no information was at hand about smoking habits. Finally, the Royal College of General Practitioners (RCGP, 1981), in a cohort study, found an increased cardiovascular risk with both age and smoking, but confidence intervals for the data on older non-smoking women were quite large. These same data were re-analyzed in a more sophisticated manner in 1989[2], and it became evident that the risk was only significant in older women who also smoked. This good news about the relative safety of the pill for non-smoking older women still awaits appreciation by the general population. Women's perceptions of the pill, all over Europe, are of health hazards rather than of benefits.

FECUNDITY

The median menopausal age in our population is 50–51 years (range 39–59 years). The perimenopausal phase, prior to the onset of menopause, is generally referred to as premenopause and is characterized by a pattern of irregular cycling and increased periods of amenorrhea, which reflect rapid hormonal changes. The length of premenopause is 4–5 years (range from less than 12 months to more than 9 years). It is also important to note that 25% of women experience premenopause at less than 43 years of age. Only 5% of premenopausal women will cycle regularly up to the age of 51 years. In those populations that are not using birth control, fertility is observed to be lost 5–10 years before the mean time of the menopause. The onset of hot flushes and decrease in bone density begin to occur prior to menopause. Therefore, fertility is probably very low in a woman who has clear signs of the perimenopause, such as hot flushes and oligomenorrhea.

Metcalf and colleagues[3] have shown that spontaneous ovulatory cycles can still occur in typically climacteric women despite raised gonadotropin levels. Experience with *in vitro* fertilization in women up to age 44 years has shown better pregnancy rates in previously amenorrheic women than in women having menstrual cycles[4]. Overall, the pregnancy rates per 100 woman years of those aged 45 years will be 10–20 and in women aged 50 years, 0–5[5]. As there are no reliable predictors of future fertile cycles, in order to prevent the increased pregnancy risk at perimenopausal age, only empirical guides can be offered[6]:

(1) In women having natural cycles, continuous birth control until there have been no periods for 1 year;

(2) In women having artificial withdrawal bleeds, if the woman is healthy and a non-smoker, continuation of a modern (third-generation) low-dose pill until 50 years of age.

Alternative options are:

(1) Change to a barrier or spermicide method of contraception and assess the menopausal state over a period of time; or

(2) Change to hormone replacement therapy using, in addition, a progestogen-only mini pill; or

(3) Take a risk.

AGE-RELATED RISKS AND MANAGEMENT STRATEGIES

The German Menopause Society organized a representative survey (Infratest, 1996) on women aged 45–64 years[7]; of these, 24% were hysterectomized and 12% bilaterally ovariectomized. About 25% of all women develop fibroids, which, due to their estrogen dependence, will reduce spontaneously following menopause. Ovarian function during perimenopause provides peripheral estrogen levels similar to those in the late follicular and preovulatory phase and far beyond the amounts of bioavailable estrogen during contraception. It is for this reason that oral contraception is partially protective against the development of these tumors; after 5 years of oral contraceptive use, the incidence of fibroids will be reduced by 17%, and after 10 years by about 13%.

Other benefits of oral contraceptive pills for women over 40 years of age, as well as prevention of pregnancy and reduction of fibroid incidence, are a 50% reduction in menorrhagia and iron deficiency anemia. These effects were demonstrated in the RCGP Oral Contraception Study which recruited women in younger age groups, but it is likely that, on theoretical grounds, the pill will reduce the menstrual flow as effectively in older women as in younger ones[8]. Finally, as 75% of all hysterectomized women had disorders of menorrhagia and fibroids, the pill could clearly reduce hysterectomy rates.

RISK OF CANCER AND ORAL CONTRACEPTIVE USE

Breast cancer

Breast cancer is the most common form of cancer in women in industrialized countries. More than 25% of all cases of breast cancer occur before the age of 50 years. A very recent collaborative re-analysis presented individual data on more than 53 000 women with breast cancer from 26 countries[9]. The studies were varied in their setting, design and timing. Similarly, the individual women included in the analyses are of variable backgrounds and have different baseline risks of breast cancer. Despite the heterogeneity of the study designs and of the subjects, the results are remarkably consistent across the various studies and for women with different characteristics.

Recency of oral contraceptive use appears to explain most of the variation in breast cancer risk. Women who are apparently using combined oral contraceptives or have used them in the past 10 years are at a slightly increased risk of having breast cancer diagnosed, although the additional cancers diagnosed tend to be localized to the breast. There is no evidence of an increase in the risk of having breast cancer diagnosed 10 or more years after cessation of use; indeed for certain groups of past users there may, if anything, be a reduction in the risk of breast cancer. In particular, there is a reduction in the risk of tumors that have spread beyond the breast associated with use of oral contraceptive preparations containing high doses of hormones.

We have to admit that there is still little information about the effects of oral contraceptive use that ceased more than 20 years ago, particularly concerning women who began use as teenagers and are now reaching an age when breast cancer is common. Such data should become available in the next decade.

Endometrial cancer

The most conclusive data were collected by the Cancer and Steroid Hormone Study[10]. In this large case–control study, 433 women aged 20–54 years with confirmed epithelial endometrial cancer were compared to 3191 controls, selected at random from the same populations. Among women using oral contraceptives for at least 12 months, as compared to non-users, the relative risk of endometrial cancer was 0.6 (95% confidence interval 0.3–0.9). No differences in risk were noted when specific oral contraceptive formulations were examined. This benefit persisted for at least 15 years after oral contraceptive use when discontinued.

Ovarian cancer

From the previously mentioned Cancer and Steroid Hormone Study cohort, 546 women aged 20–54 years with confirmed ovarian cancer, and 14 228 controls selected from the same population, were compared, to determine the risk of ovarian cancer[11]. The relative risk of developing epithelial ovarian cancer in ever users of oral contraceptives, as compared to non-users, was 0.6 (95% confidence interval 0.5–0.7). This beneficial effect was observed with oral contraceptives after only 3–6 months of use, and the benefits continued for at least 15 years after oral contraceptive use was discontinued. A number of other studies suggest a similar protection from ovarian cancer by oral contraceptive use[12,13].

The 'windows of protection' against endometrial and ovarian cancer by pill use have little effect in young women. It could, however, develop an important effect in older women through its extension into the age-related peak incidence of these reproductive tumors.

CARDIOVASCULAR RISK AND ORAL CONTRACEPTIVE USE

Epidemiological data on morbidity and mortality clearly demonstrate a fundamental difference between the use of oral contraceptives (OCs) and hormonal replacement therapy (HRT). While OCs increase the risk of cardiovascular and liver diseases, no deleterious effects are caused by treatment with natural estrogens, which may even protect from arterial diseases. As the progestogens contained in OCs are also used for HRT, it is the estrogen component which determines the extent and severity of side-effects. In 1970, in Great Britain, an association was first reported between the dose of estrogen in oral contraceptives and the risk of developing deep vein thrombosis, pulmonary embolism, cerebral thrombosis and coronary thrombosis[14]. The increase in hypertension, stroke, arterial and venous thrombosis associated with the use of OCs is based on the strong hepatic and vascular effects of ethinylestradiol, although several risk factors (smoking, obesity, diabetes, etc.) may be involved. Contrary to this, treatment with estradiol or conjugated estrogens may reduce morbidity and mortality, even in older women with cardiovascular risk factors. Accordingly, the list of contraindications for OC use is extensive, while HRT is only contraindicated in patients with existing hormone-dependent cancer or acute thrombosis.

Ethinylestradiol has a much stronger hepatic effect than estradiol in stimulating hepatic proteins, and ethinylestradiol also exerts a stronger effect on the liver metabolism than on other organs. Clinically speaking, ethinylestradiol has an unfavorable effect on:

(1) Various hepatic serum parameters;

(2) Coagulation parameters;

(3) Direct stimulatory action of platelet aggregation;

(4) Increases in risk of arterial and venous diseases;

(5) Possible unwanted pharmacological effects due to the chemical reactions of the activated ethinyl group; and

(6) Induction of hypertension (possibly caused by the direct action of ethinylestradiol on the local renin–angiotensin system in the arterial wall).

Thromboembolic disease

Oral contraceptives increase the natural incidence of venous thromboses of 1–2 per 10 000 women per year by up to 3–4-fold. Recent investigations have shown that, during intake of desogestrel- or gestodene-containing formulations, the risk is twice that shown with older, low-dose ovulation inhibitors (for review, see reference 15). During pregnancy, the incidence of thromboses rises up to 10 per 10 000 woman years and postpartum up to 40 per 10 000 woman years.

In about two-thirds of thromboses, the etiology is still unknown. Current experience suggests that, in 40% of all cases, an inherited thrombophilia is present. Among the hereditary types of thrombophilia, the resistance against activated protein C (APC resistance) represents nearly 50%, while 15–20% is based on a deficiency of antithrombin III, protein C or protein S. APC resistance, with a prevalence of 3–5% in the general population, increases the risk of thrombosis by 8-fold and in OC users by 35-fold. Protein C deficiency (prevalence 0.1–0.5%) increases the risk of thrombosis by 9-fold and in OC users by 15-fold while antithrombin III deficiency (prevalence 0.02–0.05%) enhances the risk in pill users by 8-fold. Ovulation inhibitors do not influence the risk of thrombosis in women with protein S deficiency. Antiphospholipid antibodies increase during treatment with oral contraceptives and represent a considerably enhanced risk of thrombosis.

A positive family history (before the age of 40 years) indicates an inherent thrombophilia. In these risk groups, the cost–benefit ratio of a selective screening is unfavorable as, at most, 70% of the hereditary thrombophilias can be diagnosed by laboratory analysis, and only very few patients will actually experience a thrombotic event. Only three of 1000 carriers of APC resistance will suffer from thrombosis during oral contraception[15]. On the other hand, a negative result of laboratory tests does not exclude a hereditary thrombophilic disorder which as yet cannot be substantiated. It is not yet clear whether a selective screening is superior to a careful assessment of individual and family history. A general screening cannot be justified because of the unfavorable cost–benefit ratio[15].

If we are dealing with an individual or family history presenting unfavorable laboratory parameters with an indication of an enhanced risk of thrombosis, this risk should carefully be weighed against the consequences of discontinuation of pill use. As yet we cannot identify those few individuals with risk factors who will experience a thrombosis. Therefore, in patients with thrombophilic disorders and/or other risk factors, OC use represents a high-risk situation and therefore other contraceptive methods should be considered. On the other hand, those patients with risk factors who choose to use oral contraception should be aware that, in the case of symptoms indicating a thrombosis, the physician must be consulted immediately.

Myocardial infarction and stroke

The risk factors for a myocardial infarction in women less than 50 years of age were assessed in a case–control study of 555 women who survived a myocardial infarction and 1864 controls[16]. Smoking and myocardial infarction were positively related, and this relationship was apparent at all ages and independent of other risk factors for myocardial infarction. There was no association between oral contraceptive use and myocardial infarction among non-smokers. However, the relative risk of myocardial infarction increased sharply among smokers with a current history of oral contraceptive use.

Similar findings have also been reported by others. Current evidence supports the fact that oral contraceptives, especially lower-dose formulations, are not associated with an increased incidence of myocardial infarction or stroke. The most reassuring data have come from the prospective Nurses' Health Study on 119 061 women aged between 35 and 55 years. This study was begun in 1976 and reported on follow-up of 2-year intervals[17]. The relative risk in ever users of oral contraceptives as compared to never users was 0.8 (95% confidence interval 0.6–1.0) for major coronary disease, 1.0 (95% confidence interval 0.7–1.3) for stroke and 0.9 (95% confidence interval 0.7–1.2) for death from cardiovascular disease. It was concluded that there was neither evidence of an increased risk with longer use nor any association with the time since the last use. However, any use of oral contraceptives did not increase the risk of subsequent cardiovascular disease or stroke.

An international case–control study[18] compared 153 women aged 16–44 years with a myocardial infarction event to 498 controls unaffected by myocardial infarction. The odds ratio for myocardial infarction of third- compared to second-generation oral contraceptives was estimated among all 651 study subjects. This ratio was calculated to be 0.36 (95% confidence interval 0.1–1.2) and the odds ratio for the United Kingdom and Germany alone was 0.45 (95% confidence interval 0.1–1.8). This finding from an interim analysis should, according to its authors, be interpreted with extreme caution. However, the excess risk of venous thromboembolism associated with the use of third-generation products may be balanced by the reduced risk of myocardial infarction associated with the same products.

METABOLIC EFFECTS ON BONE

Both the peak bone mass and the extent of its subsequent decrease are the key risk factors for osteoporosis. A critical decrease in bone mineral density has been consistently demonstrated following the menopause. Perimenopausal women aged 40–48 years who experienced oligomenorrhea in the 3–6 months before they entered the study were investigated by Gambacciani and colleagues[19]. Radial bone mineral density at the distal forearm, measured by dual photon absorptiometry, in conjunction with several bone metabolism markers, plasma estradiol and follicle stimulating hormone levels were repeated every 6 months for 2 years. The results suggest that premenopausal administration of OC can prevent the acceleration of bone turnover and reverse the decrease in bone density that follows the premenopausal impairment of ovarian function.

CONCLUSIONS

Definitive prospective controlled investigations on women aged 35–50 years, investigating the relationship between oral contraceptive use and thromboembolic disease, myocardial infarction, stroke, and cancers of the breast and genital organs have not been performed as yet. The clinical information hitherto presented relates to case–control studies and retrospective analyses obtained from large studies on women in all age groups. Only some data are derived from prospective case–control analyses such as the RCGP and Nurses' Health Studies. Physically and mentally healthy women of perimenopausal age certainly are at low risk when using oral contraceptives. Although thromboembolic disease, myocardial infarction and stroke are somewhat more common in older women as compared to younger women, the risk does not appear to be substantially altered in oral contraceptive users and is probably related to other risk factors for cardiovascular disease. Some questions remain about the association between breast cancer and oral contraceptive use, while oral contraceptives have proved to be protective against endometrial and ovarian cancer. The development of perimenopausal osteoporosis can be prevented. Other benign diseases such as menorrhagia, iron deficiency anemia, fibroids and benign ovarian cysts are reduced. Women with a history of particular risk factors or with pathological laboratory indices should follow stringent outpatient services.

Overall, the global effect of oral contraception at late fertile age is beneficial. 'The pill could potentially save many lives if it were in widespread use among women in their forties (without contraindications)' (James Drife at FIGO, 1994).

REFERENCES

1. Brambilla DJ, McKinlay SM, Johannes CB. Defining the perimenopause for application in epidemiologic investigations. *Am J Epidemiol* 1994; 140: 1091–5
2. Croft P, Hannaford PC. Risk factors for acute myocardial infarction in women: evidence from the RCGP oral contraception study. *Br Med J* 1989; 298: 165–8
3. Metcalf MG. Incidence of ovulatory cycles in women approaching menopause. *J Biosoc Sci* 1979; 11: 39–48
4. Kirkman RJE. From contraception to menopause. In Crosignani PG, Paoletti R, Sarrel PM, Wenger NK, eds. *Women's Health in Menopause*. London: Kluwer Academic Publishers, 1994: 207–12
5. Oral contraception in the perimenopause. *Drug Ther Bull* 1991; 29: 3–4
6. Kirkman RJE. Contraceptive options for the 'older' woman. *Eur Menopause J* 1995; 2: 10–12
7. Schneider HPG, Hauser GA. The Menopause Rating Scale (MRS II) – clusters of menopausal symptoms. Presented at the 8th International Congress on the Menopause, Sydney, 1997; abstract
8. Drife JO. The benefits of combined oral contraceptives. *Br J Obstet Gynaecol* 1989; 96: 1225–8
9. Collaborative Group on Hormonal Factors in Breast Cancer. Breast cancer in hormonal contraceptives: collaborative reanalysis of individual data on 53 297 women with breast cancer and 100 239 women without breast cancer from 54 epidemiological studies. *Lancet* 1996; 347: 1713–27
10. The Cancer and Steroid Hormone Study of the Centers for Disease Control and the National Institute of Child Health and Human Development. Combination oral contraceptive use and the risk of endometrial cancer. *J Am Med Assoc* 1987; 257: 796
11. The Cancer and Steroid Hormone Study of the Centers for Disease Control and the National Institute of Child Health and Human Development. The reduction in risk of ovarian cancer associated with oral contraceptive use. *N Engl J Med* 1987; 316: 650
12. Rosenberg L, Shapiro S, Slone D *et al.* Epithelial ovarian cancer and combination oral contraceptives. *J Am Med Assoc* 1982; 247: 3210
13. Willet PC, Bain C, Hennekens CH *et al.* Oral contraceptives and the risk of ovarian cancer. *Cancer* 1981; 48: 1684
14. Inman WHB, Vessey MP, Westerholm B *et al.* Thromboembolic disease and the steroidal content of oral contraceptives: a report to the Committee on Safety of Drugs. *Br Med J* 1970; 2: 203
15. Bauersachs R, Lindhoff-Last E, Ehrly AM, Kuhl H. The significance of hereditary thrombophilia for the risk of thrombosis associated with oral contraception. *Zbl Gynäkol* 1996; 118: 262–70
16. Rosenberg L, Kaufman DW, Helmrich SP *et al.* Myocardial infarction and cigarette smoking in women younger than 50 years of age. *J Am Med Assoc* 1985; 253: 2965

17. Stampfer MJ, Willett WC, Colditz GA *et al.* A prospective study of past use of oral contraceptive agents and risk of cardiovascular diseases. *N Engl J Med* 1988; 319; 1313
18. Lewis MA, Spitzer WO, Heinemann LAJ *et al.* Third-generation oral contraceptives and risk of myocardial infarction: an international case-control study. *Br Med J* 1996; 312: 88–90
19. Gambacciani M, Spinetti A, Cappagli B *et al.* Hormone replacement therapy in perimenopausal women with a low-dose oral contraceptive preparation: effects on bone mineral density and metabolism. *Maturitas* 1994; 19: 125–31

This paper has been reproduced from *Eur J Contracept Reprod Health Care* 1997; 2: 95–100

28 No-scalpel technique for vasectomy

M. Filshie

INTRODUCTION

It is estimated that some 60 million men have had a vasectomy worldwide and over 30 million of these have had the procedure performed in China[1]. It is also estimated that over 400 000 procedures occur in the United States annually[2] and over 50 000 cases are performed annually in the United Kingdom[3]. Acceptance of vasectomy is generally low in the developing countries but the incidence is increasing rather than decreasing. It is not surprising that much research and activity into vasectomy techniques have been undertaken, particularly in China. New experimental techniques, such as percutaneous chemical occlusion, have been investigated. These techniques are based on guiding a needle through the skin into the lumen of each vas, checking its correct placement, and then injecting the appropriate chemical. Such injections have included CABCM (a mixture of carbolic acid and *N*-butyl α-cyanoacrylate)[4], MPE (medical grade polyurethane elastoma)[5] and silicone rubber[6] which forms intravasal plugs. By far the most popular and successful technique is that of a no-scalpel vasectomy which essentially is a simple technique of vasal exposure. The technique was first introduced to China in 1975 by Dr Li Shunqiang, Director of the Chongqing Family Planning Scientific Research Institute. This technique was introduced to other countries in 1986. The technique was immediately supported by Dr Douglas Huber, the then Medical Director of the Association of Voluntary Surgical Contraception (AVSC). Both he and Dr Marc Goldsmith (representing the Population Council) organized training programs in Thailand in 1986. The largest comparative study of the Li technique versus the standard approach was conducted in Bangkok at the King's Birthday Festival on 5 December 1987[7] when 1203 patients were operated on. In 1989, the First International Symposium on the No-Scalpel Vasectomy Technique took place in Bangkok, Thailand, December 4–6. Vasectomists from all parts of the world attended and they recommended the no-scalpel technique should be used wherever possible.

The no-scalpel technique is gaining in popularity but not as much as it should. Traditional vasectomy involves a relatively large incision when compared to the no-scalpel technique, thereby making the vas easily palpable and identified and exposed. The no-scalpel vasectomy technique involves a much more subtle approach and more surgical skill and dexterity are required. Teaching and learning the technique are therefore more difficult and surgeons with poor dextrous skills will find the technique difficult and give up prematurely. Nevertheless, every effort should be made to encourage surgeons to adopt the technique. Once a surgeon has fully mastered the no-scalpel technique, he will never revert back to his previous technique.

METHODS

This technique has several important discrete steps and each has to be conducted systematically. Prior to the operation, the anterior aspect of the scrotal region should be shaved.

Instruments required

Two special instruments are required[8]. The first is the vas-grasping ring forceps and the second is the sharp curved dissection forceps (Figure l). Scissors or stitch cutters should be available. A ligation thread, e.g. Dexon, should be available to ligate the cut ends of the vas. A 10-ml syringe with 1% lignocaine is used to anesthetize the skin of the vas and this is administered through a 27 × 1.25-gauge 1.5-cm needle.

Step 1: administration of local anesthetic

The Li technique requires a totally new approach to vasal anesthesia. The anesthesia should be effective yet not produce too much anesthetic edema of the skin overlying the vas together with tissues surrounding the vas[9].

First, the first vas is identified and transfixed using a three-finger technique. This involves placement of the middle finger under the vas and the index finger and the thumb over the vas to transfix it. The vas is manipulated to lie under the mid-line. A small skin weal is made over the vas about 1–2 cm^2, utilizing only 1–1.5 ml of local anesthetic. The vas is put slightly on the stretch and a 27 × 1.25-gauge needle is angled at 45° so as to lie parallel and close to the vas towards the inguinal ring (Figure 2). Approximately 2–4 ml of 1% lignocaine is inserted around the vas by injecting either side of it. By injecting 2–4 cm there is minimal edema of the vas immediately underneath the anesthetized skin. The procedure is repeated on the opposite side.

Step 2: vasal transfixation

Using the three-finger technique, the first vas is identified and manipulated under the skin weal. The vas fixation ring clamp is opened and applied vertically to the skin over the vas. The clamp is then pressed firmly over the vas with

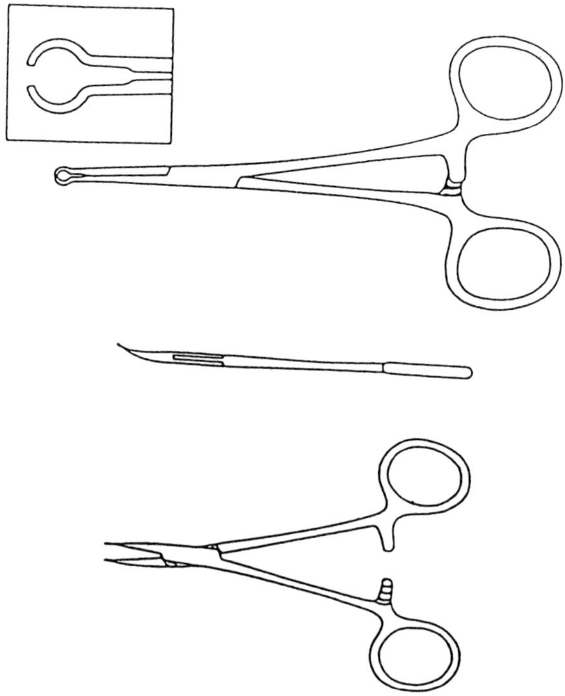

Figure 1 Instruments required

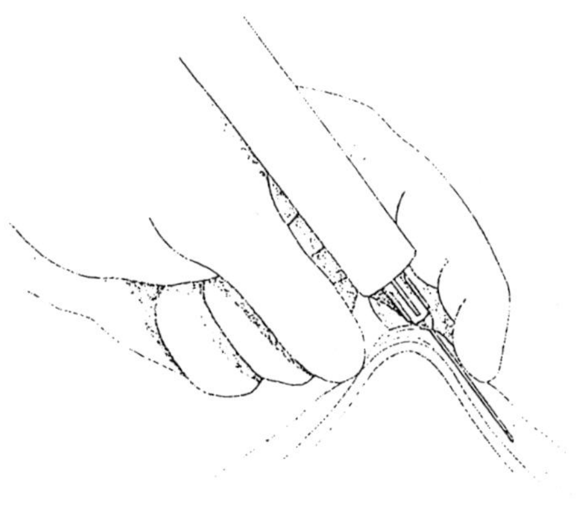

Figure 2 Application of anesthetic to the vas

counter pressure of the middle finger under the vas (Figure 3). The vas, and overlying skin, are slowly but deliberately grasped together so that the vas lies within the ring forceps. When the clamp is then depressed, the skin and underlying vas can be easily seen protruding through the clamp.

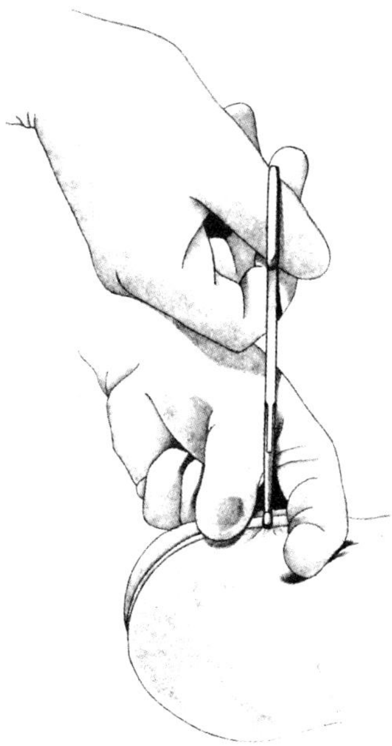

Figure 3 Grasping the vas and overlying skin

Step 3: vasal exposure

The vas is visualized by the use of the specially pointed curved dissection forceps. By opening the forceps, the skin and underlying tissues down to the vas can be punctured by one of the blades of the dissecting forceps which should be approximately at an angle of 45° to the vas (Figure 4). The blade of the forceps is then removed. The two blades are closed together and these are then inserted down the original puncture site, down to the vas itself. The forceps are then opened and the vas is usually seen clearly through the spreaded forceps (Figure 5).

Step 4: exteriorization of the vas

The vas visible through the puncture site is skewered by the right blade of the dissection forceps and the blade is then rotated through 180° slowly (Figure 6). At the same time, the vas ring clamp is slowly released so that the vas is maneuvered out of the wound. The vas clamp is then re-applied to the exteriorized vas and 2-3 cm of the vas can therefore be exposed. The dissecting forceps can also be used to strip the vessels and fascia from the vas (Figure 7).

Step 5: performing the vasectomy

The vas may be clamped and 1–2 cm removed. The ends of the vas may be cauterized and ligated and the fascial inter-position may be made between

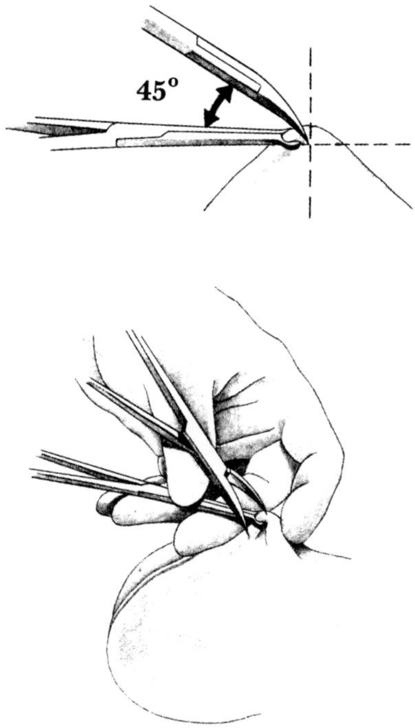

Figure 4 Puncture of skin down to the vas

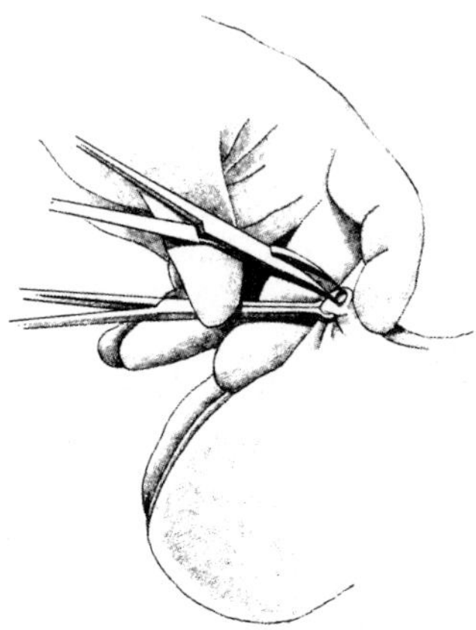

Figure 5 Insertion of dissecting forceps and spreading

the two cut ends at this time. Some surgeons like to tie the testicular end back on itself. Following the ligation procedure, the two ends are repositioned back into the scrotum and the second vas may then be located and once again maneuvered under the previous mid-line puncture. The second vas may be

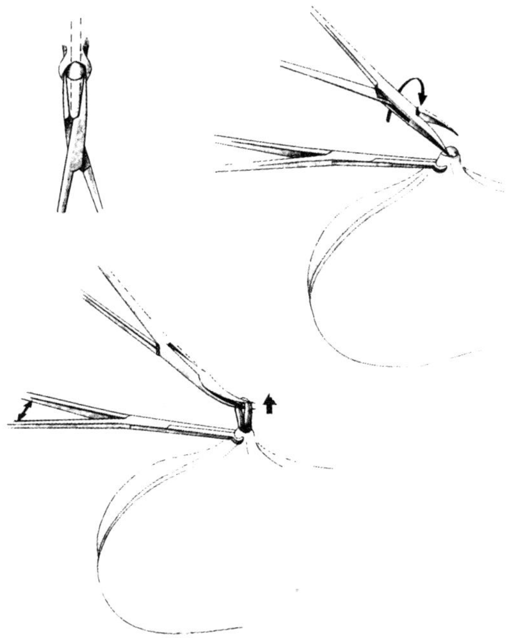

Figure 6 Exteriorizing the vas

transfixed in the same way as the first, using the same puncture site and using the ring clamp as before. If this is difficult, the ring clamp may be inserted through the puncture site and the vas may be grasped directly. Once the vas has been grasped, the exposure is completed, as with the first vas. No skin suture is usually required.

RESULTS

There are very few comparative studies relating to the no-scalpel technique. Nevertheless, the main pivotal study was conducted in Bangkok, involving randomizing the patients to either the standard technique or the no-scalpel technique. Twenty-eight physicians operated on 1203 patients. Twelve physicians utilized the no-scalpel technique, and 16 physicians used the standard technique. The mean number of procedures per physician was 57 (SD = 12) for the no-scalpel technique compared with 33 (SD = 13) for the standard procedure. Nineteen complications were reported during the 2 weeks following the operations. Sixteen occurred following the standard technique (3.1 per 100 procedures) and three occurred following the no-scalpel technique (0.4 per 100 procedures). Hemorrhage was the most common complication and two patients required surgical drainage. Nine of 11 hemorrhages (including those requiring drainage) were from patients who had undergone the standard procedure. Eight patients

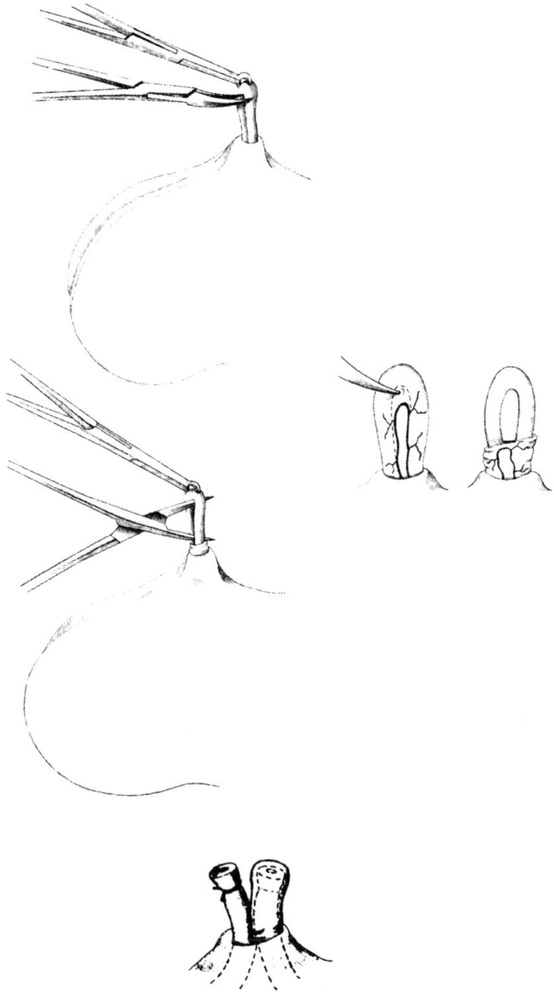

Figure 7 Stripping the vas clean

had an infection diagnosed and seven of those had received the standard technique and one the no-scalpel technique.

In a simple study of 273 patients conducted by Dr Marc Goldstein of the Newark Hospital, Cornell Medical Center, 273 men were operated on and none had hematomas or infections[10].

TEACHING THE NO-SCALPEL TECHNIQUE

This new technique needs careful teaching and the speed and rapidity of the learning depend on the dextrous skill of the trainee. Each step has to be learnt in stages. The following suggestions to facilitate teaching are recommended:

(1) The trainee should read the teaching literature and see a training video.

(2) The trainer should anesthetize the vas initially and the trainee should concentrate his/her learning on the performance of the no-scalpel technique. Once the technique is mastered, local anesthetic injection may be practised.

(3) Should the trainee find the no-scalpel technique difficult, an incision through the skin may be made similar to that performed during a standard procedure. The vas may then be more easily identified through the incision and the vas and overlying sheath can be grasped with the ring forceps. The forceps can then be depressed and the vas exposed using the Li no-scalpel technique. Once this standard puncture technique is perfected, it can then be attempted through the skin directly.

(4) The trainee will need to perform between ten and twenty vasectomies under supervision before the technique is mastered. During this time, he needs to be supported and encouraged.

CONCLUSIONS

The no-scalpel technique involves much less trauma than the standard technique. Once learnt, the operation takes almost half the time of a standard vasectomy and the number of immediate complications are approximately one-eighth of those using the standard technique. It is difficult to continue to support the use of the standard vasectomy technique based on the data to date.

A teaching booklet entitled *No Scalpel Vasectomy – an Illustrated Guide* by Betty Gonzales and Philip Shihua Li is available from the Association of Voluntary Surgical Contraception, 79 Madison Avenue, New York, NY 10016, USA. A video, instruments and teaching booklet are available from Femcare Ltd, St. Peter's Street, Nottingham, NG7 3EN, UK

ACKNOWLEDGEMENTS

The author wishes to thank Dr Douglas Huber and Betty Gonzales from the AVSC for their support and the use of their figures.

REFERENCES

1. Xiaozhang Liu, Shunqiang Li. Vasal sterilisation in China. *Contraception* 1993; 48: 255–65
2. Goldstein M, Feldberg M. *The Vasectomy Book 1982.* Los Angeles: Tarcher-Houghton Mifflin
3. Wellings K. Sterilisation trends. *Br Med J* 1986; 6527: 1029–30

4. Li SQ, Zeng WX. Toxicological evaluation of 504p: an adhesive blocking agent for vas deferens. *Reprod Contracept* (in Chinese) 1991; 2: 36
5. Zhao SC. Vas deferens occlusion by percutaneous injection of polyurethane elastomer plugs: clinical experience and reversibility. *Contraception* 1990; 4: 453
6. Zhao SC, *et al.* Intravasal injection of formed-in-place silicone rubber as a method of vas occlusion. *Int J Androl* 1992; 15: 460–4
7. Nirapathpongporn A, Huber D, Krieger JN. No-scalpel vasectomy at the King's Birthday Vasectomy Festival. *Lancet* 1990; 335: 984
8. Schlegel PN, Goldstein M. No-scalpel vasectomy. *Sem Urol* 1992; X: 252–6
9. Li Shihua P, Li S, Schlegel PN, *et al.* External spermatic sheath injection for vasal nerve block. *Urology* 1992; XXXIX: 173–6
10. Li S, Goldstein M, Zhu J, *et al.* The no-scalpel vasectomy. *J Urol* 1991; 145: 341–4

This paper has been reproduced from *Eur J Contracept Reprod Health Care* 1996; 1: 231–5

29 No scalpel vasectomy: European experience

J. M. Viladoms i Fuster and P. Shihua Li

INTRODUCTION

Vasectomy and circumcision are the most practiced urological procedures worldwide. Vasectomy is one of the fastest, simplest and most effective methods of contraception. Still far fewer vasectomies are performed than tubal ligation worldwide, although vasectomy is faster, cheaper and is associated with less morbidity than tubal ligation. No scalpel vasectomy was created and developed by Dr Shunqiang Li[1] in 1974, in the province of Sichuan, China. This method of vasectomy needs no scalpel, is associated with fewer hematomas and infections than previous methods, is faster and safer than conventional techniques and leaves a very small wound that needs no stitches. It also introduces a new local anesthetic technique that involves a deep injection alongside the vas deferens, creating a vasal nerve block.

Dr Marc Goldstein[1,2] introduced the no scalpel vasectomy technique in the United States in 1986, and it was introduced in Europe during 1993. We review our experience after performing 400 procedures and explain the technique.

MATERIALS AND METHODS

No scalpel vasectomy requires two instruments specially designed[3] to perform the procedure:

(1) Extracutaneous fixation ringed forceps, used to isolate and fix the vas deferens. The surgeon uses the ringed tip of this instrument to encircle and grasp the vas without injuring the skin (henceforth referred to as 'ringed clamp') (Figure 1).

(2) Sharpened curved hemostat, used to puncture the vas deferens, to spread the tissues, to dissect the sheath and to deliver the vas. It is similar to a curved mosquito hemostat, except that the tips are sharply pointed. Throughout this paper, the term 'dissecting forceps' will be used to refer to this instrument (Figure 2).

The remaining materials are those normally used for minor urological surgery, consisting of a 10 ml syringe used to infiltrate the local anesthetic into the skin and to effect the selective anesthetic blockade of the deferential nerves. Straight scissors used to cut the vas deferens if it is believed necessary, and ligatures. In

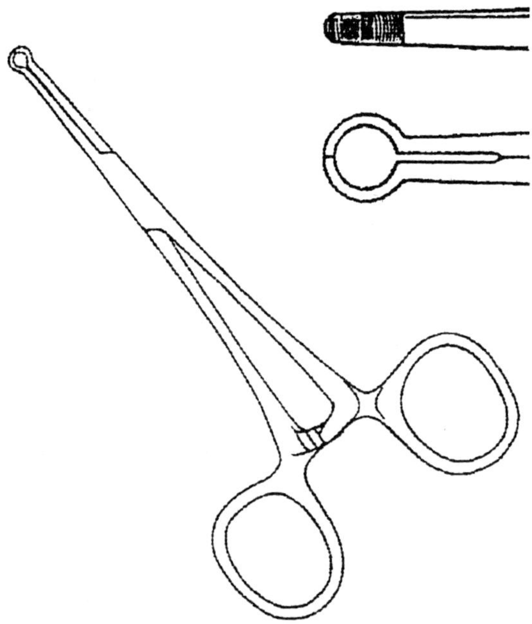

Figure 1 Ringed forceps. Extracutaneous ringed forceps used to fix the vas deferens

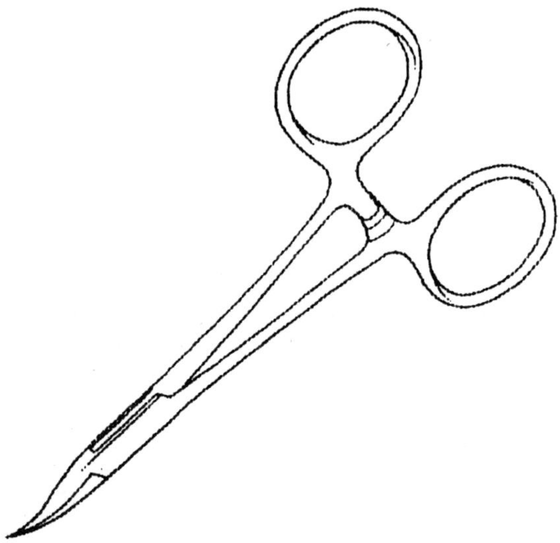

Figure 2 Dissecting forceps. Curved mosquito hemostat. Used to puncture the scrotal skin, to spread the tissues, to dissect the sheath, and to deliver the vas

addition, the following materials can be needed for vasal occlusion, depending on the surgeon's preference: thermal cautery, electrical cautery or ligature (hemoclips, etc.).

In the visit prior to the vasectomy, in addition to giving patients a questionnaire and explaining the technique and its possible complications, we examine the genitalia since most patients are included in the age group showing greater incidence of cancer of the testis. We are also interested in the existence of genital condylomata or other dermatological problems that should have been treated previously[3]. We recommend that patients come to the operating theatre with the scrotum and the inferior part of the prepuce shaved. It is important that the ambient temperature of the operating room should be increased to 20–25 °C. A warm room, by relaxing the scrotum, facilitates the following:

(1) Manipulation of the vas deferens using the three-finger technique;

(2) Fixation of the vas under the median raphe of the scrotum;

(3) Isolation of the vas from the relaxed spermatic cord;

(4) Reduction of operating time; and

(5) Reduction of complications.

The patient must sign a consent form for surgery. It must be emphasized that vasectomy is a permanent method of contraception and that vasectomy reversal is not 100% effective.

SURGICAL TECHNIQUE

Anesthesia

Good local anesthesia[4] is fundamental for an easy vasectomy for the patient and the surgeon. We use lidocaine 1% or 2% without adrenaline, and a 24- or 25-gauge needle. The selective blockade procedure of deferentiae vasa prevents the formation of a hematoma and possible direct injury to the testicular arteries and veins. The innervation of scrotal skin is separate from that of the testis and epididymis (Figure 3). The scrotal skin is supplied by fibers of the pedundal, inguinal, and ilioinguinal nerves. The internal spermatic artery (testicular) and veins are located within the internal spermatic fascia. The vas deferens runs between the internal and external spermatic fascias. The deferential artery, vein and nerves are closely related to the vas deferens. The three-finger technique of administering local anesthesia involves injection within external spermatic fascia but outside of the internal spermatic fascia, thereby minimizing the risk of hematoma and injury to the blood supply of the testis (Figure 3).

Surgical procedure

The no scalpel vasectomy technique requires skilled surgery and the figures refer to surgeons who are right-handed.

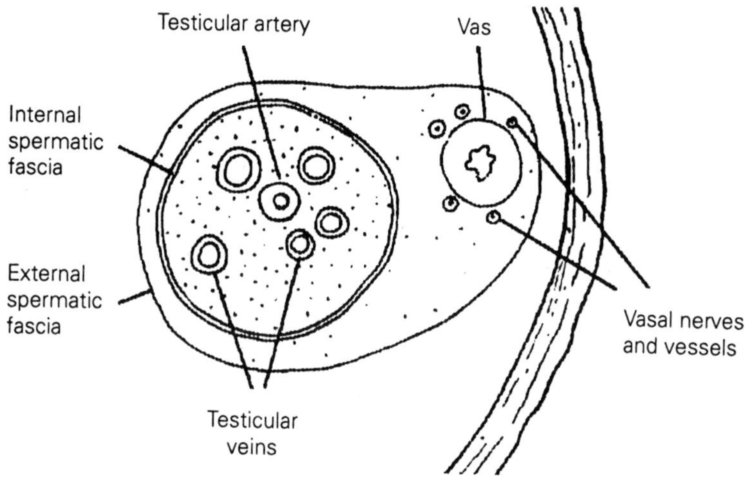

Figure 3 Schematic coronal view of the spermatic cord and internal structures. Vas deferens and its nerves are within the external spermatic fascia but outside of the internal spermatic fascia

The surgeon stands on the right side of the patient, the vas is separated from the internal spermatic vessels and is manipulated to a superficial position just under the scrotal raphe. The right vas is trapped over the middle finger, index finger and thumb (three-finger technique) (Figure 4). A minimum superficial skin wheal of 1% or 2% lidocaine is made with a needle. The needle is then advanced into the pervasal sheath to the external inguinal ring and 3–5 ml of lidocaine are injected, resulting in a vasal nerve block, at a distance from the vasectomy site (Figure 5). The same procedure, accessed through the same puncture hole, is performed for the left vas.

After the vasa are anesthetized, the right vas is mobilized again and fixed under the skin wheal using the three-finger method. The ringed clamp is grasped with the right hand and pressed perpendicularly (Figure 6) on to the scrotal skin overlying the vas. The clamp is then locked around the vas, which fixes the vas without damaging the scrotal skin. The ringed clamp is grasped in the left hand and the entrapped vas is elevated with the left index finger pressing downward to tighten the scrotal skin just ahead of the tips of the ringed clamp and over the anesthetized area.

The vas is pierced with the dissecting forceps exactly in the midline at an angle of 45° (Figure 7). A quick, sharp and single movement should be used to make a clear puncture of the skin down into the vas lumen, using, if possible, the same hole through which the anesthetic was administered. The medial blade of the forceps is advanced into the vas lumen. The left blade is withdrawn, the instrument closed and both blades are introduced through the same puncture hole at the same angle. The blades are then gently opened to spread the tissues

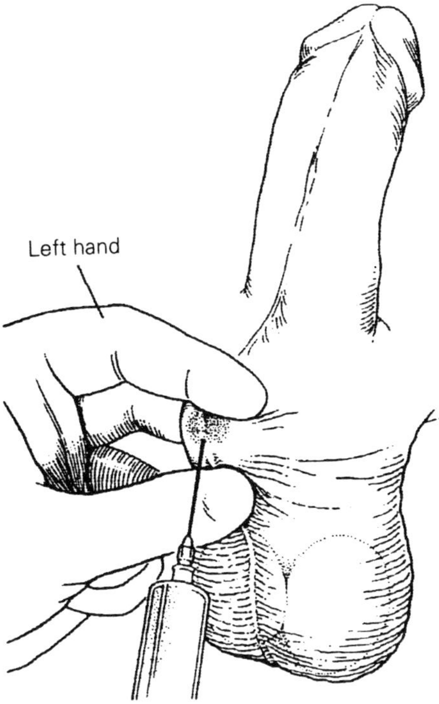

Figure 4 Fixation of the vas deferens with the three-finger technique, isolating the vas and raising the skin wheal

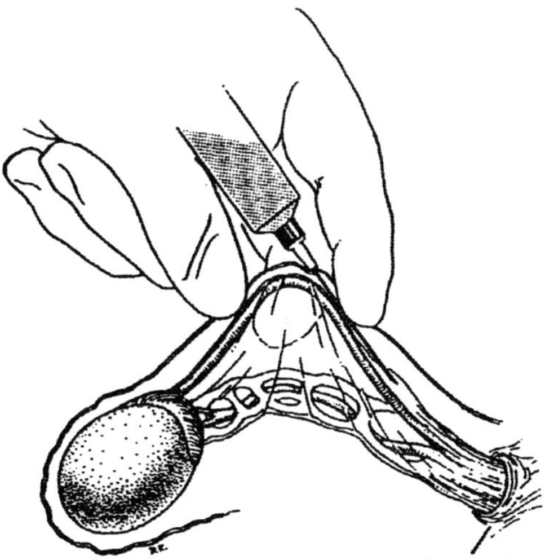

Figure 5 Advancing the needle parallel to the vas within the external spermatic fascia sheath toward the inguinal ring

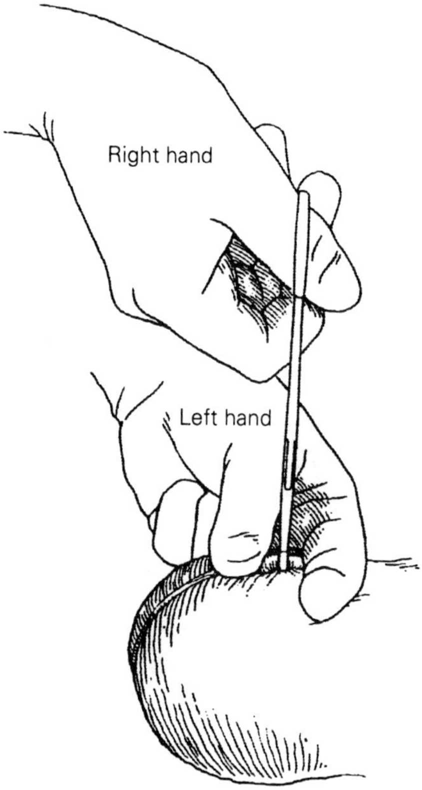

Figure 6 Pressing the tips of the ringed forceps on to the scrotal skin overlying the right vas

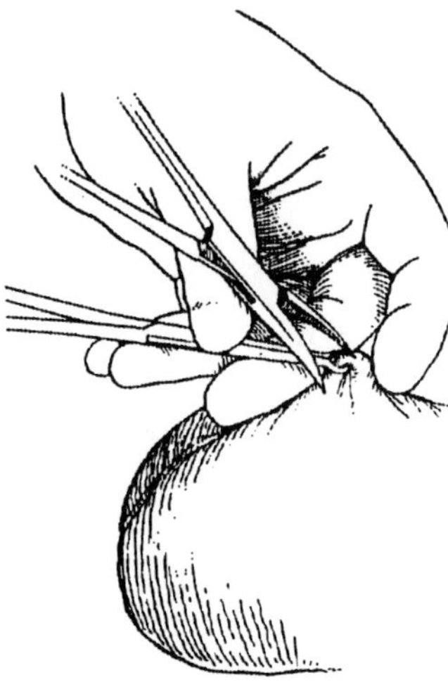

Figure 7 Pressing the index finger to tighten the scrotal skin and piercing the skin with the medial blade of the dissecting forceps

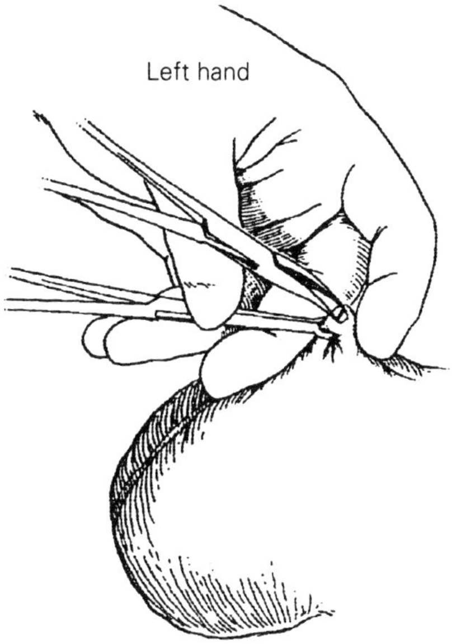

Figure 8 Inserting both tips into the puncture site and spreading the tissues to make a skin opening twice the diameter of the vas

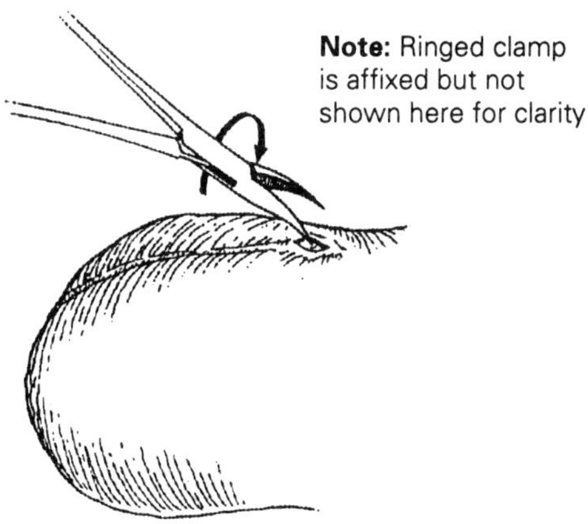

Figure 9 Piercing the wall of the vas with the lateral blade of the dissecting forceps and rotating the dissecting forceps (180°)

and to make a skin opening twice the diameter of the vas (Figure 8). Introducing the right blade of the dissecting clamp, the vas wall is skewered at a 45° angle and the dissecting clamp is rotated laterally by 180° (Figure 9). The vas is then delivered through the puncture hole, while at the same time releasing the ringed extracutaneous fixation clamp. The ring clamp is used to grasp (Figure 10) a

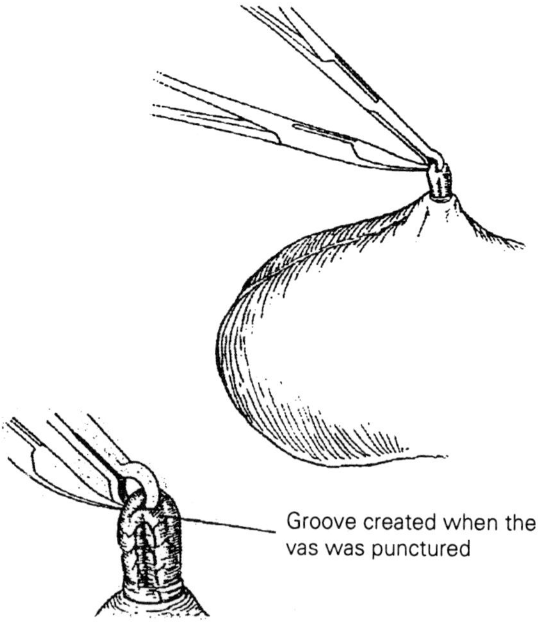

Figure 10 Grasping a partial thickness of the elevated vas deferens

partial thickness of the elevated vas and the dissecting clamp is used to puncture the sheath with one tip. This is followed by the insertion of both tips, and they are then descended to dissect at least 2 cm of the vas. Note that this is a longitudinal, not transverse motion (Figure 11). At this point the vas is divided and occlusion is effected in the preferred manner of the surgeon. Our method is to remove 1 cm of each vas, cauterized with a termal cautery of 1 cm of the vas lumen, and to seal the abdominal end segment of the vas in its sheath, with a medium titanium clip.

After returning the vas to the scrotum, the same procedure is performed on the opposite vas, accessed through the same puncture hole. In this second procedure, it is useful to put the ringed clamp into the previous hole, encircling the vas without the overlying skin. No skin sutures are necessary. The puncture hole will contract and be invisible to the patient. Antibiotic ointment is applied and a sterile dressing left in place with a scrotal support (Figure 12).

RESULTS

Since 1993[5] we have performed more than 450 non-surgical vasectomy procedures at the Hospital General de Catalunya and at Centro Médico Teknon, in Barcelona. Of the 400 most recent patients collected in this study, eight reported minor walking difficulties that disappeared within a week. The incidence of either hematoma or infection has not been appreciable. In the province of

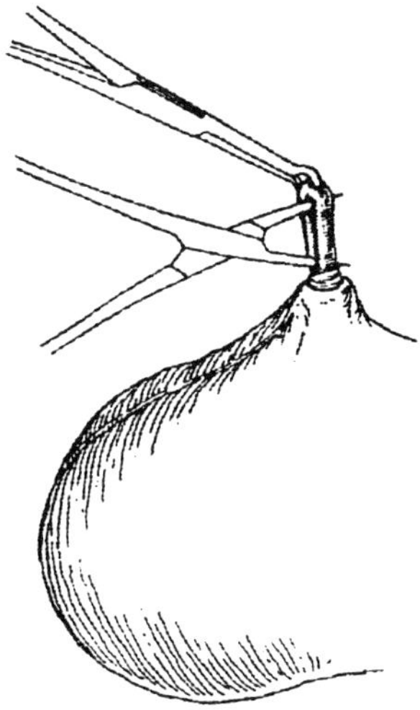

Figure 11 Inserting both tips of the dissecting forceps into the punctured sheath and opening them to strip the sheath

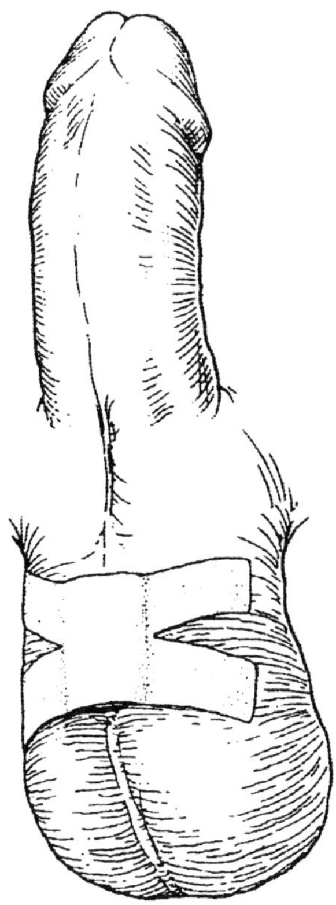

Figure 12 Dressing the wound

Table 1 Complications following no scalpel vasectomy

	Number of patients	Hematoma (n)	Infection (n)
China	179 741	160(0.09%)	1630(0.91%)
New York	238	0	0
Barcelona	400	0	0

Sichuan, China, more than 10 million non-surgical vasectomies have been performed[6]. In a study on 179 741 men, hematomas were found in 160 cases and superficial infections of the wound in 1630 cases. In New York, another study on 273 patients did not find evidence of either complication[1,2,7,8] (Table 1). The operating time for the procedures practiced in Barcelona ranged from 5 to 11 min, representing a mean time reduction of 50% compared with operating time for conventional vasectomies.

DISCUSSION

Vasectomy is safer, quicker and cheaper than tubal ligation. Despite this, many more tubal ligations are performed worldwide than vasectomies. The most frequent complications following vasectomy are hematoma and infection. With the traditional vasectomy technique, the percentage of hematomas varies between 1% and 29%, with an average of 2%. The average number of infections following traditional vasectomy is 3.4%, ranging between 2% and 38%. One death associated with scrotal gangrene has been reported. In a study carried out in Thailand[7] on 1203 men, 28 surgeons compared no scalpel vasectomy with the traditional technique (one incision in the middle of the scrotum). The percentage of complications following traditional vasectomy was found to be 3.1% while that following no scalpel vasectomy was found to be 0.4%. The no scalpel vasectomy technique took, on average, only 40% of the time taken to accomplish the incisional technique.

The method of occlusion of the vas lumen continues to be the subject of controversy[9,10]. Thermal cauterization of the deferential lumen presents a smaller failure index than that of electrosurgical cauterization. It has been suggested to leave the extreme testicular area without occlusion; interposing the deferential fascia of the cauterized abdominal extreme would favor the formation of a sperm granuloma that would reduce the intra-epididymal pressure, which would improve the forecast of vasovasostomy. Other authors corroborate this opinion, but indicate a greater percentage of recanalizations. We should not forget that the patient desires sterility more than the assurance of hypothetical reversibility.

In 1993, a study emphasized the high risk of developing prostate cancer following vasectomy[11–14].

Thereafter an expert committee was formed, comprising members from the World Health Organization, the Center for Diseases Control (CDC), the Association for Voluntary Surgical Contraception (AVSC), the John Hopkins University, the University of Harvard, etc. However, they did not find a significant association between vasectomy and prostate cancer, and concluded the following[14]:

(1) Providers should continue to offer vasectomy and to perform the procedure;

(2) Reversal of vasectomies is not warranted in order to prevent prostate cancer;

(3) Screening for prostate cancer should not be any different for men who have had a vasectomy than those who have not.

The no scalpel vasectomy technique is a refined approach for isolating and delivering the vas by use of vasal block anesthesia. It requires unique surgical skills, including new ways of handling specialized instruments and for these reasons it takes time to become proficient in the procedure. Even experienced vasectomists require hands-on training and need to carry out 15–25 procedures in order to develop proficiency.

Complications are exceptional following no scalpel vasectomy and inconvenience is reduced for the patient. The procedure of fixing the vas with the ring clamp will be useful for the techniques of percutaneous vasectomy[15], with the injection of a solution of polyurethane forming an intravasal plug that occludes the lumen of the vas deferens. In addition, the ring clamp is being used for the manipulation of the deferential extremities in vasovasostomy (vasectomy reversal).

In summary, we believe that no scalpel vasectomy is the best method of male contraception since the potential local complications are decreased. We also believe that thermal cautery is the best method for sealing the vas.

REFERENCES

1. Li S, Goldstein M, Zhu J, *et al.* The no-scalpel vasectomy. *J Urol* 1991; 145: 341–4
2. Goldstein M. Vasectomy and Vasectomy Reversal. In *Current Therapy in Endocrinology and Metabolism-3*. New York: BC Decker Inc 1988; 263–8
3. Goldstein M and Feldberg M. *The Vasectomy Book – A Complete Guide To Decision-Making*. Los Angeles: JP Tarcher Inc 1982
4. Li PS, Li S, Schlegel PN, *et al.* External spermatic sheath injection for vasal nerve block. *Urology* 1992; 39: 173–6
5. Viladoms JM, Li PS. Vasectomia sin bisturí. *Arch Esp de Urol* 1994; 47: 695–701
6. Huber D. No-scalpel vasectomy: The transfer of a refined technique from China to other countries. *Adv Contracep* 1989; 5: 217–20
7. Nirathpongporn A, Huber D and Krieger JN. No-scalpel vasectomy at the King's birthday vasectomy festival. *Lancet* 1990; 335: 894

8. Schliegel PN, Goldstein M. Vasectomy. *AUA Update Series*, lesson 13, 1992, XI: 98
9. Genniston GC. Vasectomy by electrocautery. Outcomes in a series of 2500 patients. *J Fam Practice* 1985; 21: 35–7
10. Shapiro EI, Silber SJ. Open-ended vasectomy, sperm granuloma and postvasectomy orchialgia. *Fertil Steril* 1979; 52: 546–50
11. Giovannucci E, Ashcherio A, Rimm EB, *et al.* A prospective cohort study of vasectomy and prostate cancer in US men. *J Am Med Assoc* 1993; 269: 873–7
12. Giovannucci E, Tosteson TD, Speizer FE, *et al.* A retrospective study of vasectomy and prostate cancer in US men. *J Am Med Assoc* 1993; 269: 878–82
13. Howards SS, Peterson HB. Vasectomy and prostate cancer. Chance, bias or a casual relationship? *J Am Med Assoc* 1993; 269: 914
14. Harper PB. Experts advise no change in vasectomy practice: prostate cancer link doubtful. *Assoc Vol Surg Contracep News* 1993; 31: 1–2
15. Zhao SC. Vas deferens occlusion by percutaneous injection of polyurethane elastomer plugs. Clinical experience and reversibility. *Contraception* 1990; 41: 453–5

30 Cancer and other risks of vasectomy

A. Alcaraz and O. Arango

INTRODUCTION

As a minor surgical procedure that can be performed easily under local anesthesia to induce sterilization, apparently without serious complications, vasectomy has obvious advantages for fertility control. The number of vasectomized men is increasing yearly, especially among men under 45 years. Both the number of men who have undergone the procedure (more than 50 million)[1] and their life expectancy after surgery will therefore increase, making necessary a careful examination of any report of serious long-term health risks associated with vasectomy.

The side-effects of vasectomy can be considered as short-term and long-term complications. Short-term side-effects are, in fact, the surgical complications, no one of them serious and, taken as a whole, happening in less than 4% of the patients who undergo vasectomy. Its reliability as a method of birth control must be analyzed because of the presence of late failures that are reported to occur after about 0.6% of operations and the meaning of the so-called 'special clearance' after vasectomy.

Among long-term side-effects, relevant studies have been carried out to ascertain the relationship between urological malignancies and vasectomy. Several studies in 1990, mainly hospital-based studies, raised enormous concern about an increased risk of testicular and prostate cancer among vasectomized men. Editorials in the most prestigious journals evaluated these studies and a number of other new studies, including population-based ones, which were undertaken at this date. This paper attempts to analyze these studies to clarify whether such a relationship between these urological malignancies and vasectomy is causal.

Since vasectomy mimics immunization with sperm-atozoa, different immunological disorders, including testicular atrophy, anaphylactic reactions and development of glomerulonephritis and atherosclerosis secondary to immunocomplex deposit, have been postulated. A critical review of the available data on these issues seems appropriate at this time.

SURGICAL COMPLICATIONS

Significant early postoperative complications occur in less than 4% of patients who undergo vasectomy. Infection, hematoma and orchitis are the most frequent. All of them are easily treated and *restitutio at integrum* is the usual outcome. Chronic testicular pain, a recognized complication of vasectomy, is causing interest in recent reports. Chronic testicular discomfort is a common sequela of vasectomy, occurring in around one-third of patients. Pain troublesome enough to make the patient seek further treatment and to regret vasectomy occurs in around 5%[2]. These percentages have important implications for the process of informed consent including a warning of these complications before vasectomy. When chronic testicular pain is present, ultrasound scrotal examination very often shows epididymal cysts. Histology shows dilated tubules packed with sperm and ruptured tubules with extravasation. Epididymectomy achieves complete relief of pain in almost all the cases[3].

RISK OF PREGNANCY AFTER VASECTOMY

Early failure

Vasectomy is one of the most reliable methods of birth control. When vasectomy is performed by an experienced surgeon, the rate of early failure is 0.4%[4]. Identification of early failure is easy in the postvasectomy semen analysis which shows the persistence of motile spermatozoa. Revasectomy is the treatment.

Special clearance

A second situation occurring in 2.5% of vasectomized men is the so-called 'special clearance', where there is a persistence of scanty (< 10 000/ml) sperm in two consecutively examined semen samples at least 7 months after vasectomy[4]. The trend of this semen is to azoospermia in the next 3 years[5].

The risk of pregnancy occurring in the presence of non-motile sperm has been estimated to be less than the established risk of late recanalization, according to the survey by Berger and colleagues[6]. They provide both clinical and medicolegal support so that men with a few persistent non-motile sperm after vasectomy can be issued with a special clearance, setting the risks of pregnancy in a properly documented manner so that other forms of contraception can be discontinued.

Late recanalization

In the study by O'Brien and colleagues[4] among 1000 men who had an azoospermic analysis after vasectomy, six men (0.6%) had positive semen analyses 1 year after the initial test. In all six, the sperm count was 10 000 per ml. Five of the six men produced repeat samples 1 month later, which in all five cases showed azoospermia. The authors established that the transitory reappearance of sperm following successful vasectomy occurs in about 0.6% of men. This incidence is 18 times higher than the reported pregnancy rate following successful vasectomy. Transitory reappearance of sperm following vasectomy may help to explain pregnancies occurring in the partners of apparently azoospermic men who have previously undergone vasectomy. Smith and colleagues[7] have recently reported six such cases in which paternity was proved by DNA finger-printing. Late failure of vasectomy, defined as the occurrence of pregnancy after two previous azoospermic analyses, occurs in 0.04–0.1% of vasectomized men due to recanalization, usually several years after vasectomy. Although studies in which semen analysis is performed 1 year after the previous two azoospermic analyses found a rate of 0.6% of samples with the presence of spermatozoa, the rate of pregnancies is around 1/2000 vasectomies. Clearly, the pregnancy rate does not reflect the late recanalization. All vasectomy patients and their partners should be counselled about the small possibility of late failure, and the warning of failure should be recorded.

CANCER RISK

Testicular tumor

Cale and colleagues in 1990[8] raised a new and serious worry that vasectomy increased the incidence and might accelerate the growth of testicular tumors. From a cohort of over 3000 men in Central Scotland who had undergone vasectomy, eight developed testicular cancer within 4 years of the operation compared with an expected 1.9. As the authors did not indicate the types of tumors, we do not know whether this finding was just an unfortunate coincidence (as different tumor types would suggest) or whether we should be more worried (as similar pathological appearances would suggest).

Moller and co-workers[9], after studying a cohort of 73 917 men identified in hospital discharge records and pathology registers as having had a vasectomy and comparing the cancer rates with those of the Danish population as a whole, proved that the incidence of testicular cancer in men with vasectomy is not increased. Other studies[10,11] have confirmed this lack of correlation between vasectomy and testicular cancer.

Prostate cancer

Although two previous studies[12,13] in 1990 suggested a relationship between vasectomy and prostate cancer, the cohort studies by Giovannucci and colleagues published in the *Journal of the American Medical Association* in 1993[14,15] raised enormous concern and controversy about this subject. Editorials in the most prestigious journals evaluated these studies as well as a number of other new studies which were undertaken at this date. Although the studies by Giovannucci and colleagues are highly qualified, for most prestigious epidemiologists it remains unclear whether the relationship they report on is 'causal'.

The first studies suggesting an increase in the risk of prostate cancer following vasectomy were those conducted by Rosemberg and colleagues[12] and Mettlin and co-workers[13]. Both reports were hospital-based case–control studies and both were designed to screen many possible associations between various exposures and a range of diseases, not specifically to test the hypothesis that vasectomy increases the risk of prostate cancer. Rosemberg's group studied 220 men aged 40–69 years who had been admitted to hospital from 1976 to 1988 with prostate cancer diagnosed in previous years; these patients were compared with a control group of 960 men admitted for other cancers and 571 men admitted for non-cancer reasons. They found a three- to five-fold increase in the age-adjusted risk of prostate cancer after vasectomy. However, a subsequent analysis of data collected from 1988 to 1992 found just a weak association (odds ratio, 1.2)[11]. Mettlin and colleagues compared the frequency of self-reported vasectomy at least 5 years before admission among 614 men with prostate cancer and 2588 men with other cancers. Overall, about 5% of both cases and controls reported a previous vasectomy. They found a relationship between vasectomy and prostate cancer, with the age-adjusted odds ratio of 1.7. In these studies, the association with vasectomy did not increase with age at diagnosis of prostate cancer or with time since vasectomy. This observation suggests the possibility of surveillance bias.

Giovannucci and colleagues, in order to examine the relationship between vasectomy and prostate cancer, performed two cohort studies, one retrospective[14] and the other prospective[15]. In the retrospective one, the husbands of the 14 607 married female participants of the Nurses' Health Study who reported vasectomy as the couple's form of contraception were evaluated together with the husbands of 14 607 age-matched participants whose husbands had not had a vasectomy. Vasectomy was associated with an increased risk of prostate cancer (age-adjusted risk, 1.56; $p = 0.04$). The relative risk of prostate cancer increased over time since vasectomy. In the prospective cohort study, evaluation was performed of 10 055 male members of the Health Professionals Follow-up Study, aged 40–75 years, who had had a vasectomy and 37 800 members who had not had a vasectomy. Again, vasectomy was associated with an increased risk of prostate cancer (age-adjusted risk, 1.66; $p = 0.004$); the correlation was higher when vasectomy was performed more than 20 years ago.

When risk estimates of this magnitude (odds ratio, 1.6) are derived from observational studies, they are considered weak associations[16]. To prove the causal relationship, the possibility of chance, bias or unmeasured confounding must be ruled out. *Chance* is an unlikely explanation; nevertheless, neither of these studies was initiated with the primary purpose of evaluating vasectomy as a risk factor for prostate cancer, but to evaluate many potential conditions as possible risk factors for numerous disorders. Chance will explain some study findings under those conditions and is a likely explanation for other findings from a different analysis of the Nurses' Health Study[17], in which the risk of dying from prostate cancer was not significantly increased but the risk of dying from lung cancer was. An association between vasectomy and lung cancer has not been reported previously and is implausible.

As most vasectomies are performed by urologists and most prostate cancers are diagnosed by urologists, men who have undergone vasectomy may be more likely to have their prostate cancers diagnosed. This type of *selection bias* may well account for diagnosis of prostate cancer, which, in its heterogenic behavior, shows a high rate of indolent tumors, proved both by the frequent asymptomatic tumors in necropsy studies of elderly people and by the frequent non-cancer-related deaths in non-treated people with organ-confined prostate cancer. Although the selection bias may affect some of the findings from case–control studies reported previously, it is less likely to account for findings from the cohort studies by Giovannucci and colleagues, in which the risks of both early and advanced stage prostate cancer were elevated after vasectomy. However, the fact that urologists serve as a link between vasectomy and the diagnosis of prostate cancer remains a possible explanation for the association in any United States study of vasectomy and prostate cancer.

Furthermore, Giovannucci and colleagues failed to obtain reliable information concerning the incidence of prostate cancer in their study population in a systematic manner and have therefore identified only a fraction of the clinically detectable cases of prostate cancer in their study population[18]. Index cases were identified entirely on the basis of self-reports or spousal reports, a particularly insensitive assay for the presence of a disease such as prostate cancer, which may be asymptomatic even at advanced stages. As an illustration, Labrie and colleagues[19] identified 57 cases of prostate cancer among 1002 men selected from electoral rolls giving a detection rate of 5.7%, whereas Giovannucci and co-workers identified a combined total of 396 cases of prostate cancer among 62 462 men, giving a detection rate of 0.63%. With such a large pool of undiagnosed prostate cancers, in both the vasectomy and non-vasectomy groups, any minor variation in prostate cancer screening between groups could easily result in the appearance of a significant difference in the risk of developing prostate cancer.

The most likely non-causal explanation for findings in the studies by Giovannucci and colleagues is *unmeasured confounding*. Approximately one of 11 men in western societies will develop prostate cancer and the majority of these men will not have undergone vasectomy. We simply do not know why prostate cancer is so common. Although the authors tried to control for a variety of possible risk factors for prostate cancer, the causes of prostate cancer remain unknown. It is impossible, therefore, to assume that true risk for prostate cancer is equally distributed between men who have undergone vasectomy and men who have not. The Nurses' Health Study indicated that men who underwent vasectomy had a lower total mortality than men who did not. Men who underwent vasectomy in that study must, therefore, have different characteristics from those who did not. It is entirely possible that some of these characteristics increase the risk of prostate cancer.

Furthermore, three criteria have been suggested for interpreting the likelihood of causation in epidemiological[20] studies and no one of these is fully achieved by the studies from Giovannucci and colleagues.

Strength of the association

The association is weak with an odds ratio of 1.6.

Biological plausibility

There are no known biological mechanisms to explain a causal relationship. Several hypotheses have been postulated, including a speculative greater exposure of the gland to carcinogenic factors resulting from the reduction in prostatic secretions following vasectomy; an immunological cause with no evidence of credibility; an old-fashioned hypothesis of blocking antibodies no longer accepted as a likely factor in the pathogenesis of cancer; and, finally, an alteration of the endocrine function[21].

Most available data do not support an effect of vasectomy on hormone levels[22–28]. However, there are three studies that have reported statistically significant increases in plasma concentrations of androgens. Two of them performed in the 1970s showed an increase in the levels of dihydrotestosterone (DHT)[29] and testosterone[30], respectively, in vasectomized men. The most recent study[31] found that vasectomized men had lower serum concentrations of sex hormone binding globulin (SHBG), which suggests increased tissue availability of testosterone, and a higher ratio of DHT/testosterone, implying greater conversion of testosterone to its metabolite DHT.

While some studies reported higher concentrations of testosterone or a higher ratio of testosterone to DHT among prostate cancer patients compared with controls, most studies found no increased risk of prostate cancer associated with serum testosterone or DHT[31]. Only one study suggests that increased conversion of testosterone to DHT by the enzyme 5α-reductase may be associated with increased prostate cancer risk[32].

Consistency across study findings

There is a lack of consistency across study findings. In contrast to the cohort studies by Giovannucci and colleagues, which included 300[14] and 96[15] prostate cancer cases and found significantly elevated relative risk of 1.66[14] and 1.56[15], respectively, two other cohort studies based on 135[33] and 165[9] incident cases found no association with vasectomy, and two more cohort studies[10,34] reported a decrease in the rate of prostate cancer among vasectomized men.

Case–control studies have also yielded inconsistent results. The study by Rosemberg and colleagues[12] proved only a weak association between prostate cancer and vasectomy, when a subsequent analysis of data including a longer period was performed[11].

But without doubt, the population-based case–control studies have a higher strength in proving association. The first by Hayes and colleagues[35] included 965 cases (471 black and 494 white cases) and reported a non-significant odds ratio of 1.2. The second, by John and colleagues[31] included a larger number of cases (n = 1642) with different racial and geographic populations and was the first study that attempted to exclude from the control group men with possible undiagnosed prostate cancer in order to reduce potential misclassification bias, by using exclusions on the basis of age-specific cut points for high serum concentrations of prostate-specific antigen. The authors did not find an elevated risk of prostate cancer among vasectomized men. Neither did they find differences in other subgroups previously reported as having a higher risk, such as men who had a vasectomy at a young age, men with a long time interval since vasectomy, older men and men with early stage prostate cancer.

In view of the inconsistency of the results from the various studies of vasectomy and prostate cancer, the weakness of the association in the positive studies, the failure of any study to rule out detection bias and the possibility of unidentified confounding, there is, at present, insufficient evidence to conclude that vasectomy causes prostate cancer.

IMMUNOLOGICAL DISORDERS

The hypothesis has been proven in humans and experimental animals that vasectomy mimics immunization, with spermatozoa producing the classical patterns of IgM and IgG antibody responses to the majority of the dominant sperm autoantigens. Vasovasostomy does not bring about a decrease in antisperm antibodies[36]. Some systems of protection from the autoimmune response have been identified. A free radical system has been shown to trigger instantaneous protein disposal within the granuloma cells that could be of importance in avoiding early postvasectomy autoimmune triggering[37].

Postvasectomy immunization could have adverse consequences at different levels, namely:

(1) In the recovery of fertility after vasovasostomy (irreversibility of the lesions);

(2) Sensibilizating for anaphylactic reactions to substances such as protamine;

(3) Production of non-sperm autoantibodies; and

(4) Presence and deposits of circulating immuno-complexes that could produce glomerulonephritis and atherosclerosis.

Testicular effect

There is antisperm activity in about two-thirds of vasectomized men, this being exceptional in fertile men. This antisperm sensibilization correlates with seminiferous tubule wall thickness, focal interstitial fibrosis, and the percentage composition of interstitium[38].

Bigazzi[39] and Alexander and Tung[40], working on rabbits with vasectomies, reported degeneration of seminiferous epithelium associated with immunocomplex deposition in the basement membrane; elution techniques showed that the complexes contained antisperm antibodies[41].

Anaphylactic reactions

Within a year after vasectomy, 22–30% of men develop agglutinating IgG autoantibodies against human protamine, due to the fact that commercial protamine preparations are made from the sperm of salmon and related fish species, making immunologic cross-reactivity possible between fish and human prota-mines[42].

Protamine neutralization of heparin after cardio-pulmonary bypass, cardiac catheterization, dialysis, or plasmapheresis has been associated with rare, severe and unpredictable adverse reactions, some of them life-threatening. Among the mechanisms postulated has been included complement activation because of previous sensibilization to protamine. While some authors[42] consider that vasectomized men, who have an increased incidence of protamine-specific IgG antibody in their sera, have an increased risk for life-threatening reactions to protamine, others[43] think that this is not proved, based on evidence from prospective studies of eight and 20 vasectomized men in whom any untoward responses were not detected to intraoperative protamine[44,45].

Non-sperm-specific autoantibodies

Several investigators have been concerned about the possibility that vasectomy stimulates the production of non-sperm-specific autoantibodies that cross-react with other tissues of the body. Serum samples from vasectomized men have been extensively analyzed for increased titers of other types of autoantibodies, including antinuclear antibodies, rheumatoid factor, and antibodies directed against thyroid, smooth muscle, gastric parietal cells, mitochondria and thyroglobulin. Most studies have revealed no clinically significant increase in autoantibodies in vasectomized men[46,47].

Circulating immunocomplexes

Tung[47] and Bigazzi and colleagues[48] in rabbits and Alexander and Anderson[49] in monkeys provided direct evidence of circulating immune complexes in vasectomized animals. Because immune complexes can activate serum complement, they can cause pathological lesions, particularly in the renal glomerulus and in the arteries. Deposits of immunocomplexes have been detected by immunofluorescence techniques and electron microscopy. Low pH eluates of kidneys from vasectomized rabbits have revealed the presence of antisperm antibodies[30]. Urine from certain of the long-term vasectomized rhesus monkeys has been analyzed but has not revealed proteinuria, an indication that glomerular damage is not severe in these cases. No epidemiological evidence of an increase in glomerulonephritis in vasectomized men has been reported.

In 1979, Alexander and colleagues questioned the safety of vasectomy because of an experimental study in monkeys that found an increased risk of atherosclerosis after vasectomy. They hypothesize that the vasectomy effect occurs as a result of arteritis caused by circulating immune complexes composed of sperm antigen and antisperm antibodies. At least nine epidemiological studies failed to prove such evidence[16], and later it was reported that the original findings in monkeys could not be reproduced[51].

CONCLUSION

Vasectomy as a minor surgical procedure has obvious advantages for fertility control, with a very low risk of pregnancy. Concern was raised by several studies suggesting a relationship between urological malignancies and vasectomy. On the basis of existing biological and epidemiological evidence, any causal relationship between vasectomy and risk of prostate or testicular cancer is not proved and no changes in family planning policies concerning vasectomy are justified. Information about this subject must be given to the patient, who should be counselled to follow a program for early prostate cancer detection after the age of 50.

ACKNOWLEDGEMENT

To Cristina Coder for her secretarial assistance in the writing of this manuscript.

REFERENCES

1. Population reports. Series D. March 1992, N° 5
2. McMahon AJ, Buckley J, Taylor A, *et al.* Chronic testicular pain following vasectomy. *Br J Urol* 1992; 69: 188–91
3. Selikowitz SM, Shnecd AR. A late postvasectomy syndrome. *J Urol* 1985; 134: 494–7
4. O'Brien TS, Cranston D, Ashwin P, *et al.* Temporary reappearance of sperm 12 months after vasectomy clearance. *Br J Urol* 1995; 76: 371–5
5. Davies AH, Sharp RJ, Cranston D, *et al.* The long-term outcome following 'special clearance' after vasectomy. *Br J Urol* 1990; 66: 211–12
6. Berger JR, Swami SK, Gingel JC. Persistent spermatozoa after vasectomy: a survey of British urologists. *Br J Urol* 1995; 76: 376–9

7. Smith JC, Cranston D, O'Brien D, *et al.* Fatherhood without apparent spermatozoa after vasectomy. *Lancet* 1994; 344: 30
8. Cale ARJ, Farouk M, Prescott RJ, *et al.* Does vasectomy accelerate testicular tumour? Importance of testicular examinations before and after vasectomy. *Br Med J* 1990; 300: 370–1
9. Moller H, Knudsen LB, Lynge E. Risk of testicular cancer after vasectomy: cohort of 73,000 men. *Br Med J* 1994; 309: 295–9
10. Niemhuis H, Goldacre M, Seagrott V, *et al.* Incidence of disease after vasectomy. *Br Med J* 1992; 304: 743–6
11. Rosemberg L, Palmer JR, Zamber AG, *et al.* The relation of vasectomy to the risk of cancer. *Am J Epidemiol* 1994; 140: 431–8
12. Rosemberg L, Palmer JR, Zauberg AG, *et al.* Vasectomy and the risk of prostate cancer. *Am J Epidemiol* 1990; 132: 1051–5
13. Mettlin C, Natajaran N, Huben R. Vasectomy and prostate cancer risk. *Am J Epidemiol* 1990; 132: 1056–61
14. Giovannucci E, Tosteson TD, Speizer FE, *et al.* A retrospective cohort study of vasectomy and prostate cancer in US men. *J Am Med Assoc* 1993; 269: 878–82
15. Giovannucci E, Ascherio A, Rimm EB, *et al.* A prospective cohort study of vasectomy and prostate cancer in US men. *J Am Med Assoc* 1993; 269: 873–7
16. Howards SS, Palerson HB. Vasectomy and prostate cancer: chance, bias or causal relationship. *J Am Med Assoc* 1993; 269: 913–14
17. Giovannucci E, Tosteson TD, Speizen FE, *et al.* A long term study of mortality in men who have undergone vasectomy. *N Engl J Med* 1992; 326: 1392–8
18. Morgentaler A, Dewolf WC. Vasectomy and increased risk of prostate cancer (letter). *J Am Med Assoc* 1993; 270: 705–6
19. Labrie F, Dupont A, Suburu R. Serum prostate-specific antigen as pre-screening test for prostate cancer. *J Urol* 1992, 147: 846–52
20. Smoking and Health: Report of the Advising Committee to the Surgeon General of the Public Health Service. Washington DC: US Dept. of Health, Education and Welfare, 1964. Public Health Service Publication 1103
21. Howards SS. Possible biological mechanisms for a relationship between vasectomy and prostatic cancer. *Eur J Cancer* 1993; 294: 1060-2
22. Richards IS, Davis JE, Lubell I. Current status of endocrinologic effects of vasectomy. *Urology* 1981; 18: 1–6
23. Goebelsmann U, Bernstein GS, Gale JA. Serum gonadotropic, testosterone, estradiol and estrone levels prior to and following bilateral vasectomy. In Lepow IH, ed. *Vasectomy: Immunologic and Pathophysiologic Effects in Animals and Man.* New York: Academic Press 1979; 165–81
24. Whitby RM, Gordon RD, Blair BR. The endocrine effects of vasectomy: a prospective five-year study. *Fertil Steril* 1979; 31: 518–20
25. Varma MM, Varma RR, Johanson AJ. Longterm effects of vasectomy on pituitary–gonadal function in man. *J Clin Endocrinol Metab* 1975; 40: 868-71
26. Skegg DC, Mathews JD, Guillebaud J. Hormonal assessment before and after vasectomy. *Br Med J* 1976; 1: 621–2
27. Fisch H, Laor E, Barchama N. Detection of testicular endocrine abnormalities and their correlation with serum antisperm antibodies in men following vasectomy. *J Urol* 1989; 141: 1129–32
28. Peng XS, Li FD, Miao ZR. Plasma reproductive hormones in normal and vasectomized Chinese men. *Int J Androl* 1987; 10: 471–9

29. Purvis K, Saksena SK, Cekan Z. Endocrine effects of vasectomy. *Clin Endocrinol* 1976; 5: 263–72
30. Smith KD, Tcholakian RK, Chowdhury M. Endocrine studies in vasectomized men. In Lepow IH, ed. *Vasectomy: Immunologic and Pathophysiologic Effects in Animals and Man*. New York: Academic Press 1979; 183–97
31. John EM, Whitemore AS, Wu AH, *et al.* Vasectomy and prostate cancer: results from a multiethnic case–control study. *J Natl Cancer Inst* 1995; 87: 662–95
32. Ross RK, Bernstein L, Lobo RA. 5 alpha reductase activity and risk of prostate cancer among Japanese and US white and black males. *Lancet* 1992; 339: 887–9
33. Sidney S, Quesemberry CP, Sadler MC, *et al.* Vasectomy and the risk of prostate cancer in a cohort of multiphasic health check-up examinees: second report. *Cancer Causes Control* 1991; 2: 113–16
34. Perlman JA, Spirtas R, Kelaghan J. Vasectomy and the risk of prostate cancer. *Am J Epidemiol* 1991; 34: 107–8
35. Hayes RB, Pottern LM, Greenberg R, *et al.* Vasectomy and prostate cancer in US blacks and whites. *Am J Epidemiol* 1993; 137: 263–9
36. Flickinger CJ, Howard SS, Bush LA, *et al.* Temporal recognition of sperm autoantigens by IgM and IgG autoantibodies after vasectomy and vasovasostomy. *J Reprod Immunol* 1994; 27: 135–50
37. Chattersee S, Laloraya H, Kumar GP. Free radical bombing of spermatozoa in spermatic granuloma: an attempt to prevent switch-on. *Biochem Biophys Res Commun* 1994: 201; 472–7
38. Jarrow JP, Goluboff ET, Chang TS, *et al.* Relationship between antisperm antibodies and testicular histologic changes in human after vasectomy. *Urology* 1994; 43: 521–4
39. Bigazzi P. Immunopathological findings in vasectomized rabbits. In Lepow IH, ed. *Vasectomy: Immunologic and Pathophysiologic Effects in Animals and Man*. New York: Academic Press 1979; 339–53
40. Alexander NJ, Tung KSK. Vasectomy in the rabbit: immunological and morphological effects. In Lepow IH, ed. *Vasectomy: Immunologic and Pathophysiologic Effects in Animals and Man*. New York: Academic Press 1979; 355–77
41. McDonald SW. Vasectomy and the human testis. *Br Med J* 1990; 301: 618–19
42. Adourian U, Shampaine EL, Hirschman CA, *et al.* High-titer protamine-specific IgG antibody associated with anaphylaxis: report of a case and quantitative analysis of antibody in vasectomized men. *Anesthesiology* 1993; 78: 368–72
43. Metz S. Prior vasectomy and anaphylaxis following protamine: no cause and effect. *Anesthesiology* 1993; 79: 617–18
44. Levy JH, Schwieger IA, Zaiden JR, *et al.* Evaluation of patients at risk of protamine reactions. *J Thorac Cardiovasc Surg* 1989; 98: 200-4
45. Vezina D, Sheridan P, Blain R, *et al.* Safety of protamine sulfate administration in vasectomized men. *Contraception* 1990; 41: 605–16
46. Bullock JY, Gilmore LL, Wilson JD. Autoantibodies following vasectomy. *J Urol* 1977; 118: 604
47. Tung HSK. Circulating immune complexes in vasectomy. In Lepow IH, ed. *Vasectomy: Immunologic and Pathophysiologic Effects in Animals and Man*. New York: Academic Press 1979; 205–206
48. Bigazzi PE, Kosuda LL, Hsu KG, *et al.* Immune complex orchitis in vasectomized rabbits. *J Exp Med* 1976; 143: 382–8
49. Alexander NJ, Anderson DJ. Vasectomy: consequences of autoimmunity to sperm antigens. *Fertil Steril* 1979; 32: 253–60

50. Alexander NJ, Wilson BI, Patterson BD. Vasectomy immunological effects on rhesus monkeys and men. *Fertil Steril* 1979; 32: 253–60
51. Clarkson TB, Alexander NJ, Morgan TM. Atherosclerosis of cynomologous monkeys hyper and hyporesponsive to dietary cholesterol: lack of effect of vasectomy. *Atherosclerosis* 1988; 8: 488–98

This paper has been reproduced from *Eur J Contracept Reprod Health Care* 1996; 1: 311–18

31 *Chlamydia trachomatis* detection: sensitivity, specificity and cost of testing

J. Orfila

INTRODUCTION

Chlamydia are obligate intracellular organisms that infect columnar epithelium; therefore, the specimen for testing must contain columnar epithelium. Because the endocervix is lined with columnar epithelium, it must be appropriately sampled to increase the probability that the organism will be recovered.

It is recommended that cervical specimens for *Chlamydia* be obtained after specimens for Papanicolaou smears and gonorrhea have been obtained. Swabs with plastic or wire shafts must be used because wooden shafts may contain substances that are toxic to *Chlamydia trachomatis*. Secretions and discharge should be removed from the cervical os before collection of the specimen. The swab should be rotated against the wall of the endocervical canal several times during a period of 10–30 s.

CHLAMYDIA CELL CULTURE

Chlamydia cell culture is the standard against which other tests are measured, although the sensitivity of culture is decreased by improper handling. The sensitivity of a single culture for *C. trachomatis*, determined by comparing the positivity rate of a single specimen to the positivity rate of multiple specimens collected at the same time from the same person, is 70–90%. The sensitivity may be even lower in offices in which processing of the specimens is not handled as meticulously as it is in research studies.

The main advantage of culture tests for *C. trachomatis* is that they have a specificity of 100%. This level of specificity means that, regardless of the prevalence of the disease in the population being tested, the positive-predictive value is 100%, or simply that, if the test is positive for *C. trachomatis*, the clinician can be certain that chlamydial infection is present. For this reason, cell culture is the only test that should be used in the evaluation of patients who have been sexually assaulted. The disadvantage of culture is that it is technically difficult for the laboratory to process, requires 3–7 days to obtain the result and cannot be used with some specimens such as urine and sperm.

NON-CULTURE TESTS BASED ON IMMUNOLOGICAL METHOD

These tests (based on enzyme immunoassay–immunofluoresence (EIA–IF)) for the detection of chlamydial infection have the advantage of ease of transport, and processing and require only 10 min to 4 h to obtain results. The main disadvantage of these tests is lower specificity. Cross-reactions between membrane proteins detected by the *Chlamydia* test and the membrane proteins of bacterial species other than *Chlamydia* can occur. The sensitivity of non-culture tests is between 70 and 90% when compared with a single culture.

Specificity of both the EIA and the direct fluorescent antibody test is approximately 97–99%.

A number of office-based, rapid test kits are available, including: Wampole Laboratories, Clearview Chlamydia; Abbott, Test-pack Chlamydia; and Johnson & Johnson, Surecell *Chlamydia*. All of the office-based tests are based on EIA technology. They take approximately 10–30 min to perform and require between 2 and 7 min of actual hands-on personnel time. In-office tests offer the advantage of rapid results and ease of processing; in addition, these tests are less expensive than commercial laboratory tests.

A disadvantage of the rapid tests is the paucity of data available by which to evaluate their performance, compared with laboratory-based tests, which have been extensively evaluated.

All tests for *C. trachomatis* have been less extensively studied in men than in women. The main disadvantage of urethral swab testing in men is the discomfort of the test, making it a less acceptable test in men than the cervical test in women.

Leukocyte esterase testing has been proposed as an accurate and acceptable alternative method of screening for chlamydial infection in men. In leukocyte esterase testing, the initial 10 ml of a first-void urine sample are tested with a dipstick for the presence of leukocyte esterase; the test is considered positive if trace or greater amounts are present. Leukocyte esterase testing alone has a positive-predictive value of 16% in a population with a prevalence of 7%; therefore, positive tests should be confirmed by tests that are more specific for *C. trachomatis*.

The introduction of molecular biology allowed rapid diagnosis without culture of *Chlamydia*.

Nucleic acid hybridization tests have a similar sensitivity to other non-cultured laboratory tests but may be more specific.

NUCLEIC ACID AMPLIFICATION TECHNIQUES

Several nucleic acid amplification techniques have been developed and introduced in recent years. The introduction of the polymerase chain reaction (PCR) has made possible the development of assays with keen sensitivity and specificity. Experience with PCR is quite extensive, while that with other amplification techniques, e.g. ligase chain reaction (LCR), nucleic-acid-sequence-based amplification (NASBA) and self-sustained-sequence replication (3SR) is limited. The PCR amplifies a specific DNA nucleotide sequence.

TEST SELECTION

The selection criteria of the test to be used in the laboratory should be based on public-health considerations, costs, required and existing laboratory expertise, the patient population, disease prevalence and ethics. It is difficult to weigh cost-effectiveness measurements with the individual emotional costs that may result from a false-positive test. In medicolegal cases, cases of child abuse and cases of sexual assault, a false-positive result can have major consequences. Since non-culture methods are unreliable after the use of antibiotics, isolation in cell culture, with its low false-positive results, is the method of choice. Table 2 gives the estimates of the detection limits of several assays, while Table 3 gives estimates of the sensitivities of various classes of assay based on data from the literature. It is important to consider the prevalence of *C. trachomatis* infection in the patient population. In a high prevalence population (> 5%), tests with a sensitivity between 80 and 100% can have acceptable predictive values. In a low prevalence population, the predictive values rapidly decrease. Therefore, improved detection techniques are needed when control programs become successful and the prevalence drops.

32 *Chlamydia trachomatis* screening in family planning centers: a review of cost/benefit evaluations in different countries

J. Henry-Suchet, A. Sluzhinska and D. Serfaty

INTRODUCTION

In the last 10–20 years, *Chlamydia trachomatis* infection has been recognized as one of the most widespread sexually transmitted disease (STD) organisms. It has been implicated in a wide range of genitourinary tract infections in both males and females of reproductive age. The organism has been identified as a predominant etiological agent of pelvic inflammatory diseases. Occult chlamydial infection is increasingly found to be a significant cause of tubal factor infertility and ectopic pregnancies, in addition to clinically obvious mucopurulent cervicitis, endometritis, salpingitis and Fitz–Hugh–Curtis syndrome in females. In males, infection causes urethritis, epididymitis, prostatitis and, possibly, infertility. Male chlamydial disease can remain asymptomatic or minimally symptomatic, but still results in chronic infection, which can be a major factor in sexual transmission.

Since the early 1960s, *C. trachomatis* has been diagnosed in STD centers, where its prevalence is 10–15%. During the last decade, the prevalence of *C. trachomatis* disease in apparently healthy young populations appeared to be similar to *C. trachomatis* prevalence in people visiting STD centers. It has been shown that the disease spreads among this group of uncontrolled and mostly asymptomatic young people. The analyzed studies performed during the decade 1985–95 used direct detection methods, with a possible lack of detection of 10–30% versus cultures or amplification methods (polymerase chain reaction or ligase chain reaction).

Among male and female military recruits[1–6], *C. trachomatis* prevalence is 6–12%, with one exception, Sweden, where it has been found in only in 1.3%, possibly as a consequence of long-term screening practised in the country (Table 1).

In symptomatic or asymptomatic young females from gynecological clinics and patients in general practice[7–15], chlamydial infection has been found to be

Table 1 *C. trachomatis* screening: military recruits

Reference	*Location*	*n*	*Age (years)*	*Sample*	*Method of detection*	*Percentage positive for C. trachomatis*
1	USA	448 females	17–42	cervix	DIF	10
2	USA	476 females	23	cervix	EIA	8.2
3	Austria	335 males	—	first-void urine	EIA + DIF	12.2
4	Sweden	224 males	18	first-void urine	LE + EIA/DIF	1.3
5	Norway	392 males	19–21	first-void urine	EIA	6–6.4
6	Denmark	636 males	18–23	urine + urethra	EIA + DIF	1987: 7.8 1992: 10.8

DIF, direct immunofluorescence; EIA, enzyme immunoassay; LE, leukocyte esterase test

7–20% (Table 2). Among adolescents, college girls and students, the rate of *C. trachomatis* is 6–19.8% (Table 2). (In the Katz study[10] in the USA it was 25% in 1985, but the rate dropped to 10% in 1993.) Chlamydia incidence in jailed women in New York reaches 27%[16].

In various occidental countries, the population-based studies identified *C. trachomatis* prevalence among pregnant women as being 2.8–13% (mean, 5%)[17–21]. In French Antillas, cervical *C. trachomatis* prevalence in black pregnant women reaches 27% (Table 3).

'*C. trachomatis* screening is of primary importance in populations asking for legal abortion, since most of the women wishing to interrupt their pregnancies are young, unmarried and without children. It is, therefore, important for later fertility that the abortion procedure be safe and without serious complications'[25]. In this population asking for legal abortion[22–26], prevalence is 5–18%, with age less than 20 years as the most important risk factor (Table 4). Stray-Pedersen[25] and other authors have shown that C. trachomatis cervical infection at the time of abortion is the main cause of postabortal pelvic inflammatory diseases and can be avoided by treatment (Table 5). In addition, Stray-Pedersen has shown a decrease of C. trachomatis prevalence from 15–20% to 5% at Aker Hospital, Oslo, among abortion applicants, 15–25 years of age, as a consequence of systematic C. trachomatis screening during the period 1984–92. In our experience at Hospital Saint-Louis, Paris[26], C. trachomatis prevalence evaluated by polymerase chain reaction on first-void urine is 4% in abortion applicants (8.3% in women < 20 years, 3.3% in women 20–33 years old).

According to the data from a number of scientists[23,26,27–31], among the females visiting American and Scandinavian family planning clinics, the rate of *C. trachomatis* infection is 5.2–13.3%. It is higher in urban women (6.9%) than in non-urban (5.4%) and is mostly influenced by age (< 20 years,: 7–32%; > 20 years:, 4–10%) (Table 6). In our experience at Hospital Saint-Louis, Paris[26], *C. trachomatis* prevalence evaluated by polymerase chain reaction on first-void urine is 7.5% (31.6% in women < 20 years old, 8.1% in the 21–25-year age group

Table 2 *C. trachomatis* screening: young women

Reference	Location	n	Age (years)	Sample	Method of detection	Percentage positive for C. trachomatis	Risk factor
7	Michigan USA	2303 college girls	17–40 (21)	cervix	DIF	6	leukorrhea no condom Papanicolaou + age
8	New York USA	1531 health care public	15–63 (24.5)	cervix	culture	13.6	pill > 1 contact Papanicolaou + social level
9	USA	515 college girls	18	cervix	EIA	9.5	—
10	USA	3842 adolescent women	13–18	cervix + urethra	culture	1985: 25 1993: 10	—
14	Washington USA	1804	15–34	cervix	culture + EIA/DIF	3.5	age < 25 black race social level MPC
11	USA	146 college girls	20–30 (21)	cervix	EIA	10	MPC > 2 contacts: 1 year new contact < 2 months
12	Sweden	492 young girls	17.7	cervix + first-void urine	EIA + DIF	7.9	—
13	Australia	258 students	20–26	cervix	DIF	19.8	MPC
15	Nicaragua	155	—	cervix	DIF	4	—

DIF, direct immunofluorescence; EIA, enzyme immunoassay; MPC, muco-purulent cervix

Table 3 *C. trachomatis* screening: pregnant women

Reference	Location	n	Age (years)	Sample	Method of detection	Percentage positive for C. trachomatis	Risk factor
17	USA	2100	25	cervix	EIA	5.6	—
21	USA	8000	≥ 16	cervix	culture	8.6	—
18	Germany	263		cervix	EIA	3.4	—
20	Germany Austria	20 000	—		EIA/culture	2–13	—
19	French Antillas	1411	15–39		culture	26.7	age < 20 MPC

EIA, enzyme immunoassay; MPC, muco-purulent cervix

and 2.1% in the 25–33-year age group). Contraceptive consultation is, therefore, the best opportunity for screening and treatment of this young population with high *C. trachomatis* infection prevalence. In adolescents, screening and treatment must be anonymous and free of charge.

Table 4 *C. trachomatis* screening: legal abortion

Reference	*Location*	*n*	*Age (years)*	*Sample*	*Method of detection*	*Percentage positive for C. trachomatis*	*Main risk factor*
22	Swansea UK	401	23	cervix	EIA	8	—
23	Uppsala Sweden	258	15–45 (23)	cervix urethra	EIA + culture	10	young age
24	Norway	2100	19–35	cervix	EIA	5.4	age < 19: 9% > 19: 2%
25	Norway	1193	—	cervix	culture	12	age < 20: 18% > 20: 4%
26	Paris	200	17–33	first-void urine	PCR	4	age < 20: 8% > 20: 3%

EIA, enzyme immunoassay; PCR, polymerase chain reaction

Table 5 Development of pelvic inflammatory disease after termination of pregnancy[25]

Cervical micro-organism	*Number of women (n = 1193)*	*Pelvic inflammatory disease development*	
		n	*%*
Chlamydia carriers			
treated	95	2	2.1
untreated	44	10	22.7*
Neisseria gonorrhea			
treated	10	0	—
Mycoplasma hominis			
treated	10	0	—
untreated	108	8	8.1*
Group B streptococci			
untreated	33	2	6.1*
Negative cervical culture	873	4	0.5*

*$p < 0.05$

RISK FACTORS

According to a number of authors, youth is an important risk factor (Tables 2–6). To be less than 20 years old, according to most authors[23–27,29,31], or less than 25 years old[30] is a significant risk factor in the population of family planning centers (Table 6). Multivariate analysis shows a relative risk for age less than 20 years as being 1.78[28] or 1.6[30], independent of other factors. Young age is the most predictable risk factor, according to Svensson[23].

For some others authors, there are other factors to be taken into account:

(1) Number of sexual partners > 1[8], or > 3 during the last year[27,28];

(2) Use of pill[8] and non-use of barrier methods (many authors);

(3) Existence of purulent vaginal or cervical discharge[11,27,28].

Table 6 *C. trachomatis* screening: family planning centers

Reference	Location	n	Age (years)	Sample	Method of detection	Percentage positive for C. trachomatis	Main risk factor
28	Colorado USA	11 800 total screening	23 ± 5.8 11 → 66	cervix	EIA DIF	7.7	—
29	Alaska Washington Idaho Oregon USA	72 831 selective screening	18–36 (21)	cervix	culture	9.5	age < 20: 13.3% 20–24: 9% > 24: 4% symptoms
27	Wisconsin USA	2200 selective screening	22	cervix	EIA + DIF	5.6	age < 20: 7% > 20: 4.9% symptoms
23	Uppsala Sweden	201 total screening	14–47 (24)	cervix urethra	EIA + culture col col/urethre	10.4 12.4	age < 20
30	Gothenburg Sweden	5785 total screening	14–26 (23)	cervix	culture	7.3	age 18–23: 8% > 23: 5.8%
31	Dijon France	154 total screening	15–40	cervix	DIF	17	age < 25: 19% > 25: 10%
26	Paris France	185 total screening	17–33	first-void urine	PCR	7.5	age < 20: 32% > 20: 7%

EIA, enzyme immunoassay; DIF, direct immunofluorescence; PCR, polymerase chain reaction

On the contrary, other authors[7,9,11] focus on the fact that, among young people, the symptomatic population represents only 20–25% of those affected in an epidemic.

According to Ramstedt[30], 'All risk factors analyzed are only imperfect measures of sexual behavior related to the risk of acquiring *C. trachomatis* infection.'

'The single most decisive factor is duration of the woman's present relationship. If only women whose relationship had lasted less than 1 year were screened, two-thirds of those infected would have been found by testing half of the women.'

We may regret that the sexual behavior of the sexual partner was not analyzed in these studies. In summary, age less than 20 years, probably combined with non-stable sexual relationships, seems to be the main predictive factor for *C. trachomatis* prevalence.

COST/BENEFIT EVALUATION

A cost/benefit evaluation is necessary before starting a preventive strategy for *C. trachomatis* epidemics. The results of this analysis may be different in each country. It depends mainly on:

(1) The estimated prevalence in each population (preliminary statistics are needed). Most authors agree on a systematic screening in populations with

a presumed *C. trachomatis* prevalence ≥ 5% and a selective screening for lower prevalences[31];

(2) The sensitivity of screening criteria: the lowest prevalences need the most sensitive criteria. The best criteria to date, considering feasibility, sensitivity and specificity, seem to be polymerase chain reaction or ligase chain reaction on first-void urine[33] or, according to recent studies, on autovulvovaginal sampling[34];

(3) The balance between the cost of diagnostic tests, preventive treatment and the total cost of treating complications.

According to Humphreys (Colorado, USA), *C. trachomatis* prevalence in females visiting family planning centers is 7.7%[28]. The cost of direct *C. trachomatis* detection is $5.5 and the treatment cost is $16; if the relative costs of pelvic inflammatory diseases and total or selective screening are considered (Table 7), 5 years' projection of the model yield savings of $3.81 million when universal screening is applied, and $1.25 million by means of selective screening.

Addiss and colleages[27] found, in the Wisconsin family planning population, that the overall *C. trachomatis* prevalence is 5.6%, versus 9.3% in populations with one risk factor[28]. The cost of total screening will be three times higher than the cost of selective screening. This group concluded that selective screening plus follow-up of sex partners is to be recommended.

Blackwell and colleagues in the UK[22] found that the yearly cost of hospital readmission after termination of pregnancy is above £16 000, more than twice the cost of providing routine *C. trachomatis* screening and prophylactic treatment. In Norway, Stray-Pedersen[25] recommended that, with a low rate of *C. trachomatis* infection, systematic screening should only be carried out in women < 25 years before legal abortion. In Finland, Paavonen[35] showed that the total cost of examination and treatment of complications associated with chlamydial infection (acute or subacute pelvic inflammatory disease, tubal factor infertility, ectopic pregnancy, chronic pelvic pain) was approximately six times higher than the total cost of a large-scale *C. trachomatis* screening program.

In France and a majority of the European Community countries, the cost of *C. trachomatis* direct detection (Table 8) is 4 times higher than in the USA at $20. The cost of polymerase or ligase chain reaction testing has not been estimated to date, and should be considerably higher than direct detection ($30 or more). Can we hope for a decrease of the cost when other test alternatives appear on the market? The cost of treatment, synthetic tetracycline 200 mg × 8 days or azithromycine 1 g for 1 day, is approximately $40. During the last 10 years in France, infertility has been diagnosed in approximately 10% of women 25–35 years of age. It was shown that every third infertility case was due to *C. trachomatis* infection. The cost of one infertility treatment, including surgery, hormonal treatment, antibiotics and one to four cycles of *in vitro* fertilization is $20 000. Ectopic pregnancies represent 0.5% of total pregnancies and 1% of total deliveries[36], and the treatment cost of one ectopic

Table 7 *C. trachomatis* yearly screening: cost/benefit analysis in Colorado[28]. Total screening saves $3.81 million

Cost of 1 detection: $5.5
Cost of 1 treatment: $16
Five years' projection:

Estimate	*Pelvic inflammatory disease cost*	*Screening cost*
No screening	1 370 000	0
Selective screening	1 120 000	82 500
Total screening	607 000	203 500

Table 8 Yearly *C. trachomatis* screening in family planning centers: cost/benefit analysis in France. Total cost saving by woman and year $12.5 (direct detection); $2.5 or less (PCR)

Cost of 1 detection: $20 (direct detection); ≥ $30 (PCR)
Cost of 1 treatment: $40
Ten years' projection:

Without screening (100 women)	*Cost* ($)
Tubal infertility (n = 3)	60 000
Ectopic pregnancy (n = 1)	5 000
Pelvic inflammatory disease (n = 5)	5 000
Screening	0
Total	70 000
Yearly screening (100 women) *(C. trachomatis supposed prevalence: 5%)*	*Cost* ($)
Tubal infertility (reduced 50%)	30 000
Ectopic pregnancy (reduced 50%)	2 500
Pelvic inflammatory disease (reduced 80%)	1 000
Screening	20 000–30 000 or more
Treatment of 50 women and partners	4 000
Total	57 000–67 500 or more

PCR, polymerase chain reaction

pregnancy is estimated at $5000.The prevalence of pelvic inflammatory diseases was estimated 20 years ago as 1% (ten cases per 100 women during 10 years of exposure)[37]; with its decrease from 1985 to 1995[38], we can estimate the prevalence at 0.5%, which gives five cases of pelvic inflammatory disease for 100 women in 10 years. The cost of one case of pelvic inflammatory disease is $1000 overall. A 10-year projection shows that the total cost of 'no screening' should be $70 000 for 100 women during a period of 10 years. A systematic yearly screening in family planning centers of all women from 15 to 25 years of age for 10 years will cost approximately $20 000 for 100 women by using direct detection and $30 000 or more by using polymerase chain reaction testing. The treatment of the *C. trachomatis*-positive ones and their partners will cost approximately $4000. We would prevent 50% of tubal infertility, ectopic pregnancies, and 80% of pelvic inflammatory diseases due to *C. trachomatis* infection. The total expenses of prevention and residual complications would be $57 500 (direct detection) and $67 500 (polymerase chain reaction). Even without considering the additional costs of nurses, doctors, incapacity to work and so on, the benefit would be $12 500 for 100 women in 10 years (direct detection) and $2500 by polymerase chain reaction testing. The yearly benefits for one woman would be $12.5 (direct detection) or $2.5 (polymerase chain reaction). There are 4 million women 15–25 years in France, 60% of them asking for contraceptive advice; as usual in occidental countries, it is supposed that screening would reach one-third of them or 0.8 million. The total benefit would be $10 million (FF 50 million) per year with direct detection and $2 million (FF 10 million) with polymerase chain reaction testing, if the cost of each test does not exceed $30. A reasonable choice in France and probably in Europe would be to provide total screening in family planning centers for women less than 25 years old and, possibly, selective screening of women 25–35 years of age, with risk factors evaluated as related to *C. trachomatis* frequency > 5% in this older population.

In addition, we should obtain a decrease of *C. trachomatis* prevalence, this being one of the most real benefits of screening. A decrease of *C. trachomatis* epidemics from 15–20% to 5–10% has been observed in the years 1988–95, in Scandinavian countries and in different States of the USA. In consequence of systematic or selective screening[27–29], in family planning clinics and youth clinics, a decrease of pelvic inflammatory diseases and, more recently, of ectopic pregnancies was observed in Scandinavian countries[25]. A recent prospective randomized study, with case–controls, has shown a screening for *C. trachomatis* as being significantly related to a decrease of pelvic inflammatory diseases in a screened population, during the year following detection[39].

CONCLUSION

It is believed that the prevalence of *C. trachomatis* cervical infection in females seeking contraceptive advice or legal abortion in European Community countries is considerably influenced by age: 10–20% in women less than 20 years, 5–10% in women aged 21–25 years, and 2–4% in older women. Cervical *C. trachomatis* infection causes sexual transmission and high genital tract infection with salpingitis, ectopic pregnancies and infertility as late consequences in women. It is for this reason that providing systematic yearly *C. trachomatis* screening among women less than 25 years old and selective *C. trachomatis* screening among women between 25 and 35 years of age with at least one risk factor, together with effective antibiotic treatment of the infected women and their partners, would be a reasonable and cost-saving choice.

REFERENCES

1. Orndorff GR. Screening for *Chlamydia trachomatis* by the Direct Fluorescent Antibody Test in female navy recruits. *Military Med* 1991; 156: 675–7
2. Catterson ML. Prevalence of asymptomatic chlamydial cervical infection in active duty army females. *Military Med* 1993; 158: 618–19
3. Stary A, Steyrer K, Heller-Vitouch C, Müller I, Mårdh PA. Screening for *Chlamydia trachomatis* in military personnel by urine testing. *Infection* 1991; 19: 205–7
4. Domeika MA, Bassiri M, Mårdh PA. Non-invasive sampling for detection of genital infection with *Chlamydia trachomatis* in males utilising urinary leukocyte esterase tests and immunoassays. *Infection* 1994; 22: 65–8
5. Scheel O, Anestad G, Mundal R, Berdal BP. Carriage of urethral *Chlamydia trachomatis*: EIA urinary screening in young males. In Mårdh PA, ed. *Chlamydia Research*. Bologne: Sculapio, 1992; 216
6. Jensen IP. Urinprove til screening af unge mandlige rekrutter for asymtomatisk *Chlamydia trachomatis* infektion. *Ugesker Laeger* 1993; 155: 1376–8
7. Keim J, Woodard MP, Anderson MK. Screening for *Chlamydia trachomatis* in college women on routine gynecological exams. *J Am Coll Health* 1992; 41: 17–23
8. Han Y, Morse DL, Laurence CE, Murphy D, Hipp S. Risk profile for chlamydia infection in women from public health clinics in New York State. *J Commun Health* 1993; 18: 1–9
9. Kaplan J, Meyer M, Navin J. *Chlamydia trachomatis* infection in a female college student population. *J Am College Health* 1988; 36: 3629
10. Katz BP, Blythe MJ, van der Pol B, Jones RB. Evaluation of a chlamydial control program among adolescent women. In Orfila J *et al.*, eds. *Chlamydial Infections*. 1994; 48–54
11. Sheahan SL, Coons SJ, Seabolt JP, Churchill L, Dale T. Sexual behaviour, communication, and chlamydial infections among college women. *Health Care For Women International* 1994; 15: 275–86
12. Svensson LO, Mares I, Olsson SE, Nordstrom ML. Screening for *Chlamydia trachomatis* infection in women and aspect of the laboratory diagnotics. *Acta Obstet Gynecol Scand* 1991; 70: 587–90
13. Dhupelia DK, King LG. *Chlamydia trachomatis* infections in female tertiary students. *Aust Nz Obstet Gynaecol* 1993; 33: 54–6
14. Stergachis A, Scholes D, Heidrich F, Sherer DM, Holmes KK, Stamm WE. Selective screening for *Chlamydia trachomatis* infection in a primary care population of women. *Am J Epidemiol* 1993; 138: 143–53
15. Herrmann B, Espinoza F, Egger M, Smith GD, Mårdh PA. Prevalence of cervical *Chlamydia trachomatis* infections and other STDs in female sex workers and health centers attenders in Nicaragua. In Mårdh PA, ed. *Chlamydia Research*. Bologne: Sculapio, 1992; 289
16. Holmes MD, Safyer SM, Bickell NA, Vermund SH, Hanff PA, Phillips RS. Chlamydial cervical infection in jailed women. *Am J Public Health* 1993; 83: 551–5
17. Glover DD, Gordon H, Moore G, Larsen B. *Chlamydia trachomatis* antigen prevalence among pregnant women in West Virginia. *West Virginia Med J* 1992; 88: 548–51
18. Rimbach S, Wallwienner D, Baier S, Piotrowski T, Engel K, Näher H, Bastert G. *Chlamydia trachomatis:* Screening im Rahmen der Schwangerenvorsorge und Schnell-

Nachweis bei drohender Frühgeburt. *Zentralbl Gynakol* 1993; 115: 478–82
19. Chout RT, Vaton S, Duval-Violton D, Leguyader-Despres P, Orfila J. Screening for *Chlamydia trachomatis* infection in pregnant women in Martinique. *Sex Transm Dis* 1995; 22: 221–7
20. Hoyme UB. Prevalence of *Chlamydia trachomatis* in the cervix uteri of pregnant women in Germany and Austria. In Mårdh PA, ed. *Chlamydia Research.* Bologne: Sculapio, 1992; 147
21. Rettig PJ, Mugent RP. Cervical exam correlates of *Chlamydia trachomatis* infection in a multicenter study of 8000 pregnant women. In Bowie WR, ed. *Chlamydial Infections.* Vancouver 1990; 340–3
22. Blackwell AL, Thomas PD, Wareham K, Emery SJ. Health gains from screening for infection of the lower genital tract in women attending for termination of pregnancy. *Lancet* 1993; 342: 206–9
23. Svensson LO, Mares I, Olsson SE. Detection of *Chlamydia trachomatis* by EIA in urine from women attending a youth consulting centre. *Diagnostic Tests* 1993; 217
24. Skjeldestad FE, Jerve F. *Chlamydia trachomatis* and *Neisseria gonorrhoea* among women seeking abortion in Norway. Results from a nation-wide screening. *Tidsskr-Nor-Laegeforen* 1992; 112: 2082–4
25. Stray-Pedersen B. Prevention des MST. L'expérience Norvégienne. *Contracept Fertil Sex* 1996; 24: 213–17
26. Sluzhinska A, Scieux C, Bruna N, Henry-Jorge S, Henry-Suchet J, Eyoka N, Serfaty D, Bassiri M, Mårdh PA. Urine CT screening in a family planning centre Paris. In Stary A, ed. *Chlamydia Research.* Bologne: Sculapio, 1997, in press
27. Addiss DG, Vaughn ML, Ludka D, Pfister J, Davis JP. Decreased prevalence of *Chlamydia trachomatis* infection associated with a selective screening program in FPC in Wisconsin. *Sex Transm Dis* 1993; 20: 28–35
28. Humphreys JT, Henneberry JF, Rickard RS, Beebe JL. Cost-benefit analysis of selective screening criteria for *Chlamydia trachomatis* infection in women attending Colorado family planning clinics. *Sex Transm Dis* 1992; 19: 47–53
29. Lossick J, Delisle S, Fine D, Mosure D, Lee V, Smith C. Regional Program for widespread screening for *Chlamydia trachomatis* in family planning clinics. In Bowie WR, ed. *Chlamydial Infections.* Cambridge University Press, 1990; 575–9
30. Ramstedt K, Forssman L, Giesecke J, Granath F. Risk factors for *Chlamydia trachomatis* infection in 6810 young women attending family planning clinics. *Int J STD & AIDS* 1992; 3: 117–22
31. Douvier S, Sainte-Barbe C, Oudot C, Habert F, Fritz MT. L'infection à *Chlamydia trachomatis:* Facteurs de risques. *Contracept Fertil Sex* 1996; 24: 391–8
32. Marrazzo JM, Celum CL, Fine D, Delisle S, Mosure DJ, Handsfield HH. Cost effectiveness of selective vs. universal screening for *Chlamydia trachomatis* infection in women attending family planning and STD clinics. In Orfila J, ed. *Chlamydial Infections.* Bologne: Esculapo, 1994; 63–4
33. Genç M, Mårdh PA. A cost-effectiveness analysis of screening and treatment for *Chlamydia trachomatis* infection in asymptomatic women. *Ann Intern Med* 1996; 124: 1–7
34. Stary A. DNA amplification, antigen detection test, and culture: which sample for which technique? In Stary A, ed. *3rd meeting of The European Soc. for Chlamydia Research.* Bologne: Esculapo, 1996; 251–3
35. Paavonen J. Cost-benefit analysis of *Chlamydia trachomatis* screening program in

Finland. In Henry-Suchet J, ed. *1st European Expert Workshop.* Paris, 1993
36. Job Spira N, Coste J, Aubiel-Cavalier B, Germain E, Fernandez H, Bouyer J, Pouly JL. Fréquence de la grossesse extra-utérine et caractéristiques des femmes traitées. Premiers résultats du registre d'Auvergne. *Presse Méd* 1995; 24: 351–5
37. Colvez A, Henry-Suchet J, Michel E. Les infections utéro annexielles en Médecine libérale: une situation indirecte de l'ampleur du phénomene dans la population Francaise. *J Gynecol Obstet Biol Reprod* 1983; 331–7
38. Henry-Suchet J, Tesquier L, Berthet J. Coelioscopies pour salpingites aigues et chroniques. Evolution de leur fréquence en France de 1979 à 1987 d'après une étude multicentrique. *Contracept Fertil Sex* 1992; 20: 357–62
39. Scholes D, Stergachis A, Heidrich F, Andrilla H, Holmes KK, Stamm WE. Prevention of pelvic inflammatory disease by screening for cervical chlamydial infection. *N Engl J Med* 1996; 334: 1362–6

This paper has been reproduced from *Eur J Contracept Reprod Health Care* 1996; 1: 301–9

33 Sexually transmitted disease screening in Eastern European family planning

G. Lazdane

The International Conference on Population and Development (ICPD) Plan of Action[1] states that:

> *'reproductive health . . . implies that people are able to have a satisfying and safe sex life and that they have the capability to reproduce and freedom to decide if, when and how often to do so. Implicit in this last condition are the right of men and women to be informed and to have access to safe, effective affordable and acceptable methods of family planning of their choice, as well as other methods of their choice for regulation of fertility which are not against the law, and the right of access to appropriate health care services that will enable women to go safely through pregnancy and childbirth and provide couples with the best chance of having a healthy infant . . . Reproductive health includes sexual health, the purpose of which is the enhancement of life and personal relations, and not merely counselling and care related to reproduction and sexually transmitted diseases'.*

In the Chapter 'Reproductive rights, sexual and reproductive health and family planning' of the ICPD Plan of Action, the basis for action is stated: '. . . Although the incidence of some sexually transmitted diseases has stabilised in parts of the world, there have been increasing cases in many regions'. Eastern European countries are typical examples of this trend.

There are approximately 98 million fertile women in the countries of Eastern Europe, yet the fertility rate is not high by global standards. Although this alone may not raise cause for concern, closer inspection of reproductive health services and contraceptive prevalence in Europe reveals significant differences among countries.

Based on the latest statistics compiled by the World Health Organization (WHO) Global Program on AIDS, there are currently 4.5 million AIDS cases globally[2]. Sexual transmission reportedly accounted for 70–80% of the cases of human immunodeficiency virus (HIV) infection. At present, in the newly independent states (NIS), there are only approximately 2000 cases of AIDS (Figure 1). There is concern that an increase in sexually transmitted diseases (STDs) in many countries of the Eastern European region will lead to an increase in HIV transmission.

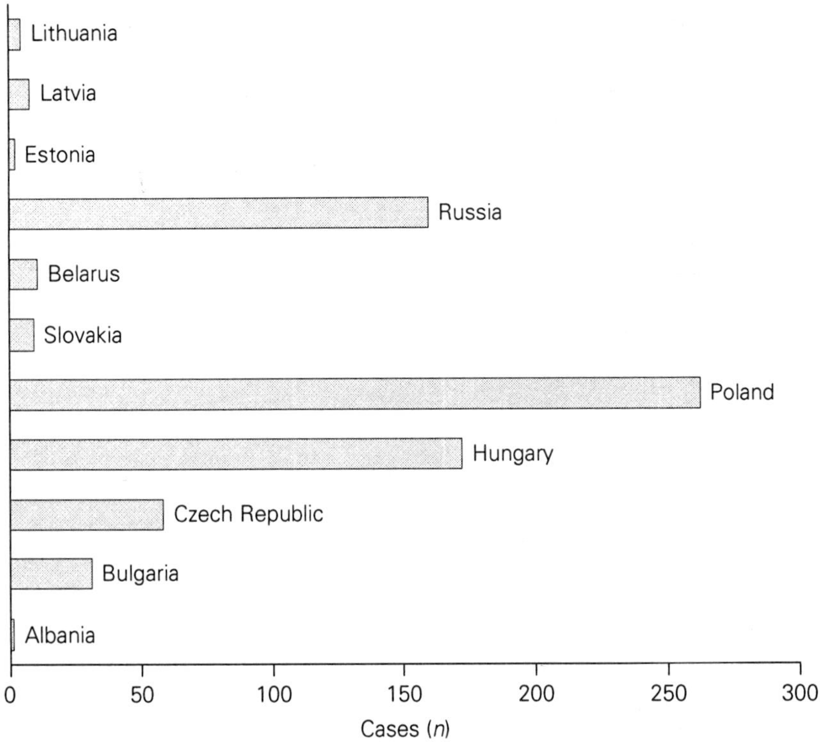

Figure 1 AIDS in Eastern Europe

The lack of epidemiological studies and reliable statistics makes the analysis of STD rate in the region difficult. An increase in the incidence of STDs has been noted in such countries as Belarus, Republic of Moldova and Ukraine[3]. A similar trend exists in the Baltic countries which have experienced an increase in cases of syphilis and chlamydia infection (Figures 2–6)[4].

Two concerns should be emphasized:

(1) Medical care in many countries of the region is in a state of flux between a centralized state-run medical system, through a mixture of state-sponsored and newly privatized government-run services, and an increased number of private medical facilities. The attitude of the private centers towards the official medical statistics is passive, especially concerning the patients with sexually transmitted diseases.

(2) The use of unspecific methods of diagnosis of STDs makes the statistical data doubtful (it mostly concerns *Chlamydia trachomatis* infection).

However, the incidence of STDs in many countries has reached a critical level. Reported cases of syphilis in Latvia have increased to 30 times higher than 5 years previously[5].

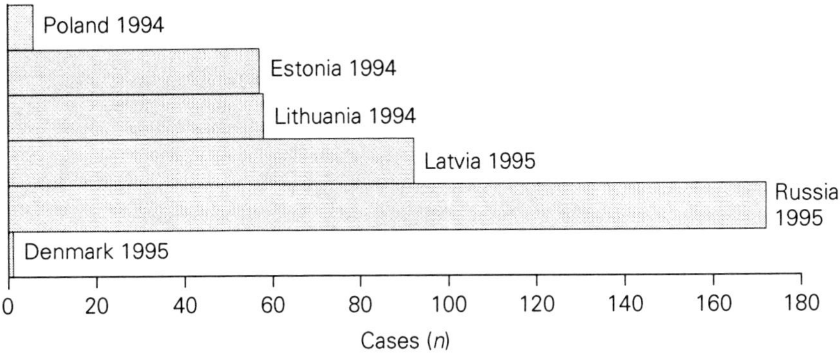

Figure 2 Syphilis incidence per 100 000 inhabitants

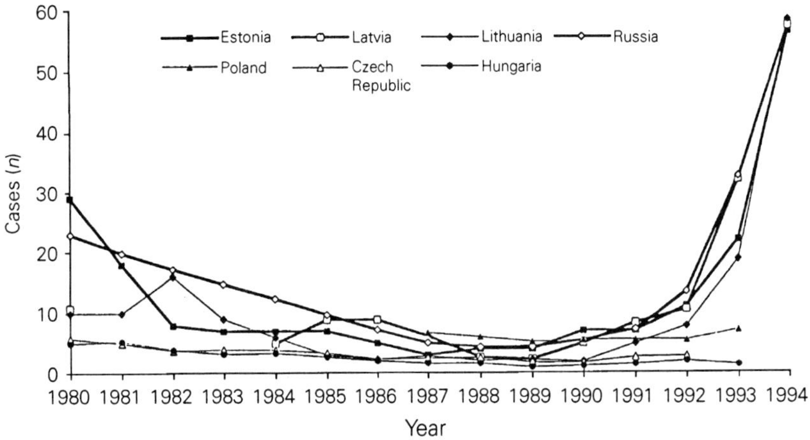

Figure 3 Syphilis incidence per year in Eastern Europe, per 100 000 inhabitants. From reference 4

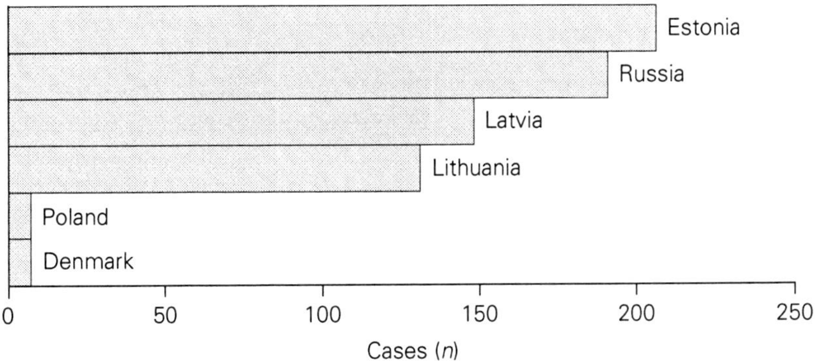

Figure 4 Gonorrhea incidence per year in Eastern Europe, per 100 000 inhabitants in 1994

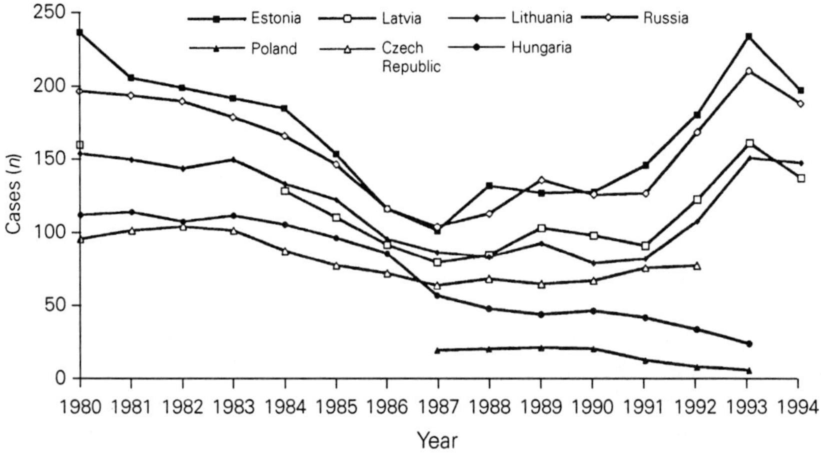

Figure 5 Gonorrhea incidence per year in Eastern Europe, per 100 000 inhabitants. From reference 4

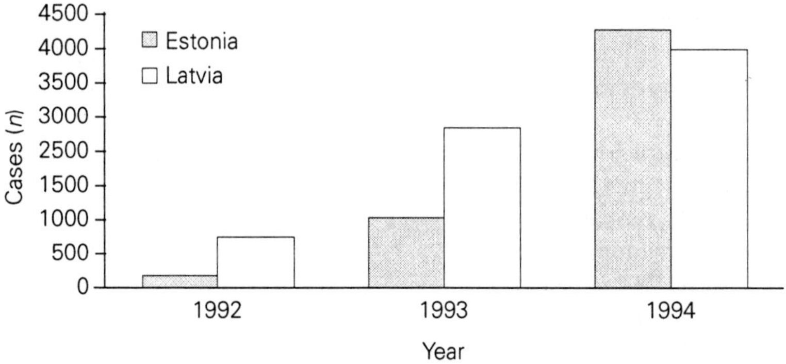

Figure 6 Morbidity with *Chlamydia trachomatis* in Baltic countries, absolute figures

This rapid increase in rates of STD infection can perhaps be explained by the delayed 'sexual revolution' occuring in Eastern European countries, which has followed the sexual taboo that existed during the previous regime. This, in combination with the current period of economic stress, has led to prostitution becoming a booming industry in recent years. Lack of specified services and education campaigns subjects women sex workers to the dangerous health consequences of STDs and AIDS.

Attitudes among the public towards one's own personal health are in a state of transition. The obligatory preventive medicine practiced during the Soviet period in the newly independent states of the former USSR created a culture in which the average person is not used to taking the responsibility for his or her personal health. People are left ill-informed about preventive medicine and, as a result, they tend to visit their doctors only with ailments that have well-advanced symptoms.

Many of the safe modern methods of contraception can also prevent anemia, STDs and some forms of benign and malignant neoplasms[6]. The choice of contraceptive method may adversely or protectively influence the risk of contracting and/or developing STD, but it is probably critical what the user does, rather than what the user uses[7].

The use of effective contraceptives is at a relatively low rate in many countries of Eastern Europe and there are no reliable statistics. Data have been collected from the medical institutions for official statistics mostly about intrauterine devices (IUDs) and hormonal pills; no relevant statistics are available about condom use and other methods of family planning (Table 1). During the 1960–70s, women's choices for controlling their fertility were limited to loop IUDs, high-dose oral contraceptives (OCs) and abortion. Condoms were available, but were not a viable choice owing to their poor quality. In addition to the above methods, withdrawal and rhythm methods were widely used to avoid unwanted pregnancy.

The induced abortion was and still remains the principal method of fertility regulation in many countries of Central and Eastern Europe (Figure 7)[8]. In several countries (Estonia, Latvia, Lithuania etc.), legal abortion is no longer free-of-charge. An examination for syphilis and gonorrhea is carried out prior to the abortion.

Since the countries of Eastern Europe regained their independence, the choice of good-quality and effective contraceptive methods is becoming broader. Pharmaceutical companies have entered the market with a range of oral contraceptives, hormonal injectable contraception and IUDs with international standard quality. Vaginal spermicides, the contraceptive sponge and a wide selection of condoms of various qualities are available.

Sterilization (currently performed almost exclusively on women) is performed, but is currently not a common choice of contraception.

Table 1 Contraceptive use (%)

Country or city	*Total*	*OC*	*IUD*	*Sterilization*	*Condoms*	*Others*
The Netherlands	71.6	39.0	2.9	21.9	6.5	—
Poland	75.0	←	26.0	→	—	49.0
Hungary	62.0	39.0	19.0	—	4.0	11.0
St. Petersburg	66.2	9.2	20.1	—	17.6	19.3
Russia	22.8	—	—	—	—	—
Czech Republic	59.0	18.7	10.17	2.0	16.0	21.0
Latvia	18.3	6.18	12.7	0.06	—	—

OC, oral contraceptive; IUD, intrauterine device

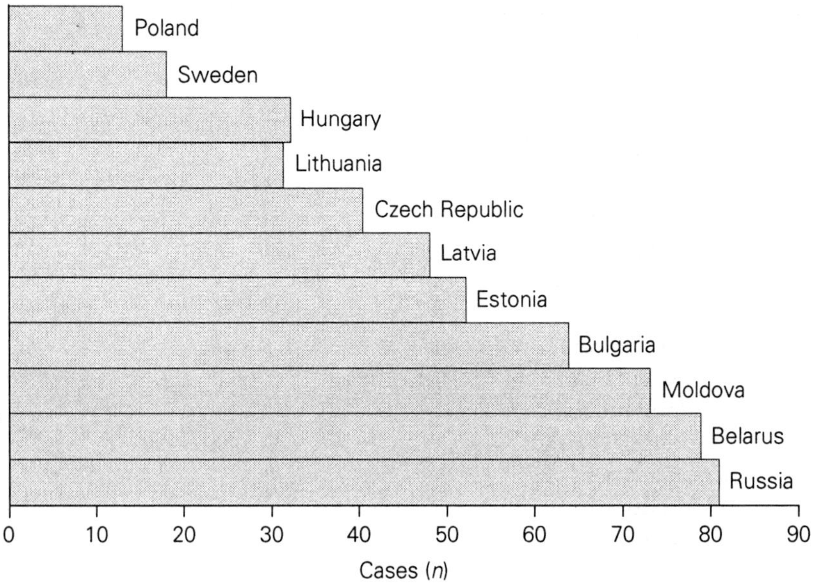

Figure 7 Number of induced abortions per 1000 women of fertile age

WHO DEALS WITH COUNSELLING AND SPREAD OF FAMILY PLANNING METHODS IN EASTERN EUROPEAN COUNTRIES?

The situation differs in the various countries. In the Baltics, the gynecologists are usually those who discuss with the woman or the couple all the available methods of contraception and perform the necessary screening. More and more family doctors or general practitioners are involved in this process, as there is the trend to create a strong network of family doctors in these countries. However, the knowledge of this group of specialists is not yet sufficient for family-planning counselling in many cases. In Hungary and some other countries, a Family Welfare Service has been created, with the task of helping to spread knowledge on contraception and family planning and to provide advice on contraception to suit the individual[9]. However, the organization of the special family-planning centers that provide medical care is a big problem owing to the lack of economic resources. In Estonia, within the framework of a pilot project, a special counselling center for youngsters was established. In this center, besides lectures and discussions on various topics related to sexual health, midwives and gynecologists provide counselling in matters such as contraception and sex life. A similar center was organized in Latvia, donated by the government, but the lack of resources decreased the financial support and now it works partly on a voluntary basis, and partly financed by the schoolchildren and students attending this center.

SHOULD STD SCREENING BE PERFORMED IN SPECIAL CONTRACEPTIVE CENTERS OR BY DOCTOR CONSULTING CLIENT ON THIS TOPIC?

The usual screening includes the medical history, clinical evaluation and bacterioscopical examination of the discharge, that will give possible information about *Trichomonas vaginalis*, *Neisseria gonorrhoeae*, candidiasis and bacterial vaginosis (including pH evaluation, KOH test etc.). If the doctor finds it to be necessary, a serological test for syphilis or HIV is carried out. The possibility of diagnosing *C. trachomatis* depends whether the patient may cover the costs of the examination. With the average monthly income in Latvia being 100 Lats (1 US$ = 0.53 Lats) in 1995, the cost of the analysis for *C. trachomatis* ranges from 2 Lats (direct immunofluorescent method and enzyme-linked immunodeficiency assay, ELISA) to 6.50 Lats (polymerase chain reaction, PCR).

Implementing STD screening and/or management services can require a significant commitment of human, laboratory and drug resources and also require additional infrastructures and funding. Most countries with a transitional economy cannot cover these expenses.

WHO PROVIDES INFORMATION ABOUT SAFE SEX AND STDs?

According to Soviet doctrine, 'there was no sex' in the Soviet Union. For 50 years, discussing sexuality in schools or in publications – indeed in public – was forbidden. As a result, when the occupied countries gained independence in 1991, the doors opened up to reveal a huge information vacuum in the area of sexuality, reproductive health and family planning.

Increasing rates of unwanted pregnancy and STDs among young women indicate the necessity for education targeted at girls and boys (Figures 8 and 9). In Estonia within the framework of the health-education program, sex education is included in the curricula of the fourth, seventh and tenth forms. In Latvia, 500 teachers have sought training to become health-education teachers. However, sex education has not yet been incorporated as a comprehensive part of the school education program, although it is being taught in one-fifth of the schools in Latvia. In Lithuania, the Catholic church has a strong influence on the government, especially on ministers of education and health care. This influence interferes with the introduction of a family-planning program and sex education, being to 'save life and moral values of society'. The teaching of family planning and sex life in schools often leaves much to be desired owing to the lack of suitable teaching materials and/or the insufficient training of the teachers.

Much is done in the field of family planning and sexual health by the non-governmental organizations in a number of Eastern and Central European countries, i.e. Albania, Bulgaria, Czech Republic, Estonia, Hungary, Latvia, Lithuania, Poland, Romania, Russia, Slovak Republic and Moldova. Many of the family-planning associations have been funded by the International Planned

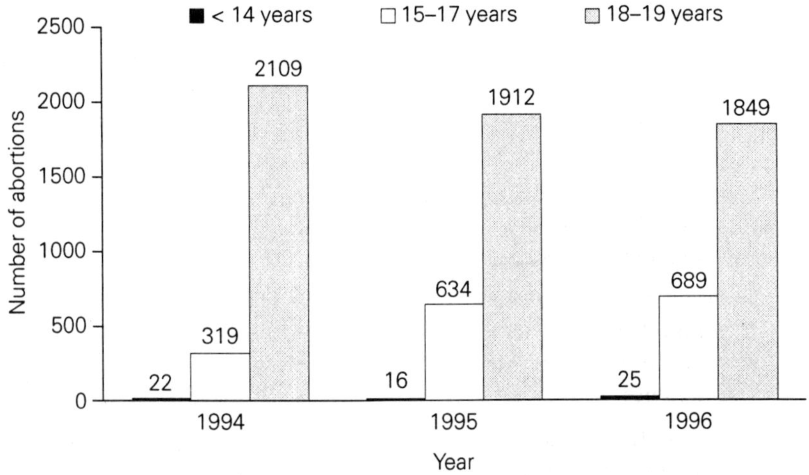

Figure 8 Induced abortions in Latvia in women aged less than 19 years (absolute figures). Data from the Bureau of Medical Statistics, Health Department of the Ministry of Welfare, Republic of Latvia

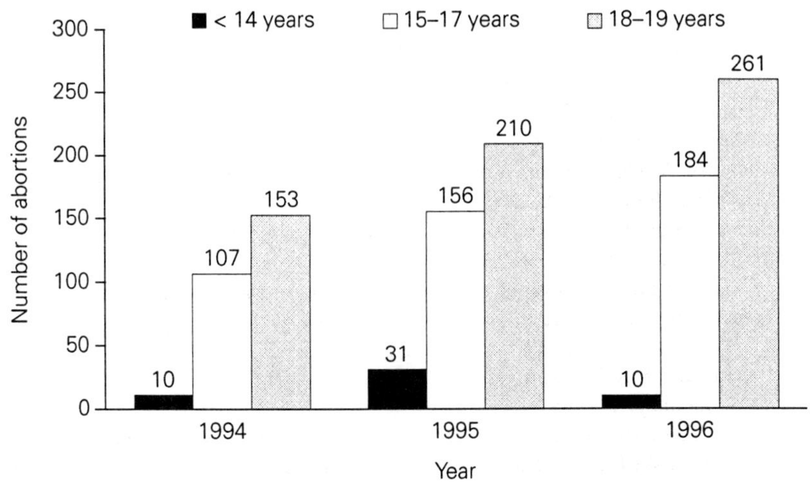

Figure 9 Incidence of syphilis among adolescents in Latvia (absolute figures). Data from the Bureau of Medical Statistics, Health Department of the Ministry of Welfare, Republic of Latvia

Parenthood Federation. In Latvia, besides the Latvia's Association for Family Planning and Sexual Health, there are the Health Education Teacher's Association, Latvia's Contraceptology Association, Latvia's Association for Sexual Equality and the HIV-positive support group whose activities are related to family planning and reproductive health. Many projects concerning information and education on STDs are performed in combination.

CONCLUSIONS

(1) Information, education and communication regarding responsible sexual behavior and prevention of STDs should be promoted by parliamentarians to school children. Sex education should be included in the school curriculum.

(2) The governments are to review the state budgets for health care and provide means to reduce STDs so that family-planning programs include STD screening and treatment.

(3) Specialized training in prevention and detection of, and counselling in STDs should be regularly organized for healthcare providers in Eastern Europe, as no up-to-date text books are available in the national languages on these topics.

(4) A unified system of data collection on STDs in Europe would be of great help in comparing the actual situations in European countries in finding out the real reasons for the huge differences in STD rates among countries.

REFERENCES

1. UN International Conference on Population and Development. *Programme of Action*, Cairo, September 1994; 113 UNDP/UNFPA/WHO/World Bank
2. *Challenges in Reproductive Health Research*. UNDP/UNFPA/WHO/World Bank special programme of research, development and research training in human reproduction binennial report, 1992–1993. 1994: 202
3. Report on WHO meeting on *Training in Reproductive Health for CCEE/NIS*, Copnhagen, June 1995, WHO Regional Office for Europe, 1996
4. Linglof T. Rapid increase of syphilis and gonorrhea in parts of the former USSR. *Sex Transm Dis* 1995; 22: 160–1
5. State Centre for the Prevention and Treatment of Sexually Transmitted Diseases. *Sexually transmitted disease statistics in Latvia*, 1996
6. UNFPA division for Arab States and Europe/WHO Regional Office for Europe Sexuality and Family Planning. *Family Planning and Reproductive Health in CCEE/ NIS*. Copenhagen, 1995
7. Hicks D. The relationship between contraception and sexually transmitted diseases. What is the risk? Presented at the *2nd Congress of the ESC*, Athens, May 1992; 57–65
8. David H. Abortion in Europe, 1920–1991: a public health perspective. *Stud Fam Plann* 1992; 23: 1–22
9. Berbik I. New Hungarian abortion act: first results. *Planned Parenthood Eur* 1994; 23: 24–25

Index